Diagnostic Tests
in Neurology

Diagnostic Tests Series

Advances in technology have placed a wide range of tests and investigations at the disposal of the clinician, and this has led to an increasing necessity for education in the selection and interpretation of these tests. These books are intended for both trainee and established clinicians as a practical guide to the investigation of patients. They are written in the belief that careful clinical examination is an essential prerequisite for the selection of appropriate investigations, and that good clinical practice entails the selection of a small number of appropriate tests rather than the application of a blanket screening programme.

The aim of these books is to describe the development, methods, and interpretation of clinical tests in various specialities, together with an evaluation of their accuracy, safety and clinical usefulness. Although some of the information will be found in standard text books, the advantage of the present series is that they are smaller and more readable, containing a comprehensive survey of clinical tests without descriptions of disease and therapy which the larger text books necessarily contain.

Due for publication in 1988 . . .
Diagnostic Tests in Respiratory Medicine *P.J. Rees*

Titles in preparation . . .
Diagnostic Tests in Gastroenterology *A.D. Beattie*
Diagnostic Tests in Cardiology *D.S. Dymond and J. Caplin*
Diagnostic Tests in Urology and Nephrology *D. Kirk and M. Allison*
Diagnostic Tests in Obstetrics and Gynaecology *D.T.Y. Liu*
Diagnostic Tests in Orthopaedics and Rheumatology *R.C. Butler and G.A. Evans*
Diagnostic Tests in Ophthalmology *W.S. Foulds*

Diagnostic Tests in Neurology

G.D. PERKIN

Department of Neurology
Charing Cross Hospital
London

SPRINGER-SCIENCE+BUSINESS MEDIA, B.V.

ISBN 978-0-412-28400-7

British Library Cataloguing in Publication Data

Perkin, G. David (George David)
  Diagnostic tests in neurology.
  1. Man. Nervous system. Tests – Manuals
  I. Title.   II. Series
  616.8′04754
ISBN 978-0-412-28400-7   ISBN 978-1-4899-3320-1 (eBook)
DOI 10.1007/978-1-4899-3320-1

Contents

Preface

In writing this book, I have attempted to provide information about the relative value of particular investigations in various neurological disorders. The book is divided into sections dealing with the methods of investigation, the investigation of particular symptoms, the investigation of specific neurological conditions and neurological emergencies. Finally, the assessment of certain disorders suggesting a particular anatomical localization, for example isolated optic atrophy, is considered.

Following an appraisal of the literature, each section ends with a recommendation regarding appropriate investigation. In some instances this is supported by an algorithm. Specific recommendations have been attempted despite the risk of producing over-dogmatic criteria for patient management. A small amount of illustrative material is included.

I am grateful to colleagues at Charing Cross Hospital who have provided some of the illustrations. Figs 1.4, 2.1 and 10.2 are reproduced from Atlas of Clinical Neurology, by G. D. Perkin *et al.*, Gower Medical Publishing, 1986, courtesy of the publishers. Fig. 3, in Chapter 4, is reproduced from Brain, vol. 2 **104**, 753–78, 1981, courtesy of the editor and Dr. R.S.J. Frackowiak. Fig. 6, in the same chapter, is reproduced from Fig. 62 in the Atlas of Positron Emission Tomography, edited by E-D. Heiss *et al.*, Springer-Verlag, 1985, courtesy of the publishers and Dr. J.C. Maziotta. Fig. 3 in Chapter 6 is reproduced from Fig. 1, Chapter 11 of Multiple Sclerosis: Immunological, diagnostic and therapeutic aspects, edited by F. Clifford Rose and R. Jones, John Libbey, 1987, courtesy of the publishers and Dr D. A. Ingram. The manuscript has been typed and re-typed by Ms Beryl Laatz, to whom I wish to extend my thanks and appreciation.

1

Methods of neurological investigation

1.1 SKULL X-RAY

Conventionally, routine skull radiography includes lateral, antero-posterior, postero-anterior and vertico-submental views. Even before the advent of modern imaging techniques, the value of skull radiography in the investigation of common neurological disorders had been questioned[1]. For example, among 100 patients with migraine, 59 had had skull films performed, all of which were normal. Similarly, in 100 patients with non-specific headache, skull X-ray was negative in all 75 in whom it was performed. A prospective study of 200 consecutive outpatients, in whom physical signs were lacking, concluded that a single lateral skull film had provided no diagnostically useful information[1]. Other than medical criteria may influence the decision to perform skull X-rays. In a study published in 1979, it was estimated that 75% of all non-hospital radiological studies in the USA were performed by non-radiologists[2]. An analysis revealed that the non-radiologist physician who owned an X-ray machine used an average of twice as many X-ray examinations as did colleagues who referred patients to radiologists. In a prospective study of skull X-rays performed over a five month period at the UCLA Emergency Medical Centre, 19% had been ordered primarily for medicolegal purposes[3]. Indeed, perhaps the sole remaining debate concerning the use of skull radiography centres on its value in the patient with head injury. Whilst an argument could be advanced for the replacement of skull radiography by CT scanning, the fact that the former was costed at some 11% of the latter in 1977 effectively eliminates that solution[4]. Amongst 1500 successive head-injured patients, skull X-ray revealed a fracture in 93[5]. Factors not associated with fracture included drowsiness, headache, seizures and the presence of a scalp haematoma; 21 factors were found to be significantly associated with a skull fracture. If the presence of any one of these factors had been made the criterion for performing skull films then only one of the 93 fractures would not have been detected. Moreover, 434 patients would not have required skull films, i.e. 29% of the total. Extrapolation for the whole of the USA suggested a potential annual saving of $15 000 000. A further argument against the universal use of skull X-ray in head injury is the poor correlation between the findings and those revealed by CT scanning. In one survey of head-injured adults, 32% with a significant intracranial abnormality on CT had normal skull films, whereas in 23% of those with a skull fracture, no significant intracranial CT change occurred[6]. Proponents of routine skull films in head injury remain, however, based on the evidence, from over 5000 cases, that the finding of a skull fracture accompanied by disorientation in a head-injured patient, by stimulating immediate CT scanning, would have identified two-thirds of all traumatic intracranial haematomas[7].

1.2 SPINAL X-RAYS

The role of spinal X-rays in the investigation of patients with chronic neck or low back pain has similarly been questioned. Here, interpretation of any abnormality has to take account of changes in the spine occurring with age in asymptomatic individuals. Radiological evidence of cervical spondylosis was found in over 80% of a population over the age of 55[8]. Although no fewer than 15 views of the cervical spine have been described, there is seldom need to exceed antero-posterior, lateral and oblique views[9], certainly for non-traumatic cases. The value of cervical spine X-rays in those with spinal injury is as debatable as the role of skull X-ray in head injury[3].

1.3 MYELOGRAPHY

The role of myelography in the diagnosis of spinal disease remains substantial, despite the advent of CT myelography and MRI (Fig. 1.1). Apart from the adverse effect of lumbar puncture (discussed below) the major problem associated with myelography is the late development of arachnoiditis. A study of patients who had required more than one myelogram found evidence, at the time of their second

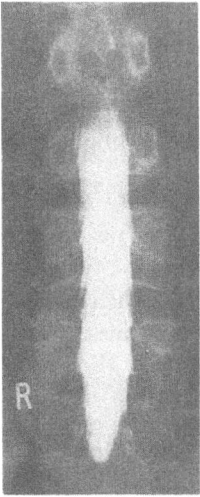

Fig. 1.1 Normal lumbar myelogram

myelogram, of thecal scarring in 74% of those in whom myodil had been the contrast medium, compared to 61% of those who had received conray [10]. The incidence of thecal scarring was higher in those who had undergone surgery in addition to myelography. In one survey of 80 cases of spinal arachnoiditis, 43 patients had had previous myelography, only one of which had been performed with a water-soluble medium [11]. Among 138 patients requiring repeat myelography, but whose first study had used metrizamide, only one showed evidence of thecal scarring and that patient had had disc surgery [12]. The incidence of headache after metrizamide myelography, in 201 cases, was 43%, with 14% of patients experiencing nausea [12]. Metrizamide myelography is not without hazard, however. Epilepsy, spinal myoclonus and psychological disturbance have been described after the procedure. Seizures are more likely if a high concentration is used, or if intracranial spill occurs [13]. Spinal myoclonus is more likely if spinal block is present. Rarer complications include asterixis and aphasia [14]. Irreversible complications have been recorded in four cases, principally composed of limb weakness[15]. Cerebral complications are diminished if a head-up posture is maintained for six hours following the procedure. The use of metrizamide should be reconsidered in patients with epilepsy, those on drugs which reduce seizure threshold, and those suspected of having spinal block.

1.4 LUMBAR PUNCTURE

In an extensive analysis of the hazards of lumbar puncture, headache was found in 0.5–36% and paraesthesiae or pain, often radicular, in 13% (persisting in 0.2%)[16]. There is general acceptance that the incidence of headache is reduced by the use of a 22 gauge needle, the figure then falling to 1.2%[17]. A 24-hour period of bed rest after the procedure appears to be without benefit[18] whereas the influence of particular postures after lumbar puncture on the subsequent development of headache appears marginal[19]. A follow-up study has been published of the complication rate of spinal anaesthetic performed in over 10 000 patients. The patients were reappraised frequently after the procedure, and then six months later[20]. No cases of arachnoiditis or sepsis were discovered. The incidence of postural headache was 14%, but lower in those who had had the lumbar puncture performed with a 24 gauge needle. Numbness in the lower limbs occurred in 0.7%, and 8 cases of abducens palsy developed. A single patient developed incapacitating neurological disease after the procedure, and was found to have a meningioma. A frequent concern is the risk of lumbar puncture in someone with a bleeding diathesis, or who is likely to receive anticoagulant therapy. In patients with thrombocytopenia, a platelet count above 40 000 is generally considered sufficient to allow the performance of lumbar puncture without hazard of haemorrhage. Spinal subarachnoid haemorrhage, epidural or subdural haematoma can appear if anticoagulation immediately follows lumbar puncture. A delay of at least 1 h before initiating therapy is generally recommended[21].

An acceptable upper limit for CSF pressure is often quoted as 180 mm of water, though this is probably too rigid a guideline. In a group of 41 obese neurologically normal individuals, the mean CSF pressure was 167, with 25% having pressures between 200 and 250[22]. From a survey of the literature, it was concluded that at least 5% of normal individuals have CSF pressures exceeding 200.

A factor which influences the CSF constituents, but to an uncertain degree, is the presence of traumatic haemorrhage. Indeed a common clinical problem is the need to distinguish the effect of a traumatic puncture from haemorrhage into the subarachnoid space. Although a decreasing red cell count in successive specimens, the presence of xanthochromia, or a colourless supernatant all favour one or other possibility, none of these factors provides an absolute distinction[23]. Spectrophotometry of the supernatant is a more valuable discriminatory procedure. An extinction value below 0.023 almost certainly excludes haemorrhage. If the extinction value is above 0.023, an absorption curve is plotted. If bilirubin is absent, haemorrhage is again excluded, whilst its presence makes haemorrhage very likely. If there is continuing uncertainty, cytology is performed – the presence of erythrophages makes haemorrhage certain. Blood-stained CSF, from a traumatic tap, can still be analysed for routine constituents. One to two white cells should be subtracted from the count for every 1000 counted red cells. A significant change in protein concentration occurs only when the erythrocyte count exceeds $16\,666/mm^3$ and the IgG/protein ratio rises by only 0.037 for every 3333 red cells[24].

Whilst many laboratories routinely measure protein and glucose concentrations together with the cell count, and then proceed to IgG ratios, the findings of one recent analysis suggest that a limited analysis of CSF suffices in most clinical settings[25]. Amongst 555 consecutive CSF examinations, a normal opening pressure, cell count and protein concentration occurred in 334 cases. Of additional tests requested, 1385, or 53%, were ordered in these cases. Of these, 1.6% were abnormal, the figure falling to 0.6% when false positive results were excluded. The findings did not alter management or diagnosis. In the 221 cases with an abnormality of opening pressure, cell count or protein, 1253 additional tests were ordered, producing true positive abnormalities in 5.6%, and leading to a new diagnosis in 13% of these patients. The authors concluded that measurement of pressure, protein concentration and cell count sufficed as a satisfactory screen for almost all neurological disorders except childhood meningitis, multiple sclerosis and those occurring in patients with immunoparesis. CSF protein concentration tends to rise with age, one study suggesting an increase of 1.6% per year[26].

An extensive literature exists on the value of other investigations performed on CSF. IgG ratios are rightly regarded as valuable screening tests in multiple sclerosis though levels can be depressed by concomitant steroid therapy[27]. Whilst agarose gel electro-phoresis is a less-sensitive technique for detecting oligoclonal bands than isoelectric focusing, it has the advantage of producing less false positive results[27]. IgM indices have been studied less frequently than IgG ratios. Rarely the IgM index is abnormal in MS in the presence of a normal IgG index[28]. Many protein, enzyme and other changes reported in the CSF are not sufficiently specific to recommend their use in clinical practice. Levels of S-100 protein, mainly located in astrocytes are raised in cerebro-vascular disease, viral infection and cord compression from tumour[29]. Complement levels of C_3 and C_4 are elevated in patients with inflammatory disorders[30]. Myelin proteolipid pro-tein is the most prominent myelin protein and it is perhaps not surprising that abnormal values in the CSF or serum follow a variety of processes which damage the CNS[31]. Elevated CSF lysozyme values have been reported in all cases of bacterial and fungal meningitis[32] but similar changes are described in other conditions, including cerebrovascular disease[33]. A variety of enzymes have been measured in the CSF from patients with tavarious neurological diseases. Altered levels of enolase, pyru-vate kinase, lactate dehydrogenase, creatine phosphokinase and aldolase are not specific, though changes in aldolase reach a specificity of 93% for cerebral tumours, higher than for any other enzyme[34]. Levels of prostaglandin $F_{2\alpha}$ in the CSF rise with many neurological diseases, particularly stroke and subarachnoid haem-orrhage[35]. Altered γ-aminobutyric acid (GABA) levels are similarly non-specific though they are particularly low in olivo-ponto-cerebellar atrophy and late-onset cortical cerebellar degen-eration[36].

1.5 PNEUMOENCEPHALOGRAPHY

Pneumoencephalography does not merit substantial discussion, as its use has virtually ceased since the advent of CT and MRI scanning. One of the reasons for its demise, quite apart from the better diagnostic capacity of these other investigations, is the high inci-dence of complications associated with it. In one study, of 50 patients, problems arising during the seven days after the procedure included headache in 78%, vomiting in a third, and an altered conscious level in 18% [37].

1.6 RADIONUCLIDE SCANNING

Between approximately 1955 and 1970, radionuclide scanning, most commonly using ^{99m}Tc pertechnetate, was regularly employed to aid the diagnosis of certain neurological disorders, particularly tumour, abscess and subdural haematoma. Patterns of abnormal uptake were recognized, though these seldom proved sufficiently specific to allow for a particular pathological correlation [38]. With the widespread availability of CT scanning, the procedure, in its original form, has virtually ceased to be used. The technique has been developed recently in order to achieve a three-dimensional image of cerebral blood flow. Following inhalation of ^{133}xenon, rotating gamma cameras detect photon emissions from three brain slices simultaneously, allowing a spatial resolution of the order of 1.7 cm [39]. The technique, single photon emission computed tomography (SPECT) has been applied to the study of cerebral blood flow in cerebrovascular disease and dementia.

1.7 ANGIOGRAPHY

Visualization of the cerebral circulation can be achieved by direct injection of contrast medium into a carotid or vertebral artery, by injection of medium via a catheter introduced from the aortic arch into the major neck vessels or, incorporating a digital subtraction technique, by the use of contrast injected into a peripheral vein or the right atrium. Conventional arteriography now largely utilizes a catheter technique with or without digital subtraction (Fig. 1.2). In a prospective study of the complication rates in 1517 consecutive cerebral angiograms, neurological complications occurred in 2.6%, and were permanent in 0.33% of cases [40]. The complication rate is probably higher in patients with cerebrovascular disease, and appears higher in training hospitals or where the procedure has been performed by junior staff members [41,42]. The realization that patients with threatening stroke may suffer a neurological event unrelated to angiography has to be used when interpreting complication rates, though a putative study of this hazard merely recorded a variety of medical complications occurring in the 48 hours before the procedure [43]. Whereas venous digital subtraction angiography (DSA) is free of hazard, in terms of neurological complication, its sensitivity for the detection of cerebrovascular disease falls considerably below that achieved by arterial injection (Fig. 1.3). The

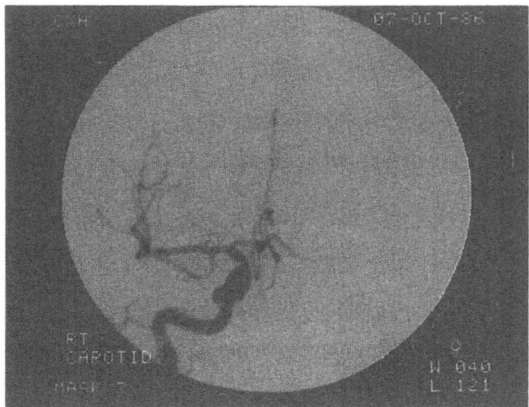

Fig. 1.2 Normal carotid angiogram. AP view. Arterial phase

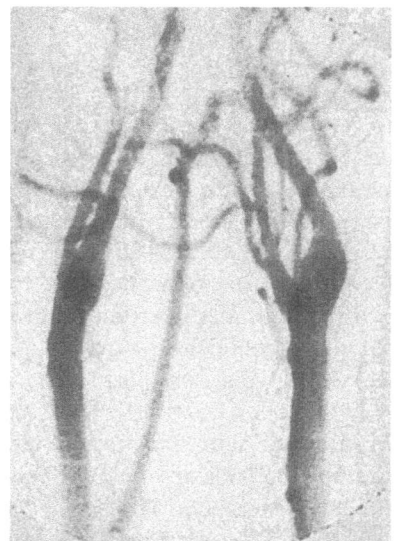

Fig. 1.3 Demonstration of neck vessels by digital subtraction angiography; left, venous study; right, arterial study

complication rate of arterial digital studies has yet to be assessed prospectively, though the fact that a smaller catheter is required, with a lower volume of contrast medium, suggests that it will prove a safer alternative to conventional angiography.

An attempt has been made to appraise the cost-effectiveness of intravenous DSA in the evaluation of suspected carotid artery disease[44]. If the investigation is followed by arterial angiography whenever a lesion is discovered, the total costs are likely to be higher than if arterial angiography is used alone. If, however, arterial studies are confined to 10% of the patients with positive venous studies, substantial savings are possible. The cost equations are complicated by the tendency for a safer technique to be applied on a wider scale than the method which it replaces.

1.8 ELECTROPHYSIOLOGY

Electroencephalography is now routinely performed with sixteen channels. Following recordings at rest, activation procedures are carried out in the form of hyperventilation and photic stimulation. Further activation by sleep, or a differing electrode montage, for example naso-pharyngeal leads, can enhance the yield of abnormal studies in patients with suspected epilepsy. A problem that continues to bedevil the interpretation of the EEG is the incidence of abnormal records in the normal population. With aging, the dominant alpha rhythm slows and low frequency activity becomes more prominent[45]. Focal sharp waves, generally correlated with a clinical diagnosis of epilepsy were encountered in 3.3% of normal adults in one series[45]. In another study of normal individuals, all of whom had passed an intensive medical training for air crew placement, 10% were found to have an abnormal EEG[46]. Indeed a polemic on the role of the investigation concluded 'the greater part of the work of most EEG departments consists of doing single records in patients referred by clinicians almost wholly ignorant of the value and limitations of the technique, and who even openly admit to using EEG as a form of supportive psychotherapy' [46].

1.8.1 Visual evoked potentials

By the use of an appropriate visual stimulus, a synchronous discharge can be excited in the visual pathways leading to a cortical potential of reproducible waveform and latency. Visual stimuli used include repetitive flashes, a reversing checkerboard pattern of light and dark squares or a pattern which appears and disappears on a background of uniform luminance. The cortical response is measured with surface electrodes over the occiput. A large positive potential (P 100) is followed by smaller negative peaks when a full field stimulus is used. The pattern response potential is influenced by the type of visual stimulus, the angle subtended by the whole stimulus and by its individual components. Normal ranges for latency vary from laboratory to laboratory. Voluntary alteration of the potential can be achieved by the subject mentally avoiding perception of the stimulus. By this means, normal subjects can obliterate the monocular pattern shift potential without any observable change in ocular fixation or attention. Other subjects can alter the latency difference between the two eyes to beyond the upper limit of normal[47]. More readily observable manoeuvres which alter amplitude and latency include continuous saccadic eye movements, switching gaze from the centre of the target or focusing on a near object. Abnormal responses are by no means confined to MS subjects. In one survey, a symmetrical increase in latency, interocular latency abnormalities, and amplitude abnormalities were as common in the non-MS group[48]. The addition of half field to central stimulation can enhance attempts at localization of the lesion.

1.8.2 Brain stem auditory evoked potentials

Monaural stimulation is usually performed with a click stimulus at 10 Hz. Click intensity is set at 65–70 dB above the hearing threshold (Fig. 1.4). A masking noise is applied to the other ear. Conventionally the response to 1000–2000 clicks is summated. The brain stem potentials are designated I to VII. Measurements utilized include interwave latencies and the wave I/V amplitude ratio. Wave I is probably the acoustic nerve action potential, wave II is derived from the cochlear nucleus, wave III from the superior olivary complex, whilst the origins of waves IV and V are less certainly identified though the latter has been attributed to the inferior colliculus. Waves VI and VII are variable. Brain stem evoked responses have been particularly applied to the diagnosis of multiple sclerosis, acoustic neuroma and the evaluation of patients in coma.

1.8.3 Somatosensory evoked potentials

With surface recording over the neck, potentials can be detected following stimulation of an upper limb peripheral nerve. Successive peaks on the negative wave are identified as P9, P11, P13 and P14. P9

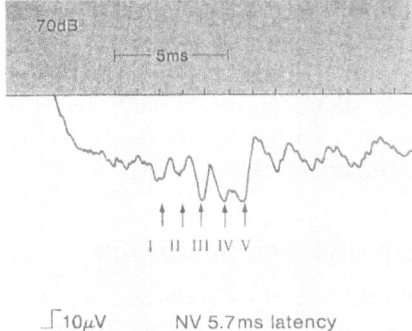

Fig. 1.4 Normal auditory evoked responses. 70 dB stimulus

is attributed to impulses in peripheral fibres proximal to the axilla, P11 to impulses in the cervical dorsal column, P13 to the cuneate nucleus, and P14 to the medial lemniscus. Following stimulation of a leg peripheral nerve, two negative responses can be recorded over the lumbosacral region, the first thought to arise from potentials ascending in the cauda equina, the second possibly generated by the dorsal horn. A cortical potential (N20) can be recorded over the contralateral sensory cortex following stimulation of the median nerve. This potential has a latency of the order of 20 ms. Late potentials can be evoked by somatosensory, visual or auditory stimuli, with latencies reaching up to 300 ms. They are influenced by the subject's state of arousal and attention.

The role of somatosensory-evoked responses in neurological investigation has been critically examined[49]. Whilst the yield of abnormal findings in MS subjects compares favourably with visual or auditory evoked responses, particularly if leg stimulation is used, serial recordings often fail to correlate with the patient's clinical status. To date, the method has proved of limited value in the evaluation of cervical spondylosis, spinal cord or head injury, the spinocerebellar degenerations and in brachial plexus lesions.

1.8.4 Central motor conduction

Percutaneous stimulation of the motor cortex by electrical or electromagnetic stimulation now allows the direct measurement of central motor conduction time. Whilst the former method can cause some discomfort, particularly when stimulation over the spinal column is attempted, the latter method is virtually painless, though at present it has not proved effective when applied over the spinal column. To date the techniques have been mainly applied to the study of patients with multiple sclerosis. The methods are capable of revealing clinically silent lesions, though probably less effectively than silent lesions in the afferent systems can be detected by evoked potential measurement[50,51].

1.8.5 Evoked responses – their present role

The status of evoked responses in the investigation of neurological disorders has been questioned. Criticisms of their value have detailed a lack of specificity, a frequent inability to achieve exact localization and an increasingly high false positive and false negative rate[52]. In relationship to multiple sclerosis, it is accepted that sequential electrophysiological studies correlate poorly with clinical developments[53]. Despite these reservations, in an analysis of 94 patients receiving 216 electrophysiological tests, only 7% of the tests were thought to have been not indicated[54].

1.9 ELECTROMYOGRAPHY AND NERVE CONDUCTION STUDIES

For the purpose of electromyography, a needle electrode is inserted into the relevant muscle, if necessary at multiple sites. Following insertion of the needle, a brief electrical discharge, the insertion activity, is seen and heard, ceasing in normal subjects within a few seconds. After cessation of this activity, electrical silence ensues disturbed, in certain pathological (and occasional physiological) states, by a number of different forms of spontaneous activity. These include fibrillation and fasciculation potentials, positive sharp waves, myotonic and high-frequency discharges. During voluntary contraction, an increasing accumulation of motor unit potentials occurs typically bi- or tri-phasic, with an amplitude reaching about 3 mV. Polyphasic potentials, defined as those with five or more phases, account for up to about 10% of the total. The duration of motor unit potentials tends to increase with age. As increasing numbers of motor units are activated, an interference pattern results which eventually, in normal subjects, submerges the contributions from individual units. The interference pattern is influenced by many factors, including the enthusiasm of the patient, so that interpretation of an incomplete pattern of slowly firing units must be cautious.

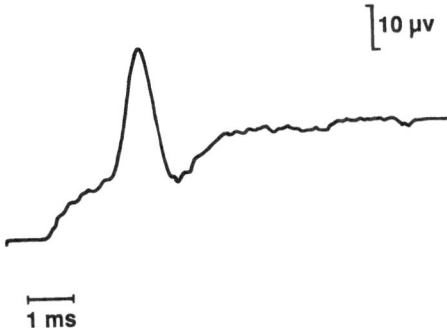

Fig. 1.5 Normal sural SAP (Sensory Action Potential). Amplitude 30 μV. Velocity to inflexion 47 m/s

Nerve conduction studies continue to provide an invaluable guide to the function of the peripheral nerve (Fig. 1.5). Slowing of conduction velocities has been reported in older patients. The decline is probably linear for median motor velocities but parabolic for other sensory and motor conduction values[55]. Velocities are equally dependent on skin temperature. Conduction velocities in sensory fibres of the median nerve decline by 2 m/s for each degree centigrade fall of temperature adjacent to the nerve[56]. Normal values for amplitude and velocity are available for all the commonly tested nerves. Where segmental demyelination occurs, slowing of conduction velocity is prominent, conventionally to a degree exceeding 40% of the normal value[57]. In an axonal neuropathy, conduction velocity is either normal or only slightly reduced. Whenever conduction values are measured, they represent the function of the most rapidly conducting fibres in that nerve. Though proximal segments of the peripheral nerves are not directly accessible, information regarding their conduction capacity can be obtained using the H reflex or F wave latency. The former is obtained by recording with a surface electrode over the soleus muscle whilst stimulating the tibial nerve. It is the electrical equivalent of a monosynaptic reflex arc, ascending via sensory fibres and descending through the anterior root. The F wave is thought to result from an antidromic stimulus ascending the motor nerve then activating the anterior horn cell. It is most readily recorded from the small hand muscles (Fig. 1.6).

Certain specialized techniques have been devised for the evaluation of the neuromuscular junction. Repetitive stimulation in

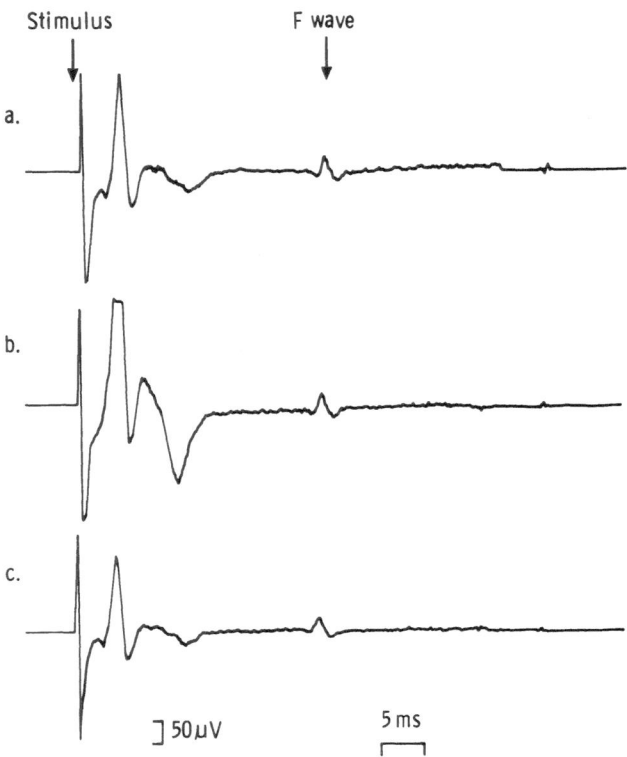

Fig. 1.6 F waves recorded from ADM (Abductor Digiti Minimi) with successive ulnar nerve stimulation at the wrist in a normal subject. Latencies range between 28 and 28.5 ms

myasthenia gravis, whether at low or high rates results in a decline in the amplitude of the compound muscle action potential which may then restabilize. In the Lambert–Eaton syndrome, with slow stimulus rates (1–10), the initial response declines then increases sometimes considerably exceeding the resting value. With higher stimulus rates (10–40) the increment begins immediately. Following a period of tetanic contraction, the compound action potential evoked by a single stimulus is increased slightly for a few seconds, but then becomes depressed for several minutes in patients with myasthenia gravis. In the Lambert–Eaton syndrome, the compound action potential rises dramatically (by at least 220%) after a 10 s period of tetanic contraction.

Single fibre electromyography is increasingly used in the diagnosis of myasthenia gravis. It allows the simultaneous recording of action potentials from two fibres belonging to the same motor unit. In normal individuals a slight variability (jitter) occurs in the time interval between the two potentials due to varying delay at the two neuromuscular junctions. In myasthenia the jitter is increased, or one junction may temporarily block completely.

1.10 CT SCANNING

Soon after the introduction of CT scanning, its effect on the practice of neurology was evident. An analysis of the first two year's experience with a scanner in the Bristol Unit was published in 1977[58]. By the last year of the analysis, 4000 scans per year were being performed. An effect on the number of arteriograms, encephalograms and radioisotope studies was immediately apparent. It was suggested that the net savings resulting from the use of the scanner, based partly on reduced expenditure on inpatient services, could amount to over £30 000 per annum. The proliferation of scanner units, particularly in the United States, was dramatic. By 1 May, 1980, there were 1471 units in the United States, compared to 45 scanners at the end of 1974[59]. By 1979, the national average for the USA was 57 scanners per million population, far ahead of the penetration achieved in Europe, where Germany, in the same year, had achieved 2.6 scanners per million, and the United Kingdom a mere 1.0 per million. By 1985, almost all hospitals in the USA with over 300 beds possessed or were served by a CT scanner[60]. An attempt to appraise the cost effectiveness of the CT scanner reviewed data on the subject up to 1981[61]. As the author pointed out, without clear data on which particular conditions were better investigated by CT scanning, attempts to appraise the cost effectiveness of the scanner were unlikely to succeed. To a certain extent, these arguments are now academic, since the intrinsic superiority of CT scanning as a radiological technique has inevitably led to its increasing installation and availability (Fig.1.7). Whether the way in which it is now utilized in many hospitals is cost effective is another matter. For certain conditions, the use of the scanner allows a reduction of hospital stay and the number of surgical procedures. For the more chronic neurological problems, for example headache, CT scanning is clearly not cost-effective[62]. The hazards of calculating the potential savings from the use of CT scanning are exemplified by studies which suggest that abnormalities

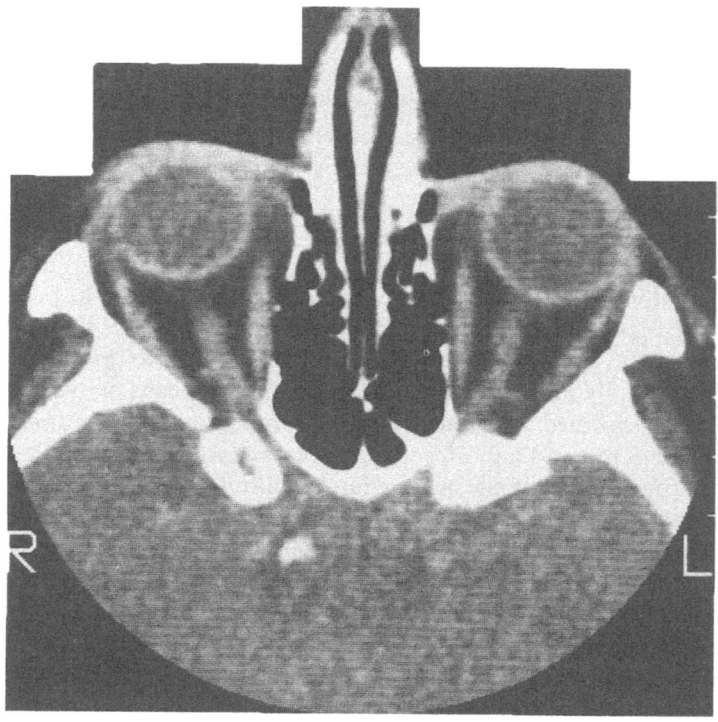

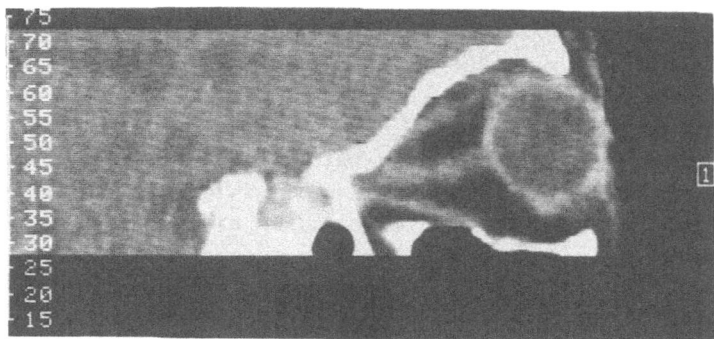

Fig. 1.7 Axial and coronal CT scans of normal orbit

in certain screening procedures can be used as a guide to the necessity for further investigation by CT. In an analysis of 136 patients with a variety of neurological disorders but no focal hemispheric signs, CT was focally abnormal in six. Of these, four had focal changes in the

EEG, the other two having diffuse abnormalities. The EEG was suggested as a screening procedure for these patients, a normal finding predicting a lack of any focal change on subsequent CT examination [63]. One thing is certain, the observer error in interpreting scans by experienced neuroradiologists is slight, certainly in terms of assessing infarction, white matter attenuation and cortical sulcal width [64].

1.11 MAGNETIC RESONANCE IMAGING (MRI) SCANNING

MRI scanning has not quite revolutionized the practice of neurology in the same way that CT scanning did in the 1970s, at least in the United Kingdom, where the number of MRI units remains extremely limited. The technique relies on the existence of minute charged particles within body tissues whose alignment can be altered by an applied magnetic field. The principle charged particle is the proton of the hydrogen atom. In the presence of an applied magnetic field (parallel to the body axis) the protons become so aligned that the majority point towards the north end of the magnet, resulting in a bulk magnetization vector whose amplitude depends on the proton density (for hydrogen imaging) and the strength of the applied magnetic field. The most commonly used magnetic strength is 0.15 T (tesla). Each tesla is 10 000 (G) gauss – by comparison, the earth's magnetic field is about 0.6 G. After the charged particles in the body have equilibrated along the north–south axis of the applied magnetic field, an electric current is passed through coils placed in such a way that the radio waves generated and their associated magnetic field are at right angles to the magnet's field. The radiofrequency field is not static, but rotates in a plane at right angles to the body at a rate equal to the radio wave frequency. According to the strength and duration of the radio pulse, the net alignment of the charged particles can be changed by 90 or 180°. After a 90° pulse is released, the disturbed nuclei will rotate around the main axis of the magnet, the rate of decay of this signal being termed the T_2 relaxation time. The time taken for the bulk magnetization vector in the north–south plane of the main magnet to be restored is termed T_1 relaxation. T_1 relaxation is measured using inversion recovery sequences, T_2 by spin–echo sequences (Fig. 1.8).

The risks of MRI scanning appear slight. Patients with pacemakers are not scanned, in view of the possible effect of the magnetic field on pacemaker function.

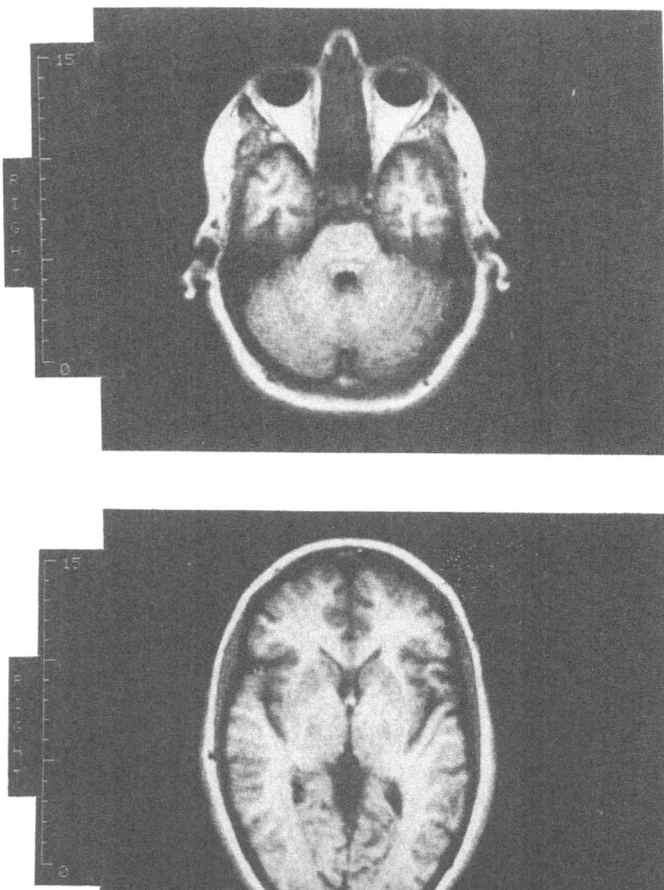

Fig. 1.8 Normal axial MRI scan at two levels

The purchase price and running costs of MRI are considerably higher than CT. In 1983, the cost of a single study was calculated to be between $180 and $382 in the United States [65]. As a consequence, penetration of the MRI scanner has been considerably slower than the penetration achieved by CT in the 1970s. At the end of 1984, there were 108 installations in the United States [60] and the average annual operating cost was calculated to be $841 500 in

1985. In comparison with CT, equipment costs were calculated to be three times higher, the space for equipment to be five times greater, and the annual technical costs to be three times higher[66]. Similar costings have been performed in the United Kingdom. Whilst a costing per patient of £49.49 was suggested for the Aberdeen installation (0.08 T) in 1985[67], an estimate for a 0.5 T magnet was £270 per patient compared to £60 per patient for CT scanning in a recent review[68]. By the end of 1987, there will be approximately 22 installations in the United Kingdom.

An estimation of the potential value of MRI scanning must remain uncertain while the technique continues to develop. The use of contrast imaging with gadolinium reveals enhancement in both inversion–recovery and spin–echo sequences[69]. By using higher strength magnets signals from other atoms, including phosphorus, can be detected. The potential exists for measuring ATP utilization and for appraising alterations in muscle metabolism[70]. Spectroscopic analysis is currently being extended to studies of carbon and fluorine bound compounds.

Experience to date indicates that certain abnormalities on MRI scanning lack specificity for a particular disease process. Indeed the frequency with which changes are found in asymptomatic individuals must be taken into account when interpreting the findings in those with neurological symptoms. In eight patients dying from non-neurological causes, subcortical white matter abnormalities (detected by post-mortem scanning) were inevitable. Histology revealed a more frequent incidence, in the abnormal areas, of dilated perivascular spaces, vascular ectasia and arteriosclerosis[71]. Scanning of the lumbar region reveals evidence of disc degeneration in over a third of asymptomatic women between the ages of 21 and 40[72].

1.12 POSITRON EMISSION TOMOGRAPHY (PET) SCANNING

During decay of certain unstable nuclei positively charged electrons (positrons) are emitted. After a short distance, the positron encounters an electron resulting in their mutual destruction. Energy is released in the form of paired photons which then travel in opposite directions. By the use of detectors ranged around the head, the origin of the signal can be located to a particular 1–2 cm tomographic slice of the brain. Reconstructed images are produced similar to those obtained by CT scanning. To date, most studies have been performed using radioisotopes of oxygen, nitrogen, carbon and fluorine. Measurements can be made of cerebral blood flow, using labelled CO_2, and local oxygen utilization (as a measure of metabolic rate) using labelled O_2. An oxygen extraction fraction, derived from these figures, represents the arterio-venous oxygen difference divided by the arterial oxygen concentration. Using a variety of other isotopes, glucose metabolism, and certain neurotransmitter systems have been investigated.

The methods have been applied to the study of cerebrovascular diseases, dementia, seizure disorders and extra-pyramidal disorders. The system is extremely expensive. By 1985, 34 centres were operational throughout the world with a further 14 centres projected [70]. Whilst the technique can, and undoubtedly will, provide information about fundamental brain mechanisms in health and disease, its role in clinical investigation will remain extremely limited.

REFERENCES

1. Bull, J.W.D. and Zilkha, K.J. (1968) Rationalizing requests for X-ray films in neurology. *Br. Med. J.*, 4, 569–70.
2. Abrams, H.L. (1979) The 'overutilization' of X-rays. *N. Engl. J. Med.*, 300, 1213–16.
3. Jergens, M.E., Morgan, M.T. and McElroy, C.E. (1977) Selective use of radiography of the skull and cervical spine. *West. J. Med.*, 127, 1–4.
4. Wagner, J.L. and Krieger, M.J. (1982) The implications of cost-effectiveness analysis of medical technology. Background paper no. 5: four common X-ray procedures: problems and prospects for economic evaluation. Congress of the United States, Office of Technology Assessment.
5. Bell, R.S and Loop, J.W. (1971) The utility and futility of radiographic skull examination for trauma. *N. Engl. J. Med.*, 284, 236–9.
6. Zimmerman, R.A., Bilaniuk, L.T., Gennarelli, T., *et al.* (1978) Cranial computed tomography in diagnosis and management of acute head trauma. *Am. J. Roentgenol.*, 131, 27–34.
7. Mendelow, A.D., Teasdale, G., Jennett, B., *et al.* (1983) Risks of intracranial haematoma in head injured adults. *Br. Med. J.*, 287, 1173–6.
8. Lord Brain (1963) Some unsolved problems of cervical spondylosis. *Br. Med. J.*, 1, 771–7.
9. Bull, J.W.D. (1948) Discussion on rupture of the intervertebral disc in the cervical region. *Proc. R. Soc. Med.*, 41, 513–16.
10. Johnson, A.J. and Burrows, E.H. (1978) Thecal deformity after lumbar

myelography with iophendylate (myodil) and meglumine iothalamate (conray 280). *B. J. Radiol.*, **51**, 196–202.
11. Shaw, M.D.M., Russell, J.A. and Grossart, K.W. (1978) The changing pattern of spinal arachnoiditis. *J. Neurol. Neurosurg. Psychiatry*, **41**, 97–107.
12. Grainger, R.G., Kendall, B.E. and Wylie, I.G. (1976) Lumbar myelography with metrizamide – a new non-ionic contrast medium. *Br. J. Radiol.*, **49**, 996–1003.
13. Killebrew, K., Whaley, R.A., Hayward, J.N. and Scatliff, J.H. (1983) Complications of metrizamide myelography. *Arch. Neurol.*, **40**, 78–80.
14. Bertoni, J.M., Schwartzman, R.J., van Hern, G. and Partin, J. (1981) Asterixis and encephalopathy following metrizamde myelography: investigations into possible mechanisms and review of the literature. *Ann. Neurol.*, **9**, 366–70.
15. Meador, K., Hamilton, W.J., El Gammal, T.A.M., *et al.* (1984) Irreversible neurologic complications of metrizamide myelography. *Neurology*, **34**, 817–21.
16. Martin, K.I. and Gean, A.D. (1986) The spinal tap: a new look at an old test. *Ann. Intern. Med.*, **104**, 840–8.
17. Tourtellotte, W.W., Henderson, W. and Tucker, R.P. (1972) A randomized double-blind clinical trial comparing the 22 vs 26 gauge needle in the production of post-lumbar puncture syndrome in normal individuals. *Headache*, **12**, 73–8.
18. Carbaat, P.A.T. and van Crevel, H. (1981) Lumbar puncture headache: controlled study on the preventive effect of 24 hours' bed rest. *Lancet, ii,* 1133–5.
19. Hilton-Jones, D., Harrad, R.A., Gill, M.W. and Warlow, C.P. (1982) Failure of postural manoeuvres to prevent lumbar puncture headache. *J. Neurol. Neurosurg. Psychiatry*, **45**, 743–6.
20. Dripps, R.D. and Vandam, L.D. (1954) Long-term follow-up of patients who received 10,098 spinal anesthetics. Failure to discover major neurological sequelae. *J. Am. Med. Assoc.*, **156**, 1486–91.
21. Ruff, R.L. and Dougherty, J.H. Jr. (1981) Complications of lumbar puncture followed by anticoagulation. *Stroke*, **12**, 879–81.
22. Corbett, J.J. and Mehta, M.P. (1983) Cerebrospinal fluid pressure in normal obese subjects and patients with pseudotumor cerebri. *Neurology*, **33**, 1386–8.
23. Buruma, O.J.S., Janson, H.L.F., den Bergh, F.A.J.T.M. and Bots, G.T.H.A.M. (1981) Blood-stained cerebrospinal fluid: traumatic puncture or haemorrhage. *J. Neurol. Neurosurg. Psychiatry*, **44**, 144–7.
24. Reske, A., Haferkamp, G. and Hopf, H.C. (1981) Influence of artificial blood contamination on the analysis of cerebrospinal fluid. *J. Neurol.*, **226**, 187–93.
25. Hayward, R.A., Shapiro, M.F. and Oye, R.K. (1987) Laboratory testing on cerebrospinal fluid. A reappraisal. *Lancet, i,* 1–4.
26. Merril, C.R. and Harrington, M.G. (1984) 'Ultrasensitive' silver stains. Their use exemplified in the study of normal human cerebrospinal fluid

proteins separated by two-dimensional electrophoresis. *Clin. Chem.,* 30, 1938–42.

27. Hershey, L.A. and Trotter, J.L. (1980) The use and abuse of the cerebrospinal fluid IgG profile in the adult: a practical evaluation. *Ann. Neurol.,* 8, 426–34.
28. Sindic, C.J.M., Cambiaso, C.L., Depré, A. *et al.* (1982) The concentration of IgM in the cerebrospinal fluid of neurological patients. *J. Neurol. Sci.,* 55, 339–50.
29. Sindic, C.J.M., Chalon, M.P., Cambiaso, C.L., *et al.* (1982) Assessment of damage to the central nervous system by determination of S-100 protein in the cerebrospinal fluid. *J. Neurol. Neurosurg. Psychiatry,* 45, 1130–5.
30. Price, P. and Cuzner, M.L. (1980) Cerebrospinal fluid complement proteins in neurological disease. *J. Neurol. Sci.,* 46, 49–54.
31. Trotter, J.L., Wegescheide, C.L. and Garvey, W.F. (1983) Immunoreactive myelin proteolipid protein-like activity in cerebrospinal fluid and serum of neurologically impaired patients. *Ann. Neurol.,* 14, 554–8.
32. Firth, G., Rees, J. and McKeran, R.O. (1985) The value of the measurement of cerebrospinal fluid levels of lysozyme in the diagnosis of neurological disease. *J. Neurol. Neurosurg. Psychiatry,* 48, 709–12.
33. Terent, A., Hällgren, R., Venge, P. and Bergström, K. (1981) Lactoferrin, lysozyme, and β_2-microglobulin in cerebrospinal fluid. Elevated levels in patients with acute cerebrovascular lesions as indices of inflammation. *Stroke,* 12, 40–6.
34. Royds, J.A., Timperley, W.R. and Taylor, C.B. (1981) Levels of enolase and other enzymes in the cerebrospinal fluid as indices of pathological change. *J. Neurol. Neurosurg. Psychiatry,* 44, 1129–35.
35. Egg, D., Herold, M., Rumpl, E. and Günther, R. (1980) Prostaglandin $F_{2\alpha}$ levels in human cerebrospinal fluid in normal and pathological conditions. *J. Neurol.,* 222, 239–48.
36. Kuroda, H., Ogawa, N., Yamawaki, Y., *et al.* (1982) Cerebrospinal fluid GABA levels in various neurological and psychiatric diseases. *J. Neurol. Neurosurg. Psychiatry,* 45, 257–60.
37. White, Y.S., Bell, D.S. and Mellick, R. (1973) Sequelae to pneumoencephalography. *J. Neurol. Neurosurg. Psychiatry,* 36, 146–51.
38. O'Mara, R.E., McAfee, J.G. and Chodos, R.B. (1969) The 'doughnut' sign in cerebral radioisotopic images. *Radiology,* 92, 581–6.
39. Paulson, O.B., Lassen, N.A., Henriksen, L., *et al.* (1983) Regional cerebral blood distribution evaluated by emission computer tomography with [133]Xenon and ^{123}I-isopropyl-amphetamine. *J. Cerebral Blood Flow Metab.,* 3, S162–3.
40. Earnest, F., IV, Forbes, G., Sandok, B.A., *et al.* (1983) Complications of cerebral angiography: prospective assessment of risk. *Am. J. Neuroradiol.,* 4, 1191–7.
41. Mani, R.L., Eisenberg, R.L., McDonald, E.J., Jr *et al.* (1978) Complications of catheter cerebral arteriography: analysis of 5,000 procedures. 1. Criteria and incidence. *Am. J. Roentgenol.,* 131, 861–5.

42. McIvor, J., Steiner, T.J., Perkin, G.D., *et al.* (1987) Neurological morbidity of arch and carotid arteriography in cerebrovascular disease. The influence of contrast medium and radiologist. *Br. J. Radiol.*, 60, 117–22.
43. Baum, S., Stein, G.N. and Kuroda, K.K. (1966) Complications of 'No arteriography'. *Radiology*, 86, 835–8.
44. Office of Technology Assessment (1985) *The cost effectiveness of digital subtraction angiography in the diagnosis of cerebrovascular disease.* Washington, DC.
45. Ingemar Petersén, K.G. and Selldén, U. (1981) On the need to collect EEG data from so-called normal individuals. *Clin. Neurophysiology* (ed. E. Stålberg and R.R. Young) Butterworths, London.
46. Matthews, W.B. (1973) The clinical value of routine electroencephalography. *J. R. Coll. Physicians*, 7, 207–12.
47. Bumgartner, J. and Epstein, C.M. (1982) Voluntary alteration of visual evoked potentials. *Ann. Neurol.*, 12, 475–8.
48. Robinson, K., Rudge, P., Small, D.G. and Storey, C.E. (1984) A survey of the pattern reversal visual evoked response (PRVER) in 1428 consecutive patients referred to a clinical neurophysiology department. *J. Neurol. Sci.*, 64, 225–43.
49. Aminoff, M.J. (1984) The clinical role of somatosensory evoked potential studies: a critical appraisal. *Muscle Nerve*, 7, 345–54.
50. Cowan, J.M.A., Rothwell, J.C., Dick, J.P.R. *et al.* (1984) Abnormalities in central motor pathway conduction in multiple sclerosis. *Lancet*, ii, 304–7.
51. Hess, C.W., Mills, K.R. and Murray, N.M.R. (1986) Measurement of central motor conduction in multiple sclerosis by magnetic brain stimulation. *Lancet*, ii, 355–8.
52. Eisen, A. and Cracco, R.Q. (1983) Overuse of evoked potentials: caution. *Neurology*, 33, 618–21.
53. Kimura, J. (1985) Abuse and misuse of evoked potentials as a diagnostic test. *Arch. Neurol.*, 42, 78–80.
54. Chiappa, K.H. and Young, R.R. (1985) Evoked responses, overused, underused, or misused? *Arch. Neurol.*, 42, 76–7.
55. Taylor, P.K. (1984) Non-linear effects of age on nerve conduction in adults. *J. Neurol. Sci.*, 66, 223–34.
56. Buchthal, F. and Rosenfalck, A. (1966) Evoked action potentials and conduction velocity in human sensory nerves. *Brain Res.*, 3, 1–122.
57. Gilliatt, R.W. (1966) Nerve conduction in human and experimental neuropathies. *Proc. R. Soc. Med.*, 59, 989–93.
58. Thomson, J.L.G. (1977) Cost-effectiveness of an EMI brain scanner. A review of a 2-year experience. *Health Trends*, 9, 16–19.
59. Office of Technology Assessment (1981) *Policy implications of the computed tomography (CT) scanner: an update.* Background paper.
60. Steinberg, E.P., Sisk, J.E. and Locke, K.E. (1985) X-ray CT and magnetic resonance imagers: diffusion patterns and policy issues. *N. Engl. J. Med.*, 313, 859–64.

61. Wagner, J.L. (1981) *The implications of cost-effectiveness analysis of medical technology. Case study no. 2: the feasibility of economic evaluation of diagnostic procedures: the case of CT scanning.* Office of Technology Assessment, Washington, DC.
62. Evans, R.G. (1984) Computed tomography – a controversy revisited. *N. Engl. J. Med.*, **310**, 1183–5.
63. Rosenberg, C.E., Anderson, D.C., Mahowald, M.W. and Larson, D. (1982) Computed tomography and EEG in patients without focal neurologic findings. *Arch. Neurol.*, **39**, 291–2.
64. Lee, D., Fox, A., Vinuela, P. *et al.* (1987) Interobserver variation in computed tomography of the brain. *Arch. Neurol.*, **44**, 30–1.
65. Office of Technology Assessment (1984) *Nuclear magnetic resonance imaging technology. A clinical, industrial, and policy analysis.*
66. Evans, R.G., Jost, R.G. and Evans, R.G. Jr (1985) Economic and utilization analysis of magnetic resonance imaging units in the United States in 1985. *Am. J. Roentgenol.*, **145**, 393–8.
67. Cherryman, G.R. (1985) Cost of operating a nuclear magnetic resonance imaging system. *Br. Med. J.*, **291**, 1437–8.
68. Hill, D.W. (1986) Making NMR cost-effective. *Br. J. Hosp. Med.*, **36**, 325.
69. Carr, D.H., Brown, J., Bydder, G.M. *et al.* (1984) Intravenous chelated gadolinium as a contrast agent in NMR imaging of cerebral tumours. *Lancet*, i, 484–6.
70. Feindel, W., Frackowiak, R.S.J., Gadian, D. *et al.* (eds) (1985) *Discussions in Neurosciences. Brain Metabolism and Imaging.* Vol. 2, No. 2. Fondation pour l'étude du Système Nerveux Central et Périphérique, Geneva.
71. Awad, I.A., Johnson, P.C., Spetzler, R.F. and Hodak, J.A. (1986) Incidental subcortical lesions identified on magnetic resonance imaging in the elderly. II. Postmortem pathological correlations. *Stroke*, **17**, 1090–101.
72. Powell, M.C., Wilson, M., Szypryt, P. *et al.* (1986) Prevalence of lumbar disc degeneration observed by magnetic resonance in symptomless women. *Lancet*, ii, 1366–7.

2

Non-specific symptoms
Encephalopathic
syndromes

2.1 HEADACHE

For many patients with headache, a confident clinical diagnosis can
be made on the basis of the history. Most patients with headache
have migraine, tension headache, a mixture of tension and migraine
headache or migrainous neuralgia. Whereas clinical criteria readily
identify patients with classical migraine and migrainous neuralgia,
overlap between the other groups sometimes defies classification [1].
Attempts to improve the accuracy of diagnosis by a computerized
system incorporating clinical data have not proved particularly
successful [1,2]. The need for investigation in patients with headache
is influenced by the results of the physical examination and the
length of history. Focal neurological signs will almost always
demand further investigation. With an increasing length of history,
the possibility of a serious pathology underlying the patient's
headache recedes.

2.1.1 Migraine

Whilst abnormalities can be discovered by certain investigative
techniques in migraine patients, they seldom, if ever, aid management. EEG changes were described in 340 of 560 migraine subjects,
focal changes correlating with the site of neurological symptoms in
classical attacks [3]. Persistent lateralized or localized EEG abnormalities are not, in themselves, an indication for further investigation. There is some evidence that the morbidity of carotid
angiography is higher in patients with migraine than in those with
other neurological disorders [4]. CT scanning is likely to reveal

evidence of infarction in patients with persistent neurological deficit, and in some patients with a history of particularly severe attacks[5]. Diagnostic problems are more likely to arise in attacks of hemiplegic migraine, particularly where a family history is lacking. Examination of the cerebrospinal fluid can further this uncertainty since, exceptionally, a pleocytosis occurs with polymorphonuclear leucocytes predominating[6]. It has been suggested that stereotyped attacks resembling hemiplegic migraine are sometimes triggered by an underlying arteriovenous malformation. In one analysis of 110 patients with such malformations, the incidence of migraine-type attacks was similar to the incidence of migraine in the general population[7].

2.1.2 Tension headache

Features supporting the diagnosis of tension headache include a protracted history, frequent pains, a diffuse distribution and descriptive terms for the pain which include tightness, pressure and band-like. The neurological examination is normal, though tenderness over scalp muscles is often prominent. Investigation is not warranted.

2.1.3 Tumour headache

In patients with tumour, the incidence of headache is unrelated to the presence of papilloedema. Whilst the distribution of the headache, for supra-tentorial tumour, correlates with the site of the growth, its characteristics hardly allow a confident diagnosis of the pathological process. The suspicion of an underlying neoplasm rests more, therefore, with the finding of focal neurological deficit, or from the development of substantial headache *de novo* in a previously headache-free individual.

2.1.4 Post-traumatic headache

Post-traumatic headache can persist for months or years after the initiating event. It does not display specific features, nor does its presence usually merit investigation. Whereas some authors have suggested that the presence of an abnormal EEG firmly establishes an organic rather than a functional basis for the headache[8], there is no justification for using any investigative technique to make such a distinction.

2.1.5 Benign exertional headache

In some individuals, a transient headache occurs in response to bending, coughing or sneezing. In one study, of 103 patients, 10 had a structural intracranial lesion, the majority located within the posterior cranial fossa [9]. An analysis of 221 cases of proven brain tumour established that five had exertional headache [9]. It is probably unreasonable to advise neuroradiological studies for all patients with exertional headache, though clearly these are indicated if there are neurological signs.

2.1.6 Cluster headache

Since cluster headache, using accepted criteria, is readily identified, and since the headache rarely, if ever, represents the effect of structural pathology, investigation is not warranted. The mean erythrocyte choline concentration is approximately half that in control patients, both during and between clusters [10]. Either air encephalography or CT scanning identifies cortical atrophy or ventricular dilatation in some patients; such findings are clearly of no significance with respect to the clinical presentation [11].

2.1.7 Cranial arteritis

Anaemia, normochromic and normocytic in character, is present in over half the patients with cranial arteritis [12]. Amongst 248 patients, haemoglobin concentrations ranged from 7.4 to 14.4 g [13]. An elevated white cell count was reported in 38% [14] and 70% [12] of cases in two series. Abnormal plasma proteins have been described in up to three-quarters of cases, with both depressed albumin and elevated globulin levels [12]. A derangement of liver function is evident in a minority of patients, including elevated alkaline phosphatase levels. Similar findings have been reported in patients with polymyalgia rheumatica [15].

The vast majority of patients with temporal arteritis have a substantial elevation of the erythrocyte sedimentation rate. In the series of 248 patients already referred to , the ESR ranged from 46 to 144 [13], whilst in an analysis of 42 cases, the median level was 96 [14]. Persistently normal levels, in biopsy proven cases, are described [16]. One study deserves comment as, since its findings are so at odds with other series, its diagnostic accuracy must be

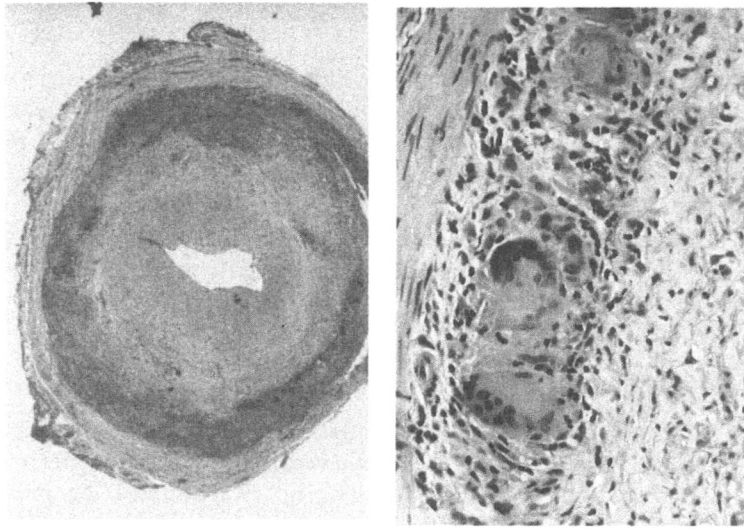

Fig. 2.1 Cranial arteritis: superficial temporal artery biopsy showing intimal thickening and medial damage (left) and giant cell with inflammatory cell infiltration at the level of the internal elastic lamina (right)

questioned. In this group of 72 cases, 8.7% had a normal ESR, and a further 45.7% had a level below 50[12]. In virtually all other reports, an ESR below 45 has been exceptional.

Though an abnormal temporal artery biopsy unequivocally establishes the diagnosis of cranial arteritis, the distribution of the pathological change can hinder histological confirmation (Fig. 2.1). Skip lesions are characteristic, with foci of arteritis as short as 330 μm sometimes occurring in an otherwise normal biopsy[17]. In some patients, biopsy from one artery is normal but typical changes are found in its fellow from the other side. Long biopsy segments of 3–7 cm are recommended, followed by analysis of multiple sections[17].

2.1.8 Recommendation

Patients presenting with headache associated with persisting focal neurological deficit require investigation though certain physical signs, for example a Horner's syndrome in association with cluster headache, are acceptable in the context of a 'benign' headache syndrome. The vast majority of patients with migraine, cluster headache and tension headache can be confidently diagnosed on the basis of the history. A normal neurological examination in such circumstances simply reinforces the diagnosis. Though exertional headache can be reasonably described as benign, some 10% of patients with this complaint have a structural brain lesion. Unless the physician resorts to universal investigation in such instances, he will be guided by the presence of neurological signs and by a failure of the headache to remit during a period of follow-up, though the problem, even when benign, can persist for years. The features of tumour headache are not sufficiently specific to signal the diagnosis. The requirement for investigation here will be triggered by an abnormal examination or the recent emergence of headache in an older individual. Since cranial arteritis carries a high morbidity, but is eminently treatable, its early identification is rightly stressed. The physician can place high, but not absolute, reliance on an elevated ESR as a screening procedure. If the ESR is normal, but the diagnosis is still seriously contemplated, a long segment temporal artery biopsy should be obtained and corticosteroid therapy initiated concurrently.

2.2 DIZZINESS

Neurological disorders including dizziness, or vertigo, amongst their catalogue of symptoms are so numerous that the first inclination, when faced with the dizzy patient, is to mount a wholesale spread of investigations to cover all diagnostic eventualities. In one evaluation, recommended investigations included, besides blood tests and radiological procedures, EEG, ECG, nerve conduction studies, ENG caloric tests, audiometry and modified psychometric evaluation. Not surprisingly, the authors had to admit that 'several of the patients found the number of appointments too inconvenient and failed to return for the entire battery of tests'[18]. The major management problem consists of the patient with a complaint of dizziness, or vertigo, in whom the initial examination has failed to reveal specific findings. At this stage, certain examination procedures, not routinely performed should be carried out, since the findings may, alone, serve to establish a firm diagnosis. Postural hypotension becomes increasingly common with advancing age. An analysis of the literature suggests that a postural systolic fall of 20 mm or more occurs in up to a quarter of elderly individuals, and a fall of 40 mm or more in perhaps 5% [19]. Dizziness was a symptom

in 13 of 15 patients in an early study of the carotid sinus
syndrome[20], a condition which will be discussed in greater detail
in the section on syncope. Dizziness, faintness, light headedness or
vertigo were mentioned by 59% of 78 patients diagnosed as having
the hyperventilation syndrome[21]. A particular type of vertigo,
benign positional vertigo, is triggered by certain head postures. The
condition can occur spontaneously, or following head injury. Head
positioning elicits a paroxysmal nystagmus which always
fatigues[22]. In a survey of 1028 dizzy patients, reported from an
ENT clinic, Meniérès disease accounted for 11% of cases. No
diagnosis was possible in 28%, and psychogenic factors were
thought to operate in 9%. In a comparable neurological outpatient
survey, 22% remained undiagnosed, but 25% were thought to have
underlying psychogenic factors (nearly half with the hyperventilation syndrome)[23].

Initial assessment of patients with dizziness, therefore, should
include measurement of postural blood pressure fall, the response to
carotid sinus pressure, the effect of hyperventilation, and the ability
of head depression with rotation to elicit vertigo and nystagmus. If
none of these manoeuvres reproduce the patient's symptoms, and the
neurological assessment is normal, the yield from further, intensive
investigation is likely to be small. Caloric testing is a valuable
screening procedure in patients with suspected Meniérè's disease or
vestibular neuronitis though the diagnostic status of the latter is open
to question[24]. None of the 125 patients seen in a dizziness clinic
proved to have an acoustic neuroma[18]. If that diagnosis is
seriously contemplated, brain stem auditory evoked responses
provide an almost infallible screening test[25]. The term disabling
positional vertigo has been used to describe patients with persistent
vertigo exacerbated by head movement in whom there is evidence of
compression of components of the vestibular nerve by vessels close
to the root entry zone into the brain-stem[26]. Brain stem auditory
evoked responses display a latency shift of wave 2 and an abnormal
amplitude and shape of wave 3.

2.2.1 Recommendation

Patients with dizziness as a major complaint, and who have no
physical signs, should be assessed for postural hypotension, carotid
sinus hypersensitivity, an adverse reaction to hyperventilation and
positional nystagmus with head depression and rotation. If these are

all negative, further investigation can probably be deferred. If there are auditory symptoms, or the dizziness amounts to persistent, posture-related vertigo, brain-stem auditory evoked responses are of value for the exclusion of acoustic neuroma and disabling positional vertigo respectively.

2.3 SYNCOPE

For many patients with syncopal attacks, the history provides sufficient clue to the diagnosis making further investigation unnecessary. Vaso-vagal attacks usually appear in adolescence, and predominate in females. The attacks occur in certain situations. Confusion with epileptic events is likely if brief twitching or tonic contraction appears in the course of a syncopal event, though neither necessarily contradicts the diagnosis. The electroencephalogram in syncopal attacks displays slow waves followed by electrical silence, clearly differentiating the attack from an epileptic event though this means of differentiation is hardly applicable in routine clinical management[27]. Syncope can appear during micturition or a prolonged bout of coughing. The associations are well recognized and do not imply significant intracranial pathology. Episodes of syncope triggered by swallowing occur in patients with glossopharyngeal neuralgia[28], and have been described rarely in individuals with a variety of cardiac or oesophageal disorders[29]. Many of the conditions causing dizziness, for example postural hypotension, can result in syncope. Conditions particularly associated with syncopal episodes include carotid sinus syncope and disorders of cardiac conduction. In the former, pressure over the relevant carotid sinus can reproduce the patient's attacks. In a review of 16 patients, six presented with vertigo, and five with syncopal attacks[30]. The syncopal attacks tend to be preceded by faintness and frequently coincide with facial pallor followed by flushing. Carotid sinus hypersensitivity is often bilateral but asymmetrical. Triggering factors, for example head rotation, or neck pressure, occur in about 25% of cases[31]. A standard technique for carotid sinus massage has been devised, stimulation insufficient to occlude pulsation in the ipsilateral superficial temporal artery being applied for 6 s under ECG control. A hypersensitive response is accepted if asystole or AV block persists for more than 3 s[32]. Perhaps in 5–10% of patients a pure vasodilator response to sinus stimulation occurs. In these, AV pacing is more successful than ventricular pacing in the relief of symptoms [32].

2.3.1 Investigations

Several studies have addressed themselves to the relative value of different investigations in the evaluation of syncopal attacks. One survey assessed 198 patients, with a mean follow up of 11 months. The final diagnostic categories were neurological (32%) cardiac (8%) metabolic or drug induced (7%) and vaso-vagal, psychogenic or postural in 40%. In 13% of the cases, no diagnosis was made. The authors achieved a diagnosis from the history and physical examination in 85% of cases [33]. They included single seizure cases in this study. It was suggested that a full blood count and metabolic screen were appropriate in all cases, though 130 full blood counts failed to reveal any evidence of occult haemorrhage, whereas, of 130 metabolic screens, only four revealed biochemical abnormalities. Skull X-ray was unhelpful. Of 63 EEGs, only three provided diagnostic information. CT scanning never resulted in the diagnosis being altered to one of a neurological basis for the event. Of 131 ECGs, four were abnormal. Despite this, the authors suggested that the ECG was the most helpful of the routine investigations performed. A similar survey, of 121 patients, though excluding those with clear-cut seizures, produced similar results [34]. In this series, EEG, skull X-rays, CT, GTT, LP, echo and cerebral angiography failed to establish a diagnosis in any of the cases in whom they were performed. A definitive diagnosis was made in 13 patients (11%), during an average hospital stay of 9 days at an average cost of $2463 per patient. A prospective analysis of syncope was subsequently published by the same group, amounting to 204 patients of whom 138 had been admitted [35]. A cause was found in 52%, five times the figure from the retrospective survey. Surprising discrepancies between the studies emerge in terms of the diagnostic yield from certain investigations. Comparable diagnostic yields for ECG monitoring were 6 and 14%. Despite their experience the authors felt unable to make a firm statement about the appropriate extent of investigation for the patient with syncope.

Most debate on the evaluation of the patient with syncope centres on the comparative value of ECG monitoring and electrophysiological studies including His bundle conduction. Among 27 patients with syncope, 24 h ECG monitoring established the presence of a significant arrhythmia in a third[36]. A leader on the subject concluded that Holter monitoring is of value for all syncopal patients where the diagnosis is in question or where an arrhythmia is suspected[37]. Others, however, have been less impressed by the diagnostic yield of this procedure, suggesting that false-positive findings may result in unjustified treatment of a presumed symptomatic arrhythmic tendency[33].

In one analysis, among 1512 tapes, only 15 coincided with syncopal events, of which only seven could be attributed to an arrhythmia[38]. Greater, though not universal, support has been given for the role of intracardiac electrophysiological recordings though in the prospective study already referred to, this technique provided diagnostic information in only 3 of 204 patients. In two early reports, over 60% of patients with syncope of unknown cause, all of whom had no clinical cardiological abnormality or abnormalities on routine ECG or Holter monitoring, had conduction abnormalities demonstrated by electrophysiological study[39,40]. In each series, appropriate arrhythmia treatment resolved attacks in over 80% of the patients. Two other studies have been rather less positive. In one, including 32 syncopal patients, intra-cardiac studies resulted in induced ventricular tachycardia in 11, and evidence of sinus nodal dysfunction in five. However, among the former, only two were without evidence of organic heart disease whereas the authors were forced to conclude, for the latter, that from follow-up information, 'it is not clear whether the observed electrophysiologic abnormalities were related to the clinical symptoms'[41]. The other report included 34 patients. Electrophysiological studies were abnormal in six, though in one the induced abnormality was not clearly symptomatic[42]. Among 15 patients with syncope with normal Holter monitoring and His bundle assessment, prolonged head-up tilt induced syncope in two-thirds with relief of symptoms subsequently by dual-chamber pacing[43].

2.3.2 Recommendation (see flow chart)

In the majority of patients with syncope, a diagnosis, if it is to be established, can be made on the basis of the history and physical examination. By these means vaso-vagal attacks, micturition and cough syncope and syncope associated with swallowing are identified. The use of hyperventilation and carotid sinus massage allow identification of attacks secondary to hyperventilation and carotid

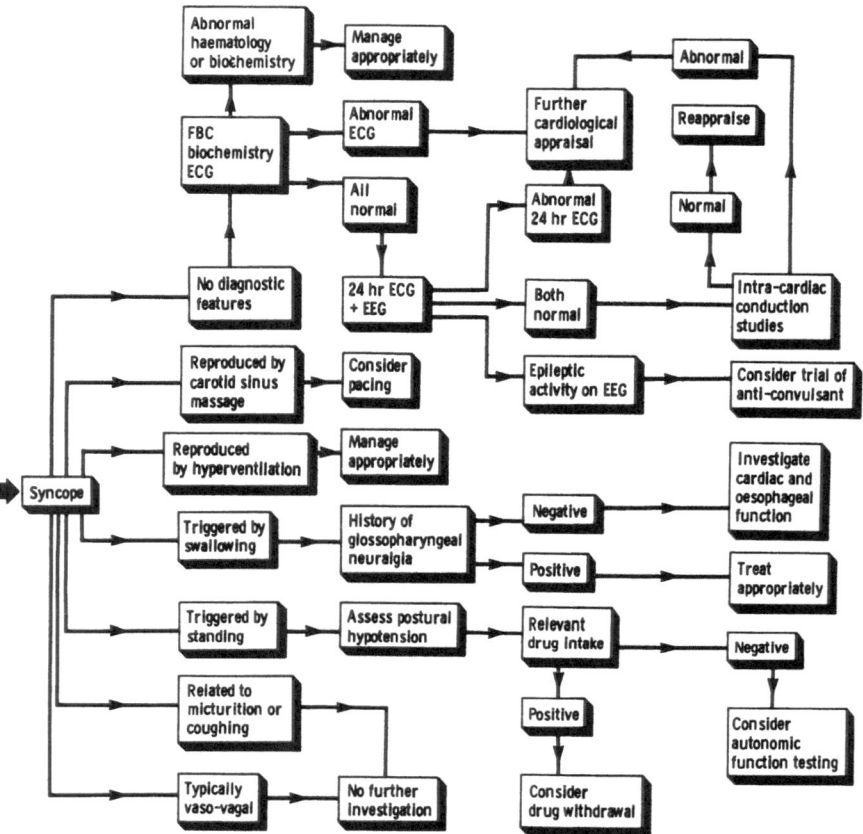

Flow chart

sinus syndrome respectively. If these procedures are unproductive, routine blood tests and ECG are indicated and may provide a diagnosis. The next investigative steps are somewhat controversial, but a combination of EEG and 24 h ECG monitoring have the merit of being relatively cheap and non-invasive. If monitoring is negative, and a primary cardiac dysrhythmia remains possible, intra-cardiac conduction studies are recommended.

2.4 DROWSINESS

Many patients who complain of excessive tiredness are found to be depressed or neurotic. More specific causes of day-time drowsiness include narcolepsy, idiopathic hypersomnolence and sleep ap-

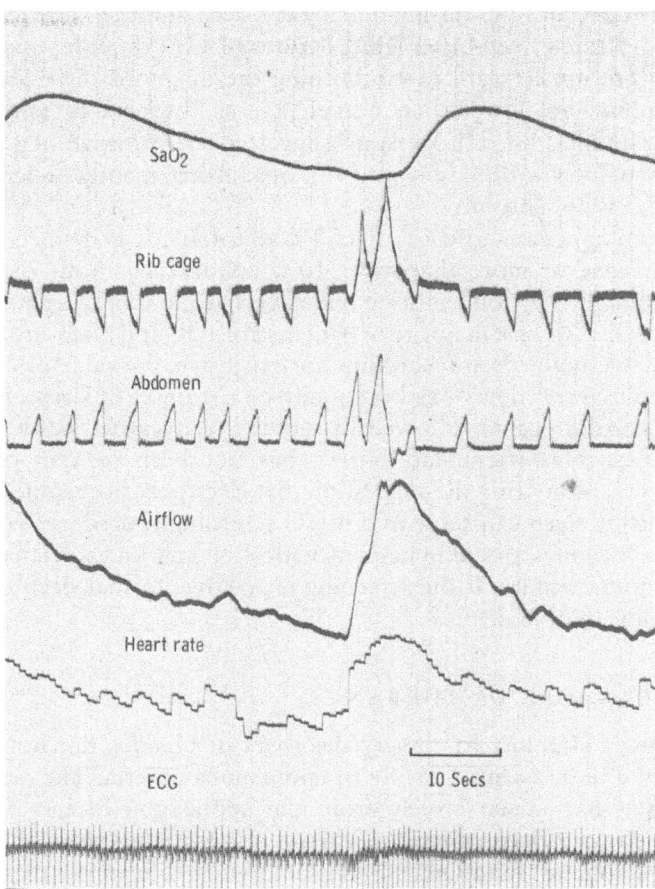

Fig. 2.2 Sleep apnoea. Antagonistic rib cage and abdominal movements cause hypoxia interspersed with brief synchronous movements producing air flow and improved oxygenation

noea [44]. The sleep episodes in hypersomnia tend to be longer and more resistible than those associated with narcolepsy. Where cataplexy accompanies narcolepsy the combination is sufficiently specific not to require further investigation [45]. Where narcolepsy occurs in isolation, the diagnosis can be confirmed by electro-encephalography, the requirement for diagnosis being REM periods occurring within 15 minutes of the onset of sleep [46]. Among 50 patients, recordings during one night's sleep and two daytime naps demonstrated sleep-onset REM periods in 42 [45]. Other investigations are unnecessary in establishing the diagnosis. CSF levels of dopamine are lowered in narcolepsy, as they are in idiopathic hypersomnia [46]. HLA testing suggested the presence of DR2 in every patient with narcolepsy [47], but further reports indicate the linkage is not absolute.

Sleep apnoea is said to affect 1% of adults. It is defined as the occurrence of more than five, 10 s, apnoeas per hour of sleep, accompanied by loud snoring and excessive daytime sleepiness [48] (Fig. 2.2). The vast majority of patients are male and many are obese. Since overnight sleep recordings are expensive, the value of various screening procedures has been analysed. At onset of sleep apnoea, bradycardia occurs followed by sudden tachycardia as breathing resumes. This particular pattern has not been seen in control subjects, prompting the suggestion that electrocardiographic analysis during sleep can serve as a useful screening procedure [49]. The phenomenon is absent in patients with sleep apnoea associated with autonomic failure. If the screening is positive, formal sleep studies are indicated [48,49].

2.5 BLADDER DISTURBANCE

Frequent attempts to classify disorders of bladder function have resulted in a confusing array of eponymous criteria. The need for revision has arisen largely from the application of increasingly sophisticated electrophysiological techniques to the study of bladder and sphincter function. A satisfactory classification, based on urodynamic study, divides bladder and sphincter activity into three categories, normal, hyperactive and inactive, producing nine combinations, one of which represents a normally functioning system [50].

The requirement for physiological analysis of bladder and sphincter function is reinforced by the poor correlation between urinary symptoms, for example in multiple sclerosis, and the findings from urodynamic study [51]. The first-introduced technique was cystometry in which recording of intravesical pressure is performed during filling of the bladder by a known volume of fluid or gas [52]. The examination can be combined with a study of the effect on pressure levels of the injection of subcutaneous urecholine. An abnormal pressure increase, reflecting denervation hypersensitivity of the detrusor muscle, should correlate with lesions at or beyond the level of the sacral outflow but, in practice, a similar reaction can occur with suprasacral lesions. In rapid cystometry, injections of 100 ml of water over a 3 s interval are performed, with analysis of pressure wave responses following each injection. Type A contractions, of low amplitude and short duration, occurring 1–2 s after injection, occur in nearly 90% of patients with cauda equina lesions [53]. Cystometry, performed in isolation, is unable to provide data on the existence or nature of any outflow obstruction.

A measure of urinary flow, or a urethral pressure profile (assessed whilst slowly withdrawing a catheter along the urethra) provides such data, but gives no information about the physiological state of the urethral sphincter. This can be obtained only by electromyography. Surface or needle electrodes have been used for this purpose. For the anal sphincter, the surface electrode is inserted in the anal canal, the needle electrode into the sphincter about 1 cm from the anal margin. For the urinary sphincter, a surface electrode can be attached to a foley catheter, or a needle electrode inserted in the midline, directed towards the apex of the prostate. In a study of spinal injury patients, abnormal units were more frequently detected from periurethral than perianal needle electrodes [54]. Among ten patients with areflexic bladders, nearly 60% had abnormally prolonged or abnormally large units in periurethral striated muscle, compared to 7% of control subjects [55]. When periurethral EMG is combined with cystometry, certain abnormal patterns of function can be defined, including uninhibited reflex sphincter relaxation, and detrusor–sphincter dyssynergia. In the latter, increasing, uninhibitable, clonic sphincter contractions develop during bladder expansion. The most frequent causes of this combination are traumatic cord lesions, myelodysplasia and multiple sclerosis [56]. Techniques have been devised, using surface electrodes attached to foley catheters, to record activity from vesical muscle during cystometry [57]. The specifity of abnormal patterns appears to be low. Methods are available for the examination of the pelvic reflex arc concerned with control of bladder function. Using a stimulating electrode applied to the dorsum of the base of the penis or clitoris, anal or urethral EMG activity can be recorded from a plug electrode in the anal canal or an electrode attached to a foley catheter within the urethra, respectively [58]. The motor element of the reflex arc can be studied separately by stimulating over the lumbar spine [59]. Application of the latter technique, along with pelvic floor EMG, has established the presence of denervation in anal or periurethral voluntary muscle in patients with idiopathic (neurogenic) faecal and urinary incontinence [60].

The data obtained from physiological studies need to be supported by radiological data. Urethrography allows detection of urethral structures or diverticulae, and assesses the state of the external sphincter. Cystography will identify trabeculation, diverticulae and vesico-ureteric reflux. Combined with urethrography during voiding, it permits evaluation of bladder neck function. Intravenous pyelography determines the state of the upper urinary tract.

2.5.1 Recommendation

Since symptomatology is unhelpful in predicting the exact balance of bladder and sphincter dysfunction in patients with a disorder of urinary control, investigation is essential if any coherent system of treatment is to be devised. Radiological assessment should include visualization of the upper urinary tract, the bladder and urethra, together with inspection of the bladder and urethra during voiding. Cystometry is seldom sufficient for an analysis of bladder performance [61]. It should be combined with EMG analysis of the periurethral striated muscle. The procedure can be usefully accompanied by X-ray video inspection of the bladder and urethra. Where a disturbance of the sacral reflex arc is suspected, measurement of evoked responses allows confirmation of abnormal conduction in the afferent or efferent pathway.

2.6 VARIOUS ENCEPHALOPATHIES

2.6.1 Wernicke's encephalopathy

Though the triad of nystagmus, ocular paresis and a disturbance of the mental state is the hallmark of Wernicke's encephalopathy, incomplete forms of the condition are reported, whilst, if the patient presents in coma, it may not be suspected. Accordingly investigation may be particularly helpful in these incomplete or atypical forms. The CSF is of no value in diagnosis, displaying at most a mild increase in the protein concentration. The EEG changes, consisting of an increase in slow activity, are non-specific and indeed may be lacking, even in patients with florid mental symptoms [62]. The most specific biochemical change in thiamine deficiency is depression of red cell transketolase activity. However, levels may be depressed in

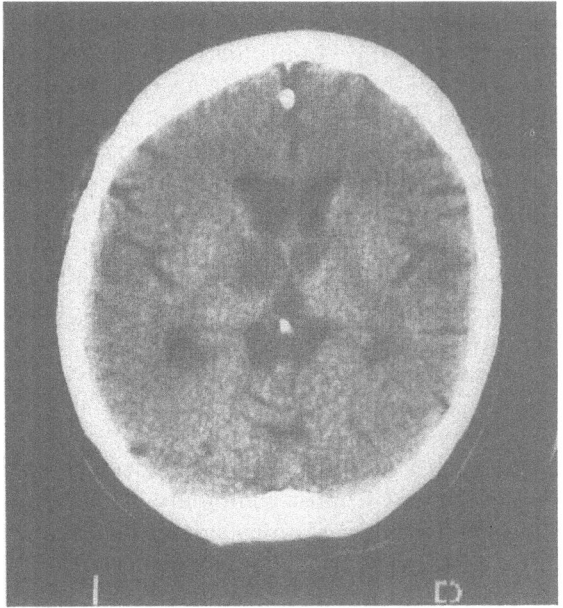

Fig. 2.3 Thalamic hypodense areas on CT in patient with Wernicke's encephalopathy

alcoholic patients without Wernicke's encephalopathy, and overlap of levels between normal individuals and patients with Wernicke's encephalopathy is found[63]. Recently electrophysiological and radiological changes have been reported. Prolongation of the I–V interval of the brain stem auditory evoked responses is found in about half the patients but can also be detected in alcoholics without neurological deficit[64]. Two studies have recorded hypodense areas in the dorsomedial nuclei of the thalamus in the acute stages of Wernicke's encephalopathy (Fig. 2.3)[65,66].

2.6.2 Whipple's disease

The most prominent neurological features of Whipple's disease include dementia, ophthalmoplegia and myoclonus. Cases with pathological changes confined to the central nervous system are recognized[67,68]. A particular movement, consisting of continuous rhythmic ocular vergence with synchronous jaw contraction is considered a pathognomonic feature [69]. The CSF protein concentration may be elevated, accompanied by abnormal IgG ratios and faint oligoclonal banding [67,68]. Electrophysiological abnormalities include evidence of a peripheral neuropathy, and abnormal central conduction, for example with brain stem or somatosensory evoked responses [68]. Epileptic activity is described in the EEG [67]. CT scanning reveals multi-focal hypodense areas with enhancement. Jejunal biopsy for PAS-positive material is diagnostic but will be negative in cases with confined CNS lesions. Characteristic sickle form, particle-containing cells are found on brain biopsy but have not been detected in CSF [70]. Definitive diagnosis of cases with pure neurological involvement requires brain biopsy.

2.6.3 Sarcoidosis

Although sarcoid has been included in this section, analysis of the literature suggests that it most commonly affects cranial or peripheral nerves [71]. Central nervous system involvement takes the form of focal cerebral hemisphere damage, cerebellar or extrapyramidal changes or disruption of the hypothalamic–pituitary axis. Where there are clear signs of involvement of other systems, the diagnosis of sarcoidosis is relatively straightforward. Difficulties arise in cases where the disease is confined to the nervous system, or where the involvement of other organs is subclinical.

Routine investigations are of limited value in such cases. The ESR is frequently normal, and abnormalities of plasma proteins or calcium levels often lacking. The CSF reveals elevated protein concentrations and lymphocyte counts in many patients, but the changes are not specific and may be absent despite clinically active disease [72]. Abnormal IgG ratios and oligoclonal IgG are described in sarcoidosis, but their presence may simply further diagnostic confusion. CSF levels of lysozyme and β_2-microglobulin are elevated in patients with neurological sarcoid but seldom where other systems alone are affected [73]. Serum levels of angiotensin-converting enzyme are elevated in 50–75% of patients with active sarcoidosis, but the abnormality is not specific to this condition. Subsequent levels, when initially elevated, correlate quite well with the clinical course in patients with pulmonary disease [74]. There is some evidence to suggest that CSF levels of the enzyme are higher in active neurosarcoidosis than in extraneural disease, correlating with disease activity [75,76].

2.6.4 Coma

Coma developing in the presence of a mass lesion is the consequence of direct compression of the ascending reticular activating system by brain-stem or cerebellar pathology, or, indirectly, as a result of transtentorial herniation secondary to cerebral hemispheric swelling. More commonly, coma is the consequence of a metabolic, toxic or diffuse process affecting brain function at multiple levels. Certain physical findings help to distinguish coma due to a mass lesion from that consequent to metabolic disease. In metabolic or toxic coma, the pupillary light reflexes are generally preserved, the eyes either rest in the midline, or roam conjugately, and abnormal motor responses tend to be confined to a diffuse increase in limb tone, sometimes merging into decorticate or decerebrate posturing[77]. Patients in metabolic coma characteristically display tremor, asterixis or generalized myoclonus. Seizures may occur and are sometimes focal. Where there is a history of drug ingestion, extensive investigation of the comatose patient, for example with CT scanning, is not warranted, though a dual pathology can operate in such cases as, for instance, in an alcoholic with a subdural haematoma. In many patients in metabolic coma, the past medical history suggests the likely mechanism. More troublesome, in terms of diagnosis, are those patients where such a history is lacking, or where focal neurological findings misleadingly suggest a structural pathology. Papilloedema can occur in respiratory failure associated with CO_2 retention[78] and in the presence of adrenal insufficiency[79]. Bilateral pyramidal signs, including extensor plantar responses, are recognized features of uraemia[80] and hepatic encephalopathy[81]. Unilateral pyramidal signs have been described in patients in hepatic failure[82] and secondary to hypoglycaemia[83]. Other metabolic, electrolyte or endocrinological disorders sometimes presenting, or associated, with coma include hyponatraemia[84], hypernatraemia, hypercalcaemia[85] and myxoedema[86]. Certain investigative findings can be misleadingly abnormal in metabolic coma. An elevated CSF protein concentration sometimes accompanies renal failure[80], and hypercalcaemia[87]. The EEG changes are rather more specific, but not sufficiently so to exclude a structural disorder. With deepening metabolic coma, the alpha rhythm is lost, the record becoming dominated by a progressively increasing slow-wave activity, sometimes in the form of bursts[80].

(a) Recommendation

Metabolic and drug-induced coma are sufficiently common to merit early exclusion in patients presenting with unexplained coma. A drug screen is recommended even where inappropriate ingestion is established, partly to assess whether more than one drug is responsible and partly to quantify the problem. Initial biochemical studies should include measurement of electrolytes, glucose, blood urea, calcium and liver function tests. The blood gases should be analysed. In older patients, thyroid function tests should be performed. Immediate CT scanning is mandatory where focal neurological deficit is found and is advisable at an early stage in the absence of focal signs if the initial metabolic and toxicology screen is negative. The EEG can contribute to the distinction of metabolic from structural causes of coma, but is not sufficiently sensitive to be considered as an essential part of the immediate investigative screen. CSF examination is warranted in comatose patients with negative CT and normal biochemistry to exclude the remote possibilities of subarachnoid haemorrhage or meningitis. In any patient, the possibility of a multifactorial basis for coma, sometimes incorporating both metabolic and structural causes, has to be considered.

2.6.5 Brain death

Extensive discussion has centred on the respective roles of neurological examination and investigation in the assessment of patients surviving cardiac arrest, and in those considered brain dead. For the former, original EEG studies concluded that individuals with normal, or near normal, records had an excellent prognosis, compared to the gloomy outlook for patients with flat, or nearly flat recordings[88]. When the EEG analysis is expanded to include 49 variables, death or survival can be predicted with a confidence exceeding 99% [89]. An argument for utilizing the EEG for this purpose can be confidently forwarded only if the clinical examination fails to provide a comparable level of discrimination. One study suggested this might be the case, indicating that more patients, with unfavourable signs at the first examination, nevertheless, achieved some degree of independence [90].

A more recent study, however, identified 93 patients surviving cardiorespiratory arrest who, at 24 hours after the event, had either absent or primitive flexor, extensor motor responses associated with spontaneous eye movements which were neither orientating nor conjugate. Of these individuals, only one regained an independent existence [91].

Debate on the role of examination and investigation in the diagnosis of brain death had been stimulated by the need to define criteria which can be applied with total confidence. Early reports of the role of the EEG in the diagnosis of brain death concluded that an isoelectric record inevitably identified a fatal outcome, providing drug ingestion had been excluded [92]. A suggestion that strictly applied clinical criteria might be of greater relevance in predicting outcome than an isoelectric EEG emerged from a clinicopathological study of 25 patients, nine of whom had had EEG recordings [93]. Amongst these nine cases, all fulfilling certain clinical criteria, one had an isoelectric EEG despite a normally appearing brain stem at autopsy, whereas two cases, with low voltage fast activity, had grossly damaged brain stems. In the light of these and other studies, criteria were formulated for diagnosing brain death in the United Kingdom which did not require confirmation by EEG or other investigative techniques [94]. Stress was placed on the need to elicit the cause of the coma, with particular emphasis on the exclusion of toxic and metabolic factors and any contribution from hypothermia. Guidelines published for clinicians working in North America were initially more circumspect, adding, to similar clinical criteria, the need to demonstrate EEG silence over a 30 minute period, not less than six hours after the onset of the coma. If any uncertainty remained, cerebral blood flow measurement was recommended [94]. In some respects, the guidelines contradicted the findings of a US collaborative study designed to examine the prognostic roles of clinical and electrophysiological examination in comatose subjects [96]. Clinical criteria consisted of coma and an apnoeic state which both failed to override the respirator during a 15 minute period, then failed to trigger ventilation over a three minute period off the respirator. An isoelectric EEG constituted the electrophysiological criterion, and it was suggested that the finding should be confirmed by further assessment, at least 24 hours later.

If absent brain-stem reflexes were included, but not the need for repeat examination, all patients fulfilling the criteria were dead within a three month period. When, however, four separate criteria for diagnosing brain death were applied retrospectively, the criteria ranging from clinical assessment alone to one including angiographic confirmation of cessation of cerebral blood flow, an individual fulfilling any of the four systems failed to survive beyond a further three months. Support for the UK Guidelines came from a report of 609 patients, all fulfilling the criteria, of whom 326 were followed rather than having their respiratory support withdrawn. All the patients subsequently died[97]. These, purely clinical, criteria continue to be applied in the UK. In the US, similar clinical appraisal is performed, though the apnoea has to be resistant to a higher PCO_2 level (60 mmHg) than the 50 mmHg thought to suffice in the UK. Moreover the United States guidelines continue to refer to the desirability of confirming the clinical criteria by the finding of EEG silence, adding that demonstration of the complete cessation of cerebral circulation in a normothermic subject for a period exceeding 10 minutes is incompatible with the survival of brain tissue[98].

Recommendation

In patients surviving a cardiorespiratory arrest, careful clinical appraisal within the first 24 hours is capable of defining a poor-risk group with a similar degree of certainty to that achieved by multivariate EEG analysis. In the diagnosis of brain death, there is no firm body of evidence to refute the use of clinical criteria as the sole arbiter of outcome, providing drug and metabolic factors are excluded and hypothermia is absent.

2.6.6 Other conditions

Most inborn errors of metabolism present in childhood but adult-onset forms of G_{M1} and G_{M2} gangliosidosis, Gaucher's disease and metachromatic leucodystrophy are recognized[99]. In adults with G_{M1} gangliosidosis, extrapyramidal features predominate[100] sometimes accompanied by myoclonus[101]. Adult Tay–Sachs disease (G_{M2} gangliosidosis) presents either as a spinocerebellar degeneration[102] or atypical motor neurone disease[103]. There may be accompanying psychotic episodes. Type 3 Gaucher's disease appears at any time from the first to the fourth decade of life[104]. Neurological findings include seizures, intellectual failure and myoclonus. Investigative findings include anaemia with thrombocytopenia, elevated serum acid phosphatase levels, Gaucher cells in the bone marrow, and depressed levels of leucocyte glucocerebrosidase. Adult-onset forms of metachromatic leucodystrophy may not be accompanied by evidence of an overt neuropathy. Clinical expression includes pyramidal and cerebellar signs, dementia and psychiatric disturbance[105]. The CSF protein concentration may be normal in such cases. Though clinical evidence of neuropathy is sometimes lacking, abnormalities of peripheral conduction are likely[106], accompanied by delay of visual and somatosensory evoked potentials. CT demonstrates symmetrical frontal and parietal non-enhancing hypodense white matter lesions[105]. The diagnosis is established by the finding of reduced levels of arylsulphatase A in leucocytes and cultured fibroblasts. Adrenoleucodystrophy can present in adult life, usually with a progressive spastic paraplegia, sometimes accompanied by peripheral neuropathy[107]. The cerebral manifestations evident in childhood cases are not encountered. Inheritance is as a sex-linked recessive. Analysis of carriers suggests that some 12% have evidence of a paraparesis[108]. Levels of very long-chain fatty acids are elevated in the serum and tissues of patients, and in all symptomatic carriers.

An autosomal dominant form of leucodystrophy has been described, beginning in the fourth or fifth decade of life, and mimicking multiple sclerosis. The cerebellar and pyramidal features, however, are accompanied by evidence of an autonomic neuropathy with orthostatic hypotension a prominent feature. CT scanning demonstrates symmetrical reduction of white matter density. Rare cases of Leigh's disease appearing in adult life have been recorded, with ataxia a more prominent feature than the dystonia found in younger cases. Other manifestations have included optic atrophy, myoclonus, epilepsy and coma[110]. The CSF can be normal or show elevated protein and globulin concentrations. In familial cases, abnormal urinary levels of inhibitory factor for thiamine diphosphate phosphoryl transferase have been recorded[110]. At times, CT scanning displays lucencies in the basal ganglia, substantia nigra, mid-brain tectum and other structures. Serial MRI scanning has been performed in one case[111]. Initial areas of increased signal intensity in the periaqueductal grey and mid-brain tectum were replaced by diffuse oedema and increased intensity signal from the substantia nigra, caudate, putamen and globus pallidus followed, in the terminal stages, by atrophy and cavitation at these sites. Though an adult case of carbamyl phosphate synthetase-1 deficiency has been described, bouts of vomiting, gait ataxia and somnolence had begun at the age of 13[112]. Investigative findings include elevated serum ammonium levels and CT evidence of hypodense white matter subcortically.

The mitochondrial myopathies have been discussed elsewhere (Section 9.4). In some patients, cerebral symptoms are prominent.

The Kearns–Sayre syndrome, which includes a progressive external ophthalmoplegia begins before the age of 15, whereas myoclonic epilepsy associated with ragged red fibres usually presents before the age of 20. Symptoms include seizures, myoclonus, ataxia and weakness. A third clinical variant includes myopathy, encephalopathy, lactic acidosis and stroke-like episodes[113].

The findings on investigation are partly influenced by the clinical subtype. Most, but not all patients show an increased blood concentration of lactic acid. A more dramatic rise in lactate levels can be triggered by exercise. CT scanning shows basal ganglia calcifications and areas of lucency, particularly in the clinical variant including stroke-like episodes.

A pure neurological presentation of systemic lupus erythematosus can affect either the peripheral or central nervous systems. The former can produce a picture suggesting Guillain–Barré syndrome (Section 8.2), manifestations of the latter include optic neuritis[114] and transverse myelitis[115]. Other neurological complications include cerebrovascular accidents, involuntary movements, particularly chorea, and disordered mental function[116]. Diagnosis is difficult when the neurological complications antedate expression of the disease in other systems. CSF changes include an abnormal protein concentration, pleocytosis and elevated IgG levels. Levels of CSF C4 are depressed in some patients with cerebral lupus. Serological studies often reveal abnormal findings even when the disease is clinically confined to the nervous system.

REFERENCES

1. Drummond, P.D. and Lance, J.W. (1984) Clinical diagnosis and computed analysis of headache symptoms. *J. Neurol. Neurosurg. Psychiatry*, **47**, 128–33.
2. Francis, J.H., Pennal, B.E. and Wadsworth, W. (1984) Development of a computer-assisted headache diagnostic and treatment system. *Headache*, **24**, 35–8.
3. Hockaday, J.M. and Whitty, C.W.M. (1969) Factors determining the electroencephalogram in migraine: a study of 560 patients, according to clinical type of migraine. *Brain*, **92**, 769–88.
4. Patterson, R.H. Jr, Goodell, H. and Dunning, H.S. (1964) Complications of carotid angiography. *Arch. Neurol.*, **10**, 513–20.
5. Hungerford, G.D., du Boulay, G.H. and Zilkha, K.J. (1976) Computerised axial tomography in patients with severe migraine: a preliminary report. *J. Neurol. Neurosurg. Psychiatry*, **39**, 990–4.

6. Bradshaw, P. and Parsons, M. (1965) Hemiplegic migraine, a clinical study. *Quart. J. Med.*, **133**, 65–85.

7. Paterson, J.H. and McKissock, W. (1956) A clinical survey of intracranial angiomas with special reference to their mode of progression and surgical treatment: a report of 110 cases. *Brain*, **79**, 233–66.

8. Denker, P.G. and Perry, G.F. (1954) Post concussion syndrome in compensation and litigation analysis of 95 cases with electroencephalographic correlations. *Neurology*, **4**, 912–18.

9. Rooke, E.D. (1968) Benign exertional headache. *Med. Clin. N. Am.*, **52**, 801–8.

10. de Belleroche, J., Cook, G.E., Das, I. *et al.* (1984) Erythrocyte choline concentrations and cluster headache. *Br. Med. J.*, **288**, 268–70.

11. Russell, D., Nakstad, P. and Sjaastad, O. (1978) Cluster headache – pneumoencephalographic and cerebral computerized axial tomography findings. *Headache*, **18**, 272–3.

12. Whitfield, A.G.W., Bateman, M. and Cooke, W.T. (1963) Temporal arteritis. *Br. J. Ophthalmol.*, **47**, 555–66.

13. Klein, R.G., Hunder, G.G., Stanson, A.W. and Sheps, S.G. (1975) Large artery involvement in giant cell (temporal) arteritis. *Ann. Intern. Med.*, **83**, 806–12.

14. Huston, K.A., Hunder, G.G., Lie, J.T. *et al.* (1978) Temporal arteritis. A 25-year epidemiologic, clinical, and pathologic study. *Ann. Intern. Med.*, **88**, 162–7.

15. Dickson, E.R., Maldonado, J.E., Sheps, S.G. and Cain, J.A. Jr (1973) Systemic giant-cell arteritis with polymyalgia rheumatica. Reversible abnormalities of liver function. *J. Am. Med. Assoc.*, **224**, 1496–8.

16. Healey, L.A. and Wilske, K.R. (1977) Manifestations of giant cell arteritis. *Med. Clin. N. Am.*, **61**, 261–70.

17. Klein, R.G., Campbell, R.J., Hunder, G.G. and Carney, J.A. (1976) Skip lesions in temporal arteritis. *Mayo Clin. Proc.*, **51**, 504–10.

18. Drachman, D.A. and Hart., C.W. (1972) An approach to the dizzy patient. *Neurology*, **22**, 323–34.

19. Blumenthal, M.D. and Davie, J.W. (1980) Dizziness and falling in elderly psychiatric outpatients. *Am. J. Psychiatry*, **137**, 203–6.

20. Weiss, S. and Baker, J.P. (1933) The carotid sinus reflex in health and disease. Its role in the causation of fainting and convulsions. *Medicine*, **12**, 297–354.

21. Perkin, G.D. and Joseph, R. (1986) Neurological manifestations of the hyperventilation syndrome. *J. R. Soc. Med.*, **79**, 448–50.

22. Barber, H.O. (1964) Positional nystagmus, especially after head injury. *Laryngoscope*, **74**, 891–944.

23, Perkin, G.D. (1986) *Basic Neurology*. Verlagsgesellschaft. Ellis Horwood. pp. 132–7.

24. Dix, M.R. and Hallpike, C.S. (1952) The pathology, symptomatology and diagnosis of certain common disorders of the vestibular system. *Proc. R. Soc. Med.*, **45**, 341–54.

25. Maurer, K. Strumpel, D. and Wende, S. (1982) Acoustic tumour

detection with early auditory evoked potentials and neuroradiological methods. *J. Neurol.*, **227**, 177–85.

26. Jannetta, P.J., Møller, M.B. and Møller, A.R. (1984) Disabling positional vertigo. *N. Engl. J. Med.*, **310**, 1700–5.

27. Gastaut, H. and Fischer-Williams, M. (1957) Electro-encephalographic study of syncope. Its differentiation from epilepsy. *Lancet*, ii, 1018–25.

28. Taylor, P.H., Gray, K., Bicknell, P.G. and Rees, J.R. (1977) Glossopharyngeal neuralgia with syncope. *J. Laryngol.*, **91**, 859–68.

29. Levin, B. and Posner, J.B. (1972) Swallow syncope. Report of a case and review of the literature. *Neurology*, **22**, 1086–93.

30. Hutchinson, E.C. and Stock, J.P.P. (1960) The carotid-sinus syndrome. *Lancet*, ii, 445–9.

31. Lown, B. and Levine, S.A. (1961) The carotid sinus. Clinical value of its stimulation. *Circulation*, **23**, 766–89.

32. Morley, C.A., Perrins, E.J., Grant, P. *et al.* (1982) Carotid sinus syncope treated by pacing. Analysis of persistent symptoms and role of atrioventricular sequential pacing. *Br. Heart J.*, **47**, 411–18.

33. Day, S.C., Cook, E.F., Funkenstein, H and Goldman, L. (1982) Evaluation and outcome of emergency room patients with transient loss of consciousness. *Am. J. Med.*, **73**, 15–23.

34. Kapoor, W.N., Karpf, M., Maher, Y. *et al.* (1982) Syncope of unknown origin. The need for a more cost-effective approach to its diagnostic evaluation. *J. Am. Med. Assoc.*, **247**, 2687–91.

35. Kapoor, W.N., Karpf, M. Wieand, S. *et al.* (1983) A prospective evaluation and follow-up of patients with syncope. *N. Engl. J. Med.*, **309**, 197–204.

36. Luxon, L.M., Crowther, A., Harrison, M.J.G. and Coltart, D.J. (1980) Controlled study of 24-hour ambulatory electrocardiographic monitoring in patients with transient neurological symptoms. *J. Neurol. Neurosurg. Psychiatry*, **43**, 37–41.

37. Critchley, E.M.R. and Wright, J.S. (1983) Evaluation of syncope. *Br. Med. J.*, **286**, 500–1.

38. Camm, A.J. and Levy, A.M. (1983) Evaluation of syncope. *Br. Med. J.*, **286**, 895.

39. Dimarco, J.P, Garan, H., Harthorne, J.W. and Ruskin, J.N. (1981) Intracardiac electrophysiologic techniques in recurrent syncope of unknown cause. *Ann. Intern. Med.*, **95**, 542–8.

40. Brandenburg, R.O. Jr, Holmes, D.R. Jr and Hartzler, G.O. (1981) The electrophysiologic assessment of patients with syncope. *Am. J. Cardiol.*, **47**, 433.

41. Hess, D.S., Morady, F. and Scheinman, M.M. (1982) Electrophysiologic testing in the evaluation of patients with syncope of undetermined origin. *Am. J. Cardiol.*, **50**, 1309–15.

42. Gulamhusein, S., Naccarelli, G.V., Ko, P.T. *et al.* (1982) Value and limitations of clinical electrophysiologic study in assessment of patients with unexplained syncope. *Am. J. Med.*, **73**, 700–5.

43. Kenny, R.A., Ingram, A., Bayliss, J. and Sutton, R. (1986) Head-up tilt: a useful test for investigating unexplained syncope. *Lancet*, i, 1352–5.
44. Parkes, J.D. (1981) Day-time drowsiness. *Lancet*, ii, 1213–18.
45. Kales, A., Cadieux, R.J., Soldatos, C.R. *et al.* (1982) Narcolepsy-cataplexy. 1. Clinical and electrophysiologic characteristics. *Arch. Neurol.*, 39, 164–8.
46. Montplaisir, J., de Champlain, J., Young, S.N. *et al.* (1982) Narcolepsy and idiopathic hypersomnia: biogenic amines and related compounds in CSF. *Neurology*, 32, 1299–302.
47. Langdon, N., Welsh, K.I., van Dam, M. *et al.* (1984) Genetic markers in narcolepsy. *Lancet*, ii, 1178–80.
48. Snoring and sleepiness. *Lancet* ii, 925–6.
49. Guilleminault, C., Connolly, S., Winkle, R. *et al.* (1984) Cyclical variations of the heart rate in sleep apnoea syndrome. Mechanisms, and usefulness of 24 h electrocardiography as a screening technique. *Lancet*, i, 126–31.
50. Raz, S. and Bradley, W.E. (1979) Neuromuscular dysfunction of the lower urinary tract, in *Campbell's Urology*, 4th edn, Vol. 2. W.B. Saunders, London, pp. 1215–70.
51. Goldstein, I. Siroky, M.B., Sax, D.S. and Krane, R.J. (1982) Neurologic abnormalities in multiple sclerosis. *J. Urol.*, 128, 541–5.
52. Lapides, J. (1967) Cystometry. *J. Am. Med. Assoc.*, 201, 618–21.
53. Susset, J.G. and Ghoniem, G.M. (1984) Rapid cystometry and sacral-evoked responses in the diagnosis of peripheral bladder and sphincter denervation. *J. Urol.*, 132, 704–7.
54. Perkash, I. (1980) Urodynamic evaluation: periurethral striated EMG versus perianal striated EMG. *Paraplegia*, 18, 275–80.
55. Fowler, C.J., Kirby, R.S., Harrison, M.J.G. *et al.* (1984) Individual motor unit analysis in the diagnosis of disorders of urethral sphincter innervation. *J. Neurol. Neurosurg. Psychiatry*, 47, 637–41.
56. Thon, W. and Altwein, J. E. (1984) Voiding dysfunction. *Urology*, 23, 323–30.
57. Takaiwa, M. and Shiraiwa, Y. (1984) A new technique of vesical electromyogram with cystometrography and urethral electromyogram. *Urol. Int.*, 39, 217–21.
58. Galloway, N.T.M., Chisholm, G.D. and McInnes, A. (1985) Patterns and significance of the sacral evoked response (the urologist's knee jerk). *Br. J. Urol.*, 57, 145–7.
59. Kiff, E.S. and Swash, M. (1984) Normal proximal and delayed distal conduction in the pudendal nerves of patients with idiopathic (neurogenic) faecal incontinence. *J. Neurol. Neurosurg. Psychiatry*, 47, 820–3.
60. Snooks, S.J., Barnes, P.R.H. and Swash, M. (1984) Damage to the innervation of the voluntary anal and periurethral sphincter musculature in incontinence: an electrophysiological study. *J. Neurol. Neurosurg. Psychiatry*, 47, 1269–73.

61. Madersbacher, H. and Dietl, P. (1984) Urodynamic practice in neuro-urological patients: techniques and clinical value. *Paraplegia*, **22**, 145–56.
62. Perkin, G.D. and Handler, C.E. (1983) Wernicke–Korsakoff syndrome. *Br. J. Hosp. Med.*, **30**, 331–4.
63. Leigh, D., McBurney, A. and McIlwain, H. (1981) Erythrocyte transketolase activity in the Wernicke–Korsakoff syndrome. *Br. J. Psychiatry*, **139**, 153–6.
64 Chan, Y-W., McLeod, J.G., Tuck, R.R. and Feary, P.A. (1985) Brain stem auditory evoked responses in chronic alcoholics. *J. Neurol. Neurosurg. Psychiatry*, **48**, 1107–12.
65. Mensing, J.W.A., Hoogland, P.H. and Slooff, J.L. (1984) Computed tomography in the diagnosis of Wernicke's encephalopathy: a radiological–neuropathological correlation. *Ann. Neurol.*, **16**, 363–5.
66. McDowell, J.R. and Le Blanc, H.J. (1984) Computed tomographic findings in Wernicke–Korsakoff syndrome. *Arch. Neurol.*, **41**, 453–4.
67. Pollock, S., Lewis, P.D. and Kendall, B. (1981) Whipple's disease confined to the nervous system. *J. Neurol. Neurosurg. Psychiatry*, **44**, 1104–9.
68. Halperin, J.J., Landis, D.M.D. and Kleinman, G.M. (1982) Whipple's disease of the nervous system. *Neurology*, **32**, 612–17.
69. Schwartz, M.A., Selhorst, J.B., Ochs, A.L. *et al.* (1986) Oculomasticatory myorhythmia: a unique movement disorder occurring in Whipple's disease. *Ann. Neurol.*, **20**, 677–83.
70. Sieracki, J.C., Fine, G., Horn, R.C. Jr and Bebin, J. (1960) Central nervous system involvement in Whipple's disease. *J. Neuropathol. Exp. Neurol.*, **19**, 70–5.
71. Jefferson, M. (1957) Sarcoidosis of the nervous system. *Brain*, **80**, 540–59.
72. Matthews, W.B. (1965) Sarcoidosis of the nervous system. *J. Neurol. Neurosurg. Psychiatry*, **28**, 23–9.
73. Oksanen, V., Grönhagen-Riska, C., Tikanoja, S. *et al.* (1986) Cerebrospinal fluid lysozyme and β_2-microglobulin in neurosarcoidosis. *J. Neurol. Sci.*, **73**, 79–87.
74. Lawrence, E.C., Teague, R.B., Gottlieb, M.S. *et al.* (1983) Serial changes in markers of disease activity with corticosteroid treatment in sarcoidosis. *Am. J. Med.*, **74**, 747–56.
75. Chan Seem, C.P., Norfolk, G. and Spokes, E.G. (1985) CSF angiotensin converting enzyme in neurosarcoidosis. *Lancet*, i, 456–7.
76. Oksanen, V., Fyhrquist, F., Grönhagen-Riska, C. and Somer, H. (1985) CSF angiotensin-converting enzyme in neurosarcoidosis. *Lancet*, i, 1050–1.
77. Plum, F. and Posner, J.B. (1980) *The Diagnosis of Stupor and Coma*, 3rd edn, F.A. Davis, Philadelphia.
78. Austen, F.K., Carmichael, M.W. and Adams, R.D. (1957) Neurological manifestations of chronic pulmonary insufficiency. *N. Engl. J. Med.*, **257**, 579–90.

79. Jefferson, A. (1956) A clinical correlation between encephalopathy and papilloedema in Addison's disease. *J. Neurol. Neurosurg. Psychiatry*, **19**, 21–7.
80. Tyler, H.R. (1968) Neurological disorders in renal failure. *Am. J. Med.*, **44**, 734–48.
81. Walshe, J.M. (1951) Observations on the symptomatology and pathogenesis of hepatic coma. *Quart. J. Med.*, **20**, 421–38.
82. Pearce, J.M.S. (1963) Focal neurological syndromes in hepatic failure. *Postgrad. Med. J.*, **39**, 653–7.
83. Montgomery, B.M. and Pinner, C.A. (1964) Transient hypoglycemic hemiplegia. *Arch. Intern. Med.*, **114**, 681–4.
84. Schwartz, W.B., Bennett, W., Curelop, S. and Bartter, F.C. (1957) A syndrome of renal sodium loss and hyponatraemia probably resulting from inappropriate secretion of antidiuretic hormone. *Am. J. Med.*, **23**, 529–42.
85. Thomas, W.C. Jr, Wiswell, J.G., Conner, T.B. and Howard, J.E. (1958) Hypercalcemic crisis due to hyperparathyroidism. *Am. J. Med.*, **24**, 229–39.
86. Forester, C.F. (1963) Coma in myxedema. *Arch. Intern. Med.*, **111**, 734–43.
87. Edwards, G.A. and Daum, S.M. (1959) Increased spinal fluid protein in hyperparathyroidism and other hypercalcemic states. *Arch. Intern. Med.*, **104**, 29–36.
88. Hockaday, J.M., Potts, F., Epstein, E. *et al.* (1965) Electroencephalographic changes in acute cerebral anoxia from cardiac or respiratory arrest. *Electroencephalogr. Clin. Neurophysiol.*, **18**, 575–86.
89. Binnie, C.D., Prior, P.F., Lloyd, D.S.L. *et al.* (1970) Electroencephalographic prediction of fatal anoxic brain damage after resuscitation from cardiac arrest. *Br. Med. J.*, **2**, 265–8.
90. Earnest, M.P., Breckinridge, J.C., Yarnell, P.R. and Oliva, P.B. (1979) Quality of survival after out-of-hospital cardiac arrest: predictive value of early neurologic evaluation. *Neurology*, **29**, 56–60.
91. Levy, D.E., Caronna, J.J., Singer, B.H. *et al.* (1985) Predicting outcome from hypoxic-ischemic coma. *J. Am. Med. Assoc.*, **253**, 1420–6.
92. Silverman, D., Saunders, M.G., Schwab, R.S. and Masland, R.L. (1969) Cerebral death and the electroencephalogram. Report of the ad hoc Committee of the American Electroencephalographic Society on EEG Criteria for Determination of Cerebral Death. *J. Am. Med. Assoc.*, **209**, 1505–10.
93. Mohandas, A. and Chou, S.N. (1971) Brain death. A clinical and pathological study. *J. Neurosurg.*, **35**, 211–18.
94. Diagnosis of brain death (1976) *Lancet*, **ii**, 1069–70.
95. Walker, A.E. (1977) An appraisal of the criteria of cerebral death. A summary statement. *J. Am. Med Assoc.*, **237**, 982–6.
96. Black, P. McL. (1978) Brain death. *N. Engl. J. Med.*, **299**, 338–44; 393–401.

97. Brain death (1981) *Lancet*, i, 363–5.
98. Guidelines for the determination of death: Report of the medical consultants on the diagnosis of death to the President's Commission for the study of ethical problems in medicine and biomedical and behavioral research (1981) *J. Am. Med. Assoc.*, **246**, 2184–6.
99. Kolodny, E.H. and Cable, W.J.L. (1982) Inborn errors of metabolism. *Ann. Neurol.*, **11**, 221–32.
100. Nakano, T., Ikeda, S-I, Kondo, K. *et al.* (1985) Adult G_{M1}-gangliosidosis: clinical patterns and rectal biopsy. *Neurology*, **35**, 875–80.
101. Mutoh, T., Sobue, I., Naoi, N. *et al.* (1986) A family with β-galactosidase deficiency. Three adults with atypical clinical patterns. *Neurology*, **36**, 54–9.
102. Willner, J.P., Grabowski, G.A., Gordon, R.E. *et al.* (1981) Chronic G_{M2} gangliosidosis masquerading as atypical Friedreich ataxia: clinical, morphologic, and biochemical studies of nine cases. *Neurology*, **31**, 787–98.
103. Mitsumoto, H., Sliman, R.J., Schafer, I.A. *et al.* (1985) Motor neuron disease and adult hexosaminidase. A deficiency in two families: evidence for multisystem degeneration. *Ann. Neurol.*, **17**, 378–85.
104. Nishimura, R.N. and Barranger, J.A. (1980) Neurological complications of Gaucher's disease, type 3. *Arch. Neurol.*, **37**, 92–3.
105. Finelli, P.F. (1985) Metachromatic leukodystrophy manifesting as a schizophrenic disorder: computed tomographic correlation. *Ann. Neurol.*, **18**, 94–5.
106. Wulff, C.H. and Trojaborg, W. (1985) Adult metachromatic leukodystrophy: neurophysiologic findings. *Neurology*, **35**, 1776–8.
107. O'Neill, B.P., Swanson, J.W., Brown, F.R. III *et al.* (1985) Familial spastic paraparesis: an adrenoleukodystrophy phenotype? *Neurology*, **35**, 1233–5.
108. Noetzel, M.J., Landau, W.M. and Moser, H.W. (1987) Adrenoleukodystrophy carrier state presenting as a chronic nonprogressive spinal cord disorder. *Arch. Neurol.*, **44**, 566–7.
109. Eldridge, R., Anayiotos, C.P., Schlesinger, S. *et al.* (1984) Hereditary adult-onset leukodystrophy simulating chronic progressive multiple sclerosis. *N. Engl. J. Med.*, **311**, 948–52.
110. Masó, E., Ferrer, I., Herraiz, J. *et al.* (1984) Leigh's syndrome in an adult. *J. Neurol.*, **231**, 253–7.
111. Kissel, J.T., Kolkin, S., Chakeres, D. *et al.* (1987) Magnetic resonance imaging in a case of autopsy-proved adult subacute necrotizing encephalomyelopathy (Leigh's disease). *Arch. Neurol.*, **44**, 563–6.
112. Call, G., Seay, A.R., Sherry, R. and Qureshi, I.A. (1984) Clinical features of carbamyl phosphate synthetase-1 deficiency in an adult. *Ann. Neurol.*, **16**, 90–3.
113. Dimauro, S., Bonilla, E., Zeviani, M. *et al.* (1985) Mitochondrial myopathies. *Ann. Neurol.*, **17**, 521–38.

114. Hackett, E.R., Martinez, R.D., Larson, P.F. and Paddison, R.M. (1974) Optic neuritis in systemic lupus erythematosus. *Arch. Neurol.*, **31**, 9–11.
115. Granger, D.P. (1960) Transverse myelitis with recovery: only manifestation of systemic lupus erythematosus. *Neurology*, **10**, 325–9.
116. Bennett, R., Hughes, G.R.V., Bywaters, E.G.L. and Holt, P.J.L. (1972). Neuropsychiatric problems in systemic lupus erythematosus. *Br. Med. J.*, **4**, 342–5.

3

Cerebrovascular disease

3.1 TIA, RIND AND STROKE WITH MINIMAL RESIDUUM

Initial classification of cerebrovascular events continues to be a clinical one based on the duration of symptomatology. Transient ischaemic attacks (TIAs) are events, thought to be based on ischaemia, which last for less than 24 hours. In reality, the majority of attacks last for a much shorter period. In one study, the median duration of carotid attacks was 14 min, and, for vertebrobasilar attacks, 8 min. For the former, 90% remitted within 6 h, for the latter, 90% remitted within 2 h [1]. Attacks exceeding 24 h in duration, but remitting in 3–4 days have been described as reversible ischaemic neurological deficits (RIND). Evidence indicates that these events, and, indeed, longer-lasting TIAs, are commonly associated with cerebral infarction, as defined by CT scanning. Indeed, the assumptions that TIAs are necessarily related to ischaemia, and unassociated with permanent structural change can be questioned. In one study of 22 patients with TIA, CT detected focal abnormalities in 32%, and MRI in 77% [2]. In another analysis comparing TIA, RIND and stroke with minimal residuum, focal ischaemic lesions, detected by CT scanning were found in 25, 25 and 35% of patients respectively [3]. Rapid recovery of neurological function, therefore, can coexist with permanent structural change as defined by CT or MRI. Many conditions, some unrelated to ischaemia, can present as TIA, including epilepsy and hypoglycaemia [4]. Similar variability, in terms of pathogenesis, is encountered in patients whose clinical presentation suggests a stroke. In an analysis of 821 patients admitted to an acute stroke unit, 13% proved to have other diagnoses, most commonly seizures, confusional states or syncope [5]. Others have claimed a higher clinical acumen, with pre- and post-CT diagnosis of stroke in agreement in 96% of cases [6]. There is universal agreement, however, that the distinction of cerebral infarction from haemorrhage based on clinical critera alone, is fraught with error. If CT scanning is used as the final arbiter, it is evident that about a quarter of all cerebral haemorrhages would have been diagnosed as infarcts if clinical criteria alone had been used [7]. In a recent population survey, where 89% of 168 strokes had had either autopsy or CT scanning, cerebral infarction was found in 76%, cerebral haemorrhage (including subarachnoid haemorrhage) in 13%, whilst 11% remained unclassified [8].

One argument for the vigorous investigation of either TIA or stroke, therefore, rests on the evidence that other pathological processes, requiring differing management, can present in this manner. It has been suggested that transient ischaemic events can occur in relationship to intracranial aneurysms, the consequence of embolic material derived from the aneurysm, though in one such example from the literature, there was evidence of a middle cerebral artery stenosis proximal to the aneurysm [9]. It is recognized that TIA may occur in association with subdural haematoma, though in some such patients, there has been evidence of co-existing extracranial carotid artery disease [10]. Since TIA is associated with a subsequent stroke risk of perhaps 5–6% per annum, investigation can reasonably be justified if it allows identification of risk factors which are then reversible. Clearly the clinical characteristics of the TIA are of very limited value in this respect. The risk is similar, in terms of subsequent completed stroke, for amaurosis fugax and other carotid events [11]. For hemispheric TIA, it has been argued that attacks of neurological dysfunction limited to one limb, or affecting speech alone are more often associated with carotid stenosis than attacks involving the arm and leg together [12]. No clear risk factors, based on the nature of the TIA, have emerged which can predict the likelihood of subsequent stroke. Investigation, therefore, is required to identify certain groups of patients with TIA in whom specific intervention, particularly surgery, is under consideration. Enthusiasm for evaluation of the carotid tree in TIA must be tempered by the knowledge that no adequate controlled trial of carotid endarterectomy has ever been undertaken. The evidence that surgery to the vertebrobasilar tree is of benefit is even less pressing. As yet there is no substantial evidence that any form of medical therapy alters outcome in completed stroke whereas the role of surgery in ischaemic stroke is unproven for carotid endarterectomy and established as ineffective in terms of extracranial–intracranial bypass. Surgical management of intracerebral haemorrhage is even more controversial.

3.1.1 Investigations

Patients with polycythaemia have a higher incidence of stroke and may present with TIA. Focal neurological deficit, including hemiplegia, can result from hypoglycaemia, most commonly occurring in diabetic patients taking insulin. The incidence of lipid abnormalities in patients with cerebrovascular disease is the subject of debate. In one study in which carotid arterial disease was identified by Doppler studies in asymptomatic individuals, a depressed ratio of high density lipoprotein concentration to cholesterol concentration was found in those with abnormal vessels [13]. Stroke incidence is higher in diabetic patients than in a control population.

3.1.2 Cerebrospinal fluid

The role of CSF examination in the diagnosis of subarachnoid haemorrhage is considered in Chapter 12. Before the introduction of CT scanning, CSF examination was considered a valuable procedure for confirmation of the diagnosis of intracerebral haemorrhage. The yield of positive findings, in proven cases, is of the order of 80% indicating that, in the remainder, the haematoma has failed to extend, at least macroscopically, into the subarachnoid space or the ventricular system. Spectrophotometric analysis, however, if performed between 24 h and 7 days after onset of symptoms reveals blood products in up to 100% of cases [14]. As is the case with subarachnoid haemorrhage, delayed lumbar puncture may reveal additional abnormalities, including an elevated white cell count and a depressed glucose concentration. In cerebral infarction, mild increases in protein concentration or cell count are encountered in a minority of patients.

If the infarct is haemorrhagic, usually the consequence of an embolic event, blood may appear in the CSF. In this respect, however, lumbar puncture is less sensitive than CT scanning for the detection of a haemorrhagic element [15]. Though the CSF in septic infarction secondary to subacute bacterial endocarditis frequently reveals a pleocytosis, the selectivity of this finding is poor, as a low-grade pleocytosis is not uncommon in aseptic cerebral infarction [16]. Oligoclonal banding is encountered in the CSF of some stroke patients, at times as a transient phenomenon[17]. A number of enzymes have been studied in the CSF after stroke. Lactate dehydrogenase levels are the most sensitive guide to cerebral damage, whilst brain creatine kinase levels correlate best with outcome[18]. Elevated concentrations of creatine kinase, glutamate oxaloacetate transaminase and lactate dehydrogenase are more likely in cortical than lacunar infarction and, for the former, correlate with the size of the infarct as determined by CT scanning[19].

3.1.3 Electroencephalography and isotope scanning

EEG is no longer performed in the evaluation of patients with acute stroke. Isotope scanning is of limited value. Serial scanning studies indicate that, for cerebral infarction, the yield of positive scans exceeds 50% if the procedure is delayed to the period between 14 and 28 days following onset. Brain-stem infarction, however, is rarely associated with positive radioisotope findings[20]. Generally a single scan sequence is performed around 30 min after injection of the radioisotope, though some studies suggest a higher yield of positive findings if delayed scans are included, carried out 2–4 hours later. Soon after the introduction of the CT scanner, a comparison of the roles of CT and radioisotope scanning in the diagnosis of cerebral infarction was made. Positive findings were noted in 55 and 69% of cases respectively[21]. Contrast injection was not included in the CT imaging, explaining, no doubt a lack of correlation of abnormal findings revealed by the two methods. Introduction of later-generation scanners has dramatically altered this early bias in favour of radioisotope scanning. Though a positive scan has been reported in up to 64% of cases of intracerebral haemorrhage[20], the yield in other series has been smaller, and the abnormalities so found are seldom distinguishable from those associated with cerebral infarction[21].

Other electrophysiological techniques can be of value in the investigation of patients with brain-stem vascular disease. In the chronic vegetative state, the brain-stem auditory evoked responses remain normal, whilst somatosensory evoked responses are likely to show prolonged central conduction times (N13–N20)[22]. Brain-stem evoked responses are likely to be abnormal in brain-stem infarction which, on clinical criteria, has involved the pons or lateral aspect of the mid brain, but is likely to be normal with medial mid-brain or medullary lesions[23]. Though the technique is more sensitive than CT for detecting brain-stem infarction, it generally simply serves to reinforce rather than initiate the clinical diagnosis.

3.1.4 Non-invasive tests

(a) Oculoplethysmography

In this procedure, ocular pulsation is recorded over each globe and the waveform analysed. Comparison is made with recordings from external carotid pulsation measured from the ear lobes. The accuracy of the procedure, in detecting an internal carotid stenosis exceeding 75%, has been reported to lie between 31 and 94% [24]. When combined with carotid phonoangiography, correct identification of stenoses exceeding 95% was achieved in 91% of cases, and of stenoses from 50 to 75% in 74% [24]. The sensitivity of either procedure is relatively limited, however, and neither is commonly employed for screening purposes.

(b) Ophthalmodynamometry

In this procedure central retinal artery pressure is measured by assessing, via an ophthalmoscope, what pressure has to be applied to the sclera to induce cessation of pulsation in retinal arterioles. The procedure has not proved to be sufficiently sensitive for it to be recommended as a sole screening procedure for carotid artery disease[25].

(c) Doppler imaging

This technique produces an image corresponding to patterns of blood flow in the vessel being examined. Both continuous-wave and pulsed systems have been used, the latter having the capability of analysing flow at differing levels of the cross-section being studied. In one report comparing continuous-wave Doppler ultrasonography with angiography[26], sensitivity for detecting carotid occlusion was 100%, with a specificity of 99%. For stenoses exceeding 50%, a sensitivity of 90% was achieved, the figure falling rapidly for less severe disease. It has been suggested that the pulsed system is capable of greater accuracy, achieving 100% sensitivity for stenoses exceeding 25% in one study [27].

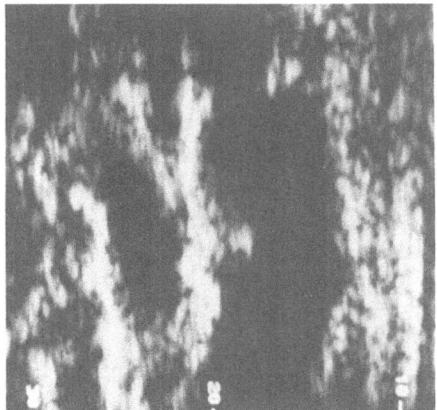

Fig. 3.1 Duplex scan showing plaques in the internal carotid artery

(d) B mode-ultrasound

Ultrasound images are formed by reflection of the ultrasound beam from tissue interfaces. The technique is relatively insensitive for the detection of severe carotid stenosis or occlusion. In one analysis, sensitivity for the detection of occlusion was only 25% [28]. Better results are achieved with less-severe disease to the point, in some series, where greater correlation with surgical findings is obtained than by conventional angiography. In a recent survey, however, in which ultrasound was compared with digital subtraction angiography, the former did not prove accurate in predicting the presence of ulcerating disease, though the latter technique hardly fared better [29].

The duplex scanner combines ultrasonic images with a pulsed Doppler system, enabling flow patterns to be measured both longitudinally and in transverse sections at selected sites of the vessel (Fig. 3.1). The system is superior to oculoplethysmography or carotid phonangiography in the detection of carotid stenoses exceeding 50% [30]. In a study of carotid disease in 117 patients, all of whom had had conventional angiography, digital subtraction angiography and duplex scanning achieved accuracies of 91% and 77% respectively [30]. Further reports have confirmed the value of duplex scanning, suggesting a comparable sensitivity to digital angiography over all the range of severity of carotid disease [31]. Non-diagnostic studies are a problem, however, occurring in 18% of the patients in the series quoted above[31]. Not surprisingly, the advent of increasingly sophisticated non-invasive studies has led to a shift in the pattern of findings on angiography, with substantial stenoses being encountered more frequently than before[32]. In general, non-invasive tests have been less-often applied to the diagnosis of disease in the vertebrobasilar system. Continuous wave doppler appeared capable, from the results of one report, of detecting vertebral or basilar artery occlusions or high-grade stenoses with considerable accuracy[33].

3.1.5 Angiography

With the advent of CT scanning, the role of angiography in the diagnosis of cerebral infarction and haemorrhage has been substantially reduced. Though angiography is capable of detecting other pathologies which sometimes mimic a stroke syndrome, it fails to provide diagnostic information in many patients with presumed infarction or haemorrhage[34]. In one study of 32 patients with haemorrhage in the region of the basal ganglia, the anterior cerebral artery remained undisplaced in 34%, whereas the lenticulostriate arteries were either poorly visualized, or undisplaced, in 35%. Lateral displacement of the middle cerebral artery was evident in the majority, however, and shift of the internal cerebral vein in all[35]. If CT scanning suggests a typical hypertensive haemorrhage, particularly if sited in the putamen, thalamus, cerebellum or pons, angiography is rarely indicated. If the individual is normotensive, and the haemorrhage is lobar, then angiography may be required to exclude tumour or arteriovenous malformation[36].

Conventional angiography is generally now performed via a catheter rather than by direct puncture of the vessel (Fig. 3.2). Its relevance in patients with ischaemic cerebrovascular disease, lies in its capacity to detect atheroma at particular sites of the vascular tree of which the most relevant, at least in terms of potential surgical intervention, is the carotid bifurcation. Whereas stenotic or occlusive disease at the bifurcation is readily detected using standard projections, the addition of oblique views leads to a significant increase in the diagnosis of irregular or ulcerating plaques[37].

The main limiting factor in the use of conventional angiography is its morbidity. One review has suggested that the cerebral complication rates of direct carotid puncture and catheter angiography, based on data from the literature, are 8 and 7% respectively[38].

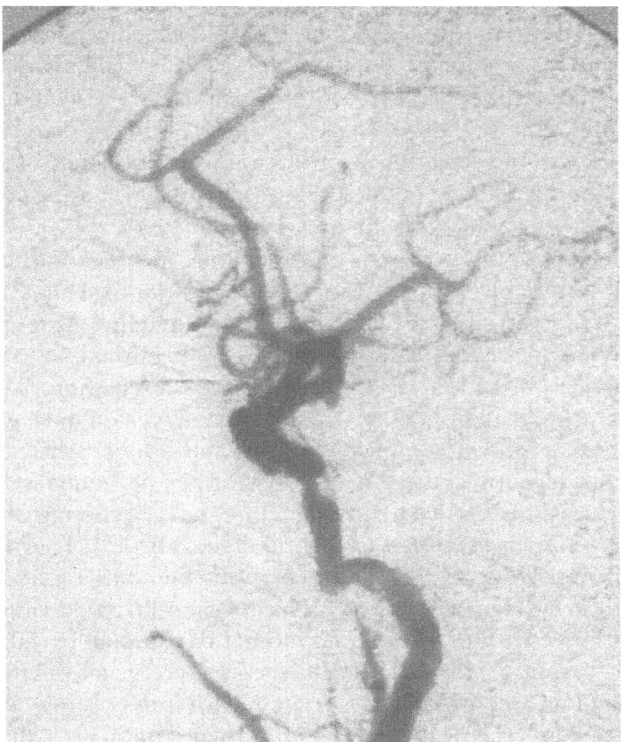

Fig. 3.2 Angiogram demonstrating stenosis immediately below the carotid siphon

The risk can be eliminated by the use of digital subtraction angiography in which venous injection of contrast is performed. In an early study of this technique, in 100 patients, inadequate visualization of one or both carotid vessels occurred in 40[39]. Where visualization had been good or excellent, the technique, compared to conventional arterial catheter studies, achieved a sensitivity of 95% and a specificity of 99%[39]. These figures fell sharply where the quality of the images was poorer. It was noted that the film costs for this procedure were less than 10 dollars, compared to a figure of 68 to 190 dollars for conventional angiography.

Digital angiography in general has performed rather better than Doppler in the detection of carotid bifurcation disease[40,41], though one study whilst confirming the advantage, concluded that this did not result in a clear gain in terms of patient management [42]. As indicated earlier, duplex scanning probably achieves a comparable sensitivity to digital angiography for the demonstration of carotid bifurcation disease [31]. A recent review concluded that digital angiography achieved sensitivity and specificity rates between 89 and 93% in the detection of carotid stenoses exceeding 60% [43], whereas another study obtained a sensitivity of 84% and a specificity of 93% when dealing with stenoses exceeding 30% [44].

Problems encountered with this technique include a difficulty in defining carotid ulceration, a problem differentiating a tight internal carotid stenosis from an occlusion and poor imaging of the external carotid. The procedure is far inferior to conventional angiography for the demonstration of the intracranial circulation. For this purpose, arterial angiography remains necessary, a digital technique here allowing a lower volume of contrast and a finer catheter [43]

Angiography, of course, may reveal other pathologies besides atherosclerosis. Certain diagnostic features have been suggested that allow a confident diagnosis of carotid dissection [45]. They include irregular narrowing of the internal carotid extending to the base of the skull (string sign), a tapering occlusion, smooth narrowing over a short distance with or without an intimal flap and an extraluminal pouch of contrast. Extracranial dissections are usually within the media and are commonly associated with pre-existing vascular disease. Though classically associated with ipsilateral neck and facial pain, together with a Horner's syndrome, both features may be lacking. Intracranial dissections, most commonly in the middle cerebral artery, occur in young people, in the sub-intimal plane and are seldom associated with evidence of pre-existing vascular disease. Angiography in these cases often simply shows an occluded vessel [46].

3.1.6 CT scanning

In cases of cerebral infarction, there is often little or no detectable abnormality in scans performed within 24 hours of onset. Subsequently a low-density area appears, with associated oedema a prominent feature, in the first week, in perhaps 20% of cases. In haemorrhagic infarction there is a mixed density pattern, with the higher density usually central. Contrast enhancement is found in about 70% of cerebral infarcts [47]. It is never found within the first 24 h, reaches a maximum incidence at about 14 days and then

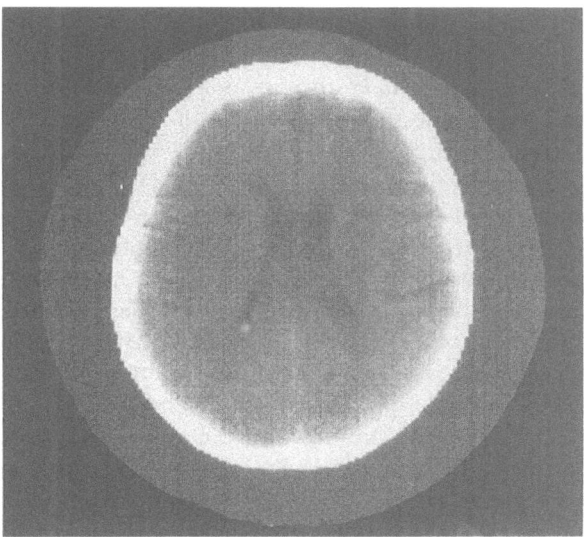

Fig. 3.3 CT scan showing bilateral lacunar infarction

diminishes. Rarely it can persist for several weeks. Enhancement is almost inevitable with cortical infarction. Sometimes, despite florid enhancement, pre-contrast studies are negative. The pattern of enhancement varies, with patchy, ring, homogeneous and cortical variants [47]. The pattern of infarction can generally be correlated with a particular arterial territory. Cerebellar infarction is rarer than cerebral and is found most often in the distribution of the posterior inferior cerebellar artery, usually consequent to vertebral artery occlusion. Infarction in the territory of the superior cerebellar artery is commonly associated with distal basilar artery occlusion [48]. Rarely, intraluminal clotted blood is revealed on scanning by a diffuse high density area within the artery on pre-contrast films [49]. Lacunar infarcts are found in particular sites, including the putamen, caudate, thalamus, pons and the internal capsule. They range in size form 2 cm to 0.3 cm. The smaller lesions are thought to result from occlusion of penetrating branches of the large cerebral arteries by lipohyalinosis, whereas the larger infarcts may be the consequence of occlusions due to atheroma or embolus [50]. A number of clinical syndromes are described according to the site of infarction. CT scanning reveals low density, non-enhancing lesions without mass effect[51] (Fig. 3.3). The incidence of extracranial atherosclerotic disease in patients with lacunar infarction is unsettled. It has been reported to be absent by some[52] but prominent by others[51,53].

Intracerebral haemorrhage appears as an area of increased density surrounded by a zone of low attenuation. A mass effect maybe observed for as long as 9 weeks, and enhancement, usually ring-shaped, can persist for a similar duration[54]. In some cases the scan eventually returns to normal, in others an area of low attenuation persists. The availability of CT scanning has allowed precise clinicopathological correlations to be made for haemorrhages occurring at particular sites, for example within the thalamus[55]. Furthermore, previously considered atypical presentations of intracerebral haemorrhage are now recognized to be more common. For example, progression of disability after onset is not infrequent[56], whereas rupture into the ventricular system is no longer regarded as being of particular relevance in terms of outcome. At times a lacunar syndrome is the consequence of haemorrhage rather than infarction[57]. A major management decision in patients with intracerebral haemorrhage is whether angiography is necessary to exclude the presence of angioma or berry aneurysm. Where the individual is hypertensive, and the lesion is in a typical site for hypertensive haemorrhage, angiography is rarely indicated[36]. Sometimes, CT provides certain clues suggesting the likely origin of intracerebral blood. For caudate haemorrhages, those secondary to carotid artery aneurysms tend to be contiguous with the frontal horn of the lateral ventricle, whereas hypertensive-related haemorrhages are contiguous with the anterior part of the body of the lateral ventricle, frequently extending into it[58]. It is recommended that brain-stem haemorrhage in young, normotensive individuals, merits angiography in order to exclude an arterio-venous malformation[56]. If CT reveals blood in both the fourth ventricle and the basal cisterns, an underlying angioma or aneurysm is highly likely to be responsible[56]. Between 4 and 10% of intracerebral haemorrhage is secondary to cerebral amyloid angiopathy[59]. The diagnosis is suggested if CT demonstrates cortical or subcortical haemorrhage, frequently extending into the subarachnoid space, and commonly multifocal[59,60].

3.1.7 Magnetic resonance imaging

As yet the exact role of MRI in stroke, and its possible advantage

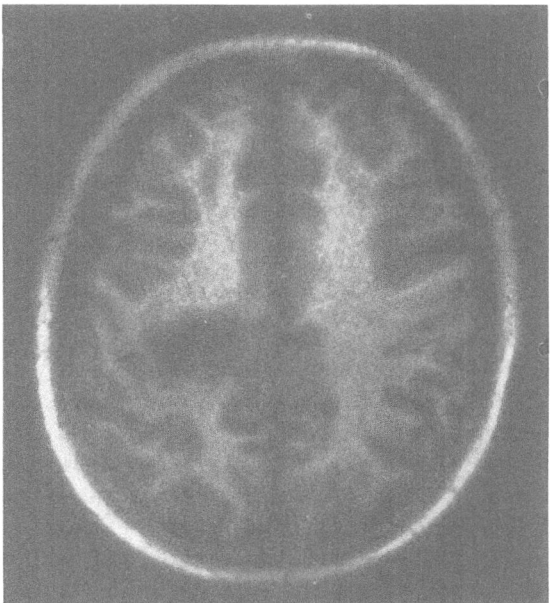

Fig. 3.4 MRI scan showing left hemisphere infarct

over CT is in the process of definition. Early reports indicated that MRI could reveal abnormalities in ischaemic stroke within six hours of onset[61]. Embolic or thrombotic infarcts have been associated with areas of reduced image intensity (prolonged T_1) on inversion–recovery sequences, whereas lacunar infarcts have produced small, circular areas of prolonged T_1 [62]. Cerebral haemorrhage has been reported to show a central zone of longer T_1, but a rim of shorter T_1. A recent survey has, in general, confirmed the earlier studies. In early infarction, inversion–recovery sequences display subtle alteration in the interface between grey and white matter with prolongation of both T_1 and T_2 (Fig. 3.4). The procedure is at least as sensitive as CT scanning in the detection of ischaemic infarction, and more so for cases scanned within 24 hours of onset[63]. It is particularly valuable for the detection of lesions confined to the brain stem or cerebellum[64]. Lacunar infarcts, displaying prolonged T_1 and T_2 are better displayed than by CT scanning. Sequential scanning in cases of intracerebral haemorrhage shows an initial prolonged T_1 evolving into a shorter T_1 with a surrounding zone, due to cerebral oedema, of long T_1 [65]. CT scanning is generally superior for the demonstration of intracerebral haemorrhage when scanning is performed several days after onset of disability [63]. Periventricular lesions are found frequently in older subjects, though the majority of these have had stroke-like events, or possess risk factors relevant for the development of cerebrovascular disease. The pattern appears consistent with the pathological changes described in subcortical arteriosclerotic encephalopathy [66].

3.1.8 Cardiological investigations

Stroke, or transient ischaemia, may be the manifestation of a primary cardiological disorder. Among 125 patients with infective endocarditis, 18% presented with stroke [67], whereas 25% of cases of atrial myxoma, in one series, had a neurological event as a major early symptom [68]. Mitral valve prolapse has been reported to be more common in patients with cerebral ischaemic events [69], particularly those under the age of 45 [70]. In 117 successive patients with episodes of transient cerebral or retinal ischaemia, structural cardiac defects were found twice as commonly as in age- and sex-matched controls [71]. A considerable literature has accumulated on the value of echocardiography and prolonged ECG monitoring in patients with episodes of cerebral ischaemia. Whatever the cardiac disease being sought, two-dimensional echocardiography is a more sensitive technique than M-mode echocardiography [72,73]. Its ability to detect atrial thrombi, particularly those located in the appendage is, however, low, whilst it is estimated that only 43–79% of proven valvular lesions associated with infective endocarditis are visualized [74]. In unselected stroke patients, echocardiography detected structural cardiac disease in 36.9% [73] and 37.1% [75] in two series, and in 34.3% of a group of 132 stroke patients under the age of 46 years [76]. If, however, patients with known, or clinically overt cardiac disease, and those with a history of arrhythmia are excluded, routine echocardiography can scarcely be justified as a screening procedure in patients with stroke [72–75], except, perhaps, in younger individuals [76]. It has been suggested that the finding of an increased AP diameter of the left atrium on two-dimensional echocardiography is far more likely in patients with atrial fibrillation and cardiac thrombus than in those with atrial fibrillation alone [77].

The role of routine prolonged ECG monitoring in patients with stroke is similarly questionable. In one study, of 263 patients with suspected cerebral embolism Holter monitoring was performed in 150[73]. Atrial fibrillation was detected in 15 (paroxysmal in four). All had a history of atrial fibrillation, or had been found to have it on routine ECG. Others have suggested a better yield from performing prolonged ECG monitoring compared to routine studies[78,79], though in one of these reports, of 10 patients with carotid ischaemic events and haemodynamically significant arrhythmias, six had ipsilateral carotid stenosis on angiography[79].

3.1.9 Other investigations

Indium labelling of platelets has been performed in the hope of predicting, from foci of abnormal activity, the likelihood of subsequent ischaemic events in that arterial territory. The method has a low sensitivity (43%) for the detection of arteriographic abnormalities, and positive findings do not allow the prediction of subsequent TIA or completed stroke in the relevant territory[80]. Although a considerable body of information is available regarding the changes of blood flow and regional metabolic activity in stroke, as obtained by positron emission tomography, the scarcity and cost of the procedure do not allow for its routine application in the investigation of stroke patients[81].

3.1.10 Recommendation

(a) TIA, RIND and stroke with minimal residuum (see flow chart)

Certain haematological and biochemical investigations are appropriate, including a full blood count, ESR, glucose studies and, for younger patients, serological tests to exclude meningovascular syphilis. CSF examination is not necessary nor are lipid studies relevant unless the subject is young, or has clinical features suggesting hyperlipidaemia.

If there is no clinical evidence of cardiac disease, and no history of arrhythmia, together with a normal routine ECG, neither echocardiography nor prolonged ECG monitoring can be justified.

Where the clinical event can be clearly localized to the brain stem, there is seldom need to proceed to either CT or MRI studies. Exception should be made for younger subjects with a completed

Flow chart

brain-stem stroke in case the finding of a brain-stem haemorrhage suggests the need for angiography.

CT or MRI scan is likely to be abnormal in most patients with stroke, and in many TIA cases where the attack has been prolonged. If scanning establishes the presence of a haemorrhage of a typical 'hypertensive' distribution, no further studies are warranted unless there are multifocal haemorrhages suggesting the possibility of a bleeding diathesis. Where the haemorrhage is not in a site commonly associated with hypertension, and particularly when the individual is normotensive, angiography may be required to exclude an aneurysmal or angiomatous source. If radiological studies suggest brain-stem infarction, or lacunar infarction, angiography is unlikely to alter further management. For carotid territory events, where there is a giant lacune, or a carotid territory infarct, or the scan is normal, investigation of the carotid bifurcation is appropriate as a possible source of embolic material. Duplex scanning, if available, is the most sensitive of the non-invasive tests and can be used as a screening procedure. If negative, further investigation can be postponed unless ischaemic episodes recur. If they do, or duplex scanning suggests significant bifurcation disease, then formal angiography is appropriate to delineate the bifurcation in detail. At the same time, visualization of the intracranial circulation will be necessary to appraise the terminal carotid and its anterior and middle cerebral branches. If duplex scanning is unavailable, digital venous angiography can be used in its place, with comparable results.

(b) Stroke with substantial residuum

It is difficult, indeed unwise, to make dogmatic statements regarding the necessity of radiological investigation of stroke. The matter is influenced by the physician's concept of the role of medical and surgical intervention, and also by the availability of a scanning facility. Even the most enthusiastic would pause, I trust, before submitting a 90 year old with a disabling hemiplegia to a scanning procedure which will have no influence on management. Younger patients, on the other hand, certainly those under the age of 50 merit a more aggressive approach, even if it is recognized that the findings may not lead to specific therapeutic intervention. If the possibility of surgical intervention, in terms of endarterectomy, is being contemplated, then clearly carotid strokes justify a more intensive appraisal than those occurring in vertebrobasilar territory. Certainly scanning has a major advantage in that, if performed at an appropriate time

after onset, it can successfully distinguish infarction from haemorrhage and assist, therefore, in a more rational management though,
even then, the most important risk factor requiring control is the
same for both conditions, namely hypertension.

Haematological and biochemical investigations are similar to
those used for the TIA patient. CSF examination is not warranted in
the stroke patient (excluding the patient with subarachnoid haemorrhage, discussed elsewhere). Haemorrhagic infarction is more
readily diagnosed by CT scanning.

3.2 CEREBRAL VENOUS THROMBOSIS

A recent review described the clinical manifestations of cerebral
venous thrombosis in 38 patients[82]. In this series, the diagnosis
was accepted if there was angiographic evidence of partial or total
lack of filling of at least one dural sinus on two projections. There
were two groups of patients, one with intracranial hypertension
alone, the second with focal symptoms and signs. Headache
occurred in three-quarters of the cases, but less than a third had
seizures. Many predisposing factors have been described, including
pregnancy, the use of an oral contraceptive, local infection and
trauma. Thrombosis of the dural sinuses or the cavernous sinus can
occur in isolation but the former is generally complicated by
evidence of cortical vein thrombosis.

3.2.1 Investigations

In the series already referred to, an elevated ESR (exceeding 20) was
found in 59% of the cases. The EEG tends to show diffuse rather
than focal activity and can be normal, particularly in those with
intracranial hypertension alone[82]. The CSF changes are non-
specific, with an increased protein concentration and a lymphocytic
pleocytosis being common. Among 32 patients, five had normal
CSF, though three of these had presented with intracranial hypertension alone[82]. Technetium scanning can be of value, with incomplete visualization of the superior sagittal or lateral sinuses. The CT
findings are non-specific. Some patients have normal studies, even in
the presence of focal symptomatology. Others show small rather
than large ventricles, often associated with evidence of hemispheric
swelling. Focal changes include areas of infarction, sometimes
haemorrhagic. Gyral enhancement is frequent in those with focal

lesions. An area of increased density may be apparent within the superior sagittal or straight sinus on pre-contrast films, contrasting with a filling defect within the sinus on post-contrast studies (the delta sign)[83]. More specific changes, including abnormalities of the orbit, have been reported in cavernous sinus thrombosis[84]. Magnetic resonance imaging, in cavernous sinus thrombosis, is able to detect, on T_1 weighted images, high signal abnormalities in the sinus and the superior ophthalmic vein[85].

Definitive diagnosis depends on angiography whose findings include occlusion of dural sinuses and non-visualization of cerebral veins or their delayed emptying with evidence of a collateral circulation involving cortical veins.

3.2.2 Recommendation

The diagnosis of cortical venous thrombosis requires a high index of suspicion. The changes on routine blood testing, EEG examination and CSF analysis are non-specific, though any CSF abnormality in the setting of a picture suggesting benign intracranial hypertension should alert the physician to the possibility of the diagnosis. Technetium scanning, in some hands, has served as a sensitive screening procedure[82], though allowance has to be made for the normal variability of the structure and disposition of the intracranial sinuses. CT should be performed, followed, if the diagnosis is still considered possible, by angiography.

3.3 ARTERIO-VENOUS MALFORMATION

Pathological entities within this umbrella include, besides arterio-venous malformation (AVM), telangiectasiae and cavernous and venous malformations. Arteriovenous malformations most commonly consist of cavernous spaces supplied by arteries from any of the carotid or vertebrobasilar branches and draining through normal, though possibly dilated, venous channels. The majority are single. It has been suggested that bleeding from these malformations accounts for about 1% of all strokes. There is no doubt that a proportion (the figure is debated) of AVM remain asymptomatic in life. The most common clinical presentation is with intraparenchymal or subarachnoid haemorrhage, the former predominating. In some cases there is an association with berry aneurysms. Other presentations include epilepsy, often focal, and focal, or global,

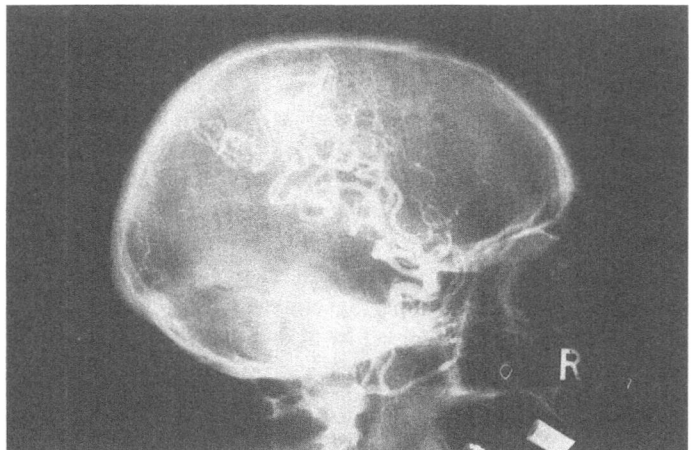

Fig. 3.5 Carotid angiogram showing right parietal arterio-venous malformation

neurological deficits, thought to result partly from steal of circulation into the malformation. There remains debate as to whether an association exists between AVM and headache.

3.3.1 Investigation

Calcification of AVM, on skull X-ray, has been reported in 29.5% of cases in one series[86]. Less commonly, altered vascular channels and enlarged carotid or vertebral arteries (visible because calcified) have been described. Technetium scanning is highly successful in detecting AVM, best demonstrated as a focal increase in radioactivity in the earliest phase of sequential studies[87]. Angiography allows definition of the angioma itself together with its supply vessels and draining veins (Fig. 3.5). Certain characteristics differentiate the vessels from those associated with malignant tumour, the former being regular and uniform, the latter irregular and separated by tumour spaces[88]. Rarely, thrombus formation within the AVM prevents its demonstration by angiography[89].

CT scanning is highly successful in the diagnosis of AVM[90]. Pre-contrast studies demonstrate, most commonly, a mixed-density lesion, sometimes containing areas of calcification. A proportion of AVM are not seen on precontrast films. Following contrast injection there is enhancement of the vascular channels, often showing a typically serpiginous pattern. Occasionally, enhancement is lacking or is a clue, in cases of parenchymal haematoma that the aetiology is AVM. MRI demonstrates the vascularity of these lesions together with associated parenchymal change [62].

3.3.2 Recommendation

CT scanning is the most appropriate investigation in suspected AVM, and may declare the diagnosis when performed in patients with a stroke syndrome. Dynamic technetium scanning is a valuable screening procedure if CT is not immediately available. MRI is likely to have a similar sensitivity to CT. If scanning suggests an AVM, and particularly if surgical intervention is contemplated, then angiography should be performed.

REFERENCES

1. Dyken, M.L., Conneally, P.M., Haerer, A.F. *et al.* (1977) Cooperative study of hospital frequency and character of transient ischemic attacks. 1. Background, organization, and clinical survey. *J. Am. Med. Assoc.*, **237**, 882–6.
2. Awad, I., Modic, M., Little, J.R. *et al.* (1986) Focal parenchymal lesions in transient ischemic attacks: Correlation of computed tomography and magnetic resonance imaging. *Stroke*, **17**, 399–403.
3. Calandre, L., Gomara, S., Bermejo, F. *et al.* (1984) Clinical-CT correlations in TIA, RIND, and strokes with minimum residuum. *Stroke*, **15**, 663–6.
4. Reggia, J.A., Tabb, D.R., Price, T.R. *et al.* (1984) Computer-aided assessment of transient ischemic attacks. A clinical evaluation. *Arch. Neurol.*, **41**, 1248–54.
5. Norris, J.W. and Hachinski, V.C. (1982) Misdiagnosis of stroke. *Lancet*, i, 328–31.
6. Britton, M., Hindmarsh, T., Murray, V. and Tydén, S.A. (1984) Diagnostic errors discovered by CT in patients with suspected stroke. *Neurology*, **34**, 1504–7.
7. Drury, I., Whisnant, J.P. and Garraway, W.M. (1984) Primary intracerebral hemorrhage: impact of CT on incidence. *Neurology*, **34**, 653–7.
8. Incidence of stroke in Oxfordshire: first year's experience of a community stroke register. Oxfordshire community stroke project. (1983) *Br. Med. J.*, **287**, 713–7.
9. Fisher, M., Davidson, R.I. and Marcus, E.M. (1980) Transient focal cerebral ischemia as a presenting manifestation of unruptured cerebral aneurysms. *Ann. Neurol.*, **8**, 367–72.
10. Moster, M.L., Johnston, D.E. and Reinmuth, O.M. (1983) Chronic

subdural hematoma with transient neurological deficits: a review of 15 cases. *Ann. Neurol.*, **14**, 539–42.

11. Parkin, P.J., Kendall, B.E., Marshall, J. and McDonald, W.I. (1982) Amaurosis fugax: some aspects of management. *J. Neurol. Neurosurg. Psychiatry*, **45**, 1–6.

12. Harrison, M.J.G., Iansek, R. and Marshall, J. (1986) Clinical identification of TIAs due to carotid stenosis. *Stroke*, **17**, 391–2.

13. van Merode, T., Hick, P., Hoeks, A.P.G. and Reneman, R.S. (1985) Serum HDL/total cholesterol ratio and blood pressure in asymptomatic atherosclerotic lesions of the cervical carotid arteries in men. *Stroke*, **16**, 34–7.

14. Kjellin, K.G. and Söderström, C.E. (1974) Diagnostic significance of CSF spectrophotometry in cerebrovascular diseases. *J. Neurol. Sci.*, **23**, 359–69.

15. Ruff, R.L. and Dougherty, J.H. Jr (1981) Evaluation of acute cerebral ischemia for anticoagulant therapy: computed tomography or lumbar puncture? *Neurology*, **31**, 736–40.

16. Sörnäs, R., Östlund, H. and Müller, R. (1972) Cerebrospinal fluid cytology after stroke. *Arch. Neurol.*, **26**, 489–501.

17. Roström, B. and Link, H. (1981) Oligoclonal immunoglobulins in cerebrospinal fluid in acute cerebrovascular disease. *Neurology*, **31**, 590–6.

18. Vaagenes, P., Urdal, P., Melvoll, R. and Valnes, K. (1986) Enzyme level changes in the cerebrospinal fluid of patients with acute stroke. *Arch. Neurol.*, **43**, 357–62.

19. Donnan, G.A., Zapf, P., Doyle, A.E. and Bladin, P.F. (1983) CSF enzymes in lacunar and cortical stroke. *Stroke*, **14**, 266–9.

20. Welch, D.M., Coleman, E., Hardin, W.B. and Siegel, B.A. (1975) Brain scanning in cerebral vascular disease: a reappraisal. *Stroke*, **6**, 136–41.

21. Gado, M.H., Coleman, E., Merlis, A.L. *et al.*(1976) Comparison of computerized tomography and radionuclide imaging in 'stroke'. *Stroke*, **7**, 109–13.

22. Hansotia, P.L. (1985) Persistent vegetative state. Review and report of electrodiagnostic studies in eight cases. *Arch. Neurol.*, **42**, 1048–52.

23. Faught, E. and Oh, S.J. (1985) Brainstem auditory evoked responses in brainstem infarction. *Stroke*, **16**, 701–5.

24. Kapsch, D., Cook, L., Lichti, E. and Silver, D. (1981) Use of combined oculoplethysmography, carotid phonoangiography and doppler in the non-invasive diagnosis of extracranial carotid occlusive disease. *Stroke*, **12**, 317–21.

25. Sanborn, G.E., Miller, N.R., McGuire, M. and Kumar, A.J. (1981) Clinical-angiographic correlation of ophthalmodynamometry in patients with suspected carotid artery disease: a prospective study. *Stroke*, **12**, 770–4.

26. Humphrey, P.R.D. and Bradbury, P.G. (1984) Continuous wave doppler ultrasonography in the detection of carotid stenosis and occlusion. *J. Neurol. Neurosurg. Psychiatry*, **47**, 1128–30.

27. Russell, D., Lindegaard, K-F., Nakstad, P. *et al.* (1984) Detection of carotid occlusive disease by pulsed doppler spectral analysis. *J. Neurol. Neurosurg. Psychiatry*, **47**, 1307–13.
28. Anderson, D.C., Loewenson, R., Yock, D. *et al.* (1983) B-mode, real-time carotid ultrasonic imaging. Correlation with angiography. *Arch. Neurol.*, **40**, 484–8.
29. Fischer, G.G., Anderson, D.C., Farber, R. and Lebow, S. (1985) Prediction of carotid disease by ultrasound and digital subtraction angiography. *Arch. Neurol.*, **42**, 224–7.
30. Keagy, B.A., Pharr, W.F., Thomas, D. and Bowes, D.E. (1982) Comparison of oculoplethysmography/carotid phonoangiography with duplex scan/spectral analysis in the detection of carotid artery stenosis. *Stroke*, **13**, 43–5.
31. Zwiebel, W.J., Strother, C.M., Austin, C.W. and Sackett,, J.F. (1985) Comparison of ultrasound and IV-DSA for carotid evaluation. *Stroke*, **16**, 633–43.
32. O'Leary, D.H., Clouse, M.E., Potter, J.E. and Wheeler, H.G. (1985) The influence of non-invasive tests on the selection of patients for carotid angiography. *Stroke*, **16**, 264–7.
33. Ringelstein, E.B., Zeumer, H. and Poeck, K. (1985) Non-invasive diagnosis of intracranial lesions in the vertebrobasilar system. A comparison of doppler sonographic and angiographic findings. *Stroke*, **16**, 848–55.
34. Bull, J.W.D., Marshall, J. and Shaw, D.A. (1960) Cerebral angiography in the diagnosis of the acute stroke. *Lancet*, **i**, 562–5.
35. Huckman, M.S., Weinberg, P.E., Kim, K.S. and Davis, D.O. (1970) Angiographic and clinico-pathologic correlates in basal ganglionic hemorrhage. *Radiology*, **95**, 79–82.
36. Ojemann, R.G. and Heros, R.C. (1983) Spontaneous brain hemorrhage. *Stroke*, **14**, 468–75.
37. Fisher, M., Ahmadi, J., Zee, C-S. *et al.* (1985) Arteriography of the carotid bifurcation: oblique projections. *Neurology*, **35**, 1201–4.
38. Faught, E., Trader, S.D. and Hanna, G.R. (1979) Cerebral complications of angiography for transient ischemia and stroke: prediction of risk. *Neurology*, **29**, 4–15.
39. Chilcote, W.A., Modic, M.T., Paulicek, W.A. *et al.* (1981) Digital subtraction angiography of the carotid arteries: a comparative study in 100 patients. *Radiology*, **139**, 287–95.
40. Little, J.R., Furlan, A.J., Modic, M.T. *et al.* (1982) Intravenous digital subtraction angiography in brain ischemia. *J. Am. Med. Assoc.*, **247**, 3213–16.
41. Celesia, G.G., Strother, C.M., Turski, P.A. *et al.* (1983) Digital subtraction arteriography. A new method for evaluation of extracranial occlusive disease. *Arch. Neurol.*, **40**, 70–4.
42. Guidotti, M., Landi, G., Scotti, G. and Scarlato, G. (1985) Digital subtraction angiography in patients with cerebral ischaemic attacks and normal continuous wave doppler studies. *J. Neurol. Neurosurg. Psychiatry*, **48**, 39–43.

43. Pelz, D.M., Fox, A.J. and Vinuela, F. (1985) Digital subtraction angiography: current clinical applications. *Stroke*, 16, 528–36.
44. Tans, J.Th.J., Hoogland, P.H. and Jonkman, E.J. (1985) The role of venous digital subtraction angiography of the carotid bifurcation in the evaluation of patients with reversible ischemic attacks or stroke. *Stroke*, 16, 435–40.
45. Hart, R.G. and Easton, J.D. (1983) Dissections of cervical and cerebral arteries. *Neurol. Clin.*, 1, 155–82.
46. O'Connell, B.K., Towfighi, J., Brennan, R.W. *et al.* (1985) Dissecting aneurysms of head and neck. *Neurology*, 35, 993–7.
47. Hornig, C.R., Busse, O., Buettner, T. *et al.* (1985) CT contrast enhancement on brain scans and blood CSF barrier disturbances in cerebral ischemic infarction. *Stroke*, 16, 268–73.
48. Kase, C.S., White, J.L., Joslyn, J.N. *et al.* (1985) Cerebellar infarction in the superior cerebellar artery distribution. *Neurology*, 35, 705–11.
49. Gacs, G., Fox, A.J., Barnett, H.J.M. and Vinuela, F. (1983) CT visualization of intracranial arterial thromboembolism. *Stroke*, 14, 756–62.
50. Fisher, C.M. (1982) Lacunar strokes and infarcts: A review. *Neurology*, 32, 871–6.
51. Wiseberg, L.A. (1982) Lacunar infarcts. Clinical and computed tomographic correlations. *Arch. Neurol.*, 39, 37–40.
52. Rascol, A., Clanet, M., Manelfe, C. *et al.* (1982) Pure motor hemiplegia: CT study of 30 cases. *Stroke*, 13, 11–17.
53. Nelson, R.F., Pullicino, P., Kendall, B.E. and Marshall, J. (1980) Computer tomography in patients presenting with lacunar syndromes. *Stroke*, 11, 256–61.
54. Herold, S., Kummer, R.V. and Jaeger, Ch. (1982) Follow-up of spontaneous intracerebral haemorrhage by computed tomography. *J. Neurol.*, 228, 267–76.
55. Kawahara, N., Sato, K., Muraki, M. *et al.* (1986) CT classification of small thalamic hemorrhages and their clinical implications. *Neurology*, 36, 165–72.
56. Weisberg, L.A. (1986) Primary pontine haemorrhage: clinical and computed tomographic correlations. *J. Neurol. Neurosurg. Psychiatry*, 49, 346–52.
57. Mori, E., Tabuchi, M. and Yamadori, A. (1985) Lacunar syndrome due to intracerebral hemorrhage. *Stroke*, 16, 454–9.
58. Wiseberg, L.A. (1984) Caudate hemorrhage. *Arch. Neurol.*, 41, 971–4.
59. Rees Cosgrove, G., Leblanc, R., Meagher-Villemure, K. and Ethier, R. (1985) Cerebral amyloid angiopathy. *Neurology*, 35, 625–31.
60. Gilbert, J.J. and Vinters, H.V. (1983) Cerebral amyloid angiopathy: incidence and complications in the aging brain. 1. Cerebral hemorrhage. *Stroke*, 14, 915–23.
61. Sipponen, J.T., Kaste, M., Ketonen, L. *et al.* (1983). Serial nuclear magnetic resonance (NMR) imaging in patients with cerebral infarction. *J. Comput. Assist. Tomogr.*, 7, 585–9.

62. Dewitt, L.D., Buonanno, F.S., Kistler, J.P. *et al.* (1984) Nuclear magnetic resonance imaging in evaluation of clinical stroke syndromes. *Ann. Neurol.*, **16**, 535–45.
63. Dewitt, L.D. (1986) Clinical use of nuclear magnetic resonance imaging in stroke. *Stroke*, **17**, 328–31.
64. Ross, M.A., Biller, J., Adams, H.P. Jr and Dunn, V. (1986) Magnetic resonance imaging in Wallenberg's lateral medullary syndrome. *Stroke*, **17**, 542–5.
65. Sipponen, J.T., Sepponen, R.E. and Sivula, A. (1983) Nuclear magnetic resonance (NMR) imaging of intracerebral hemorrhage in the acute and resolving phases. *J. Comput. Assist. Tomogr.*, **7**, 954–9.
66. Gerard, G. and Weisberg, L.A. (1986) MRI periventricular lesions in adults. *Neurology*, **36**, 998–1001.
67. Pelletier, L.L. Jr and Petersdorf, R.G. (1977) Infective endocarditis: A review of 125 cases from the University of Washington Hospitals, 1963–1972. *Medicine*, **56**, 287–313.
68. Sandok, B.A., Estorff, I.V. and Giuliani, E.R. (1980) CNS embolism due to atrial myxoma. Clinical features and diagnosis. *Arch. Neurol.*, **37**, 485–8.
69. Sandok, B.A. and Giuliani, E.R. (1982) Cerebral ischemic events in patients with mitral valve prolapse. *Stroke*, **13**, 448–50.
70. Scharf, R.E., Hennerici, M., Bluschke, V. *et al.* (1982) Cerebral ischemia in young patients: Is it associated with mitral valve prolapse and abnormal platelet activity *in vivo*? *Stroke*, **13**, 454–8.
71. de Bono, D.P. and Warlow, C.P. (1981) Potential sources of emboli in patients with presumed transient cerebral or retinal ischaemia. *Lancet*, **i**, 343–6.
72. Donaldson, R.M., Emanuel, R.W. and Earl, C.J. (1981) The role of two-dimensional echocardiography in the detection of potentially embolic intracardiac masses in patients with cerebral ischaemia. *J. Neurol. Neurosurg. Psychiatry*, **44**, 803–9.
73. Come, P.C., Riley, M.F. and Bivas, N.K. (1983) Roles of echocardiography and arrhythmia monitoring in the evaluation of patients with suspected systemic embolism. *Ann. Neurol.*, **13**, 527–31.
74. Knopman, D.S., Anderson, D.C., Asinger, R.W. *et al.* (1982) Indications for echocardiography in patients with ischemic stroke. *Neurology*, **32**, 1005–11.
75. Nishide, M., Irino, T., Gotoh, M. *et al.* (1983) Cardiac abnormalities in ischemic cerebrovascular disease studied by two-dimensional echocardiography. *Stroke*, **14**, 541–5.
76. Biller, J., Johnson, M.R., Adams, H.P. Jr *et al.* (1986) Echocardiographic evaluation of young adults with nonhemorrhagic cerebral infarction. *Stroke*, **17**, 608–12.
77. Caplan, L.R., D'Cruz, I., Hier, D.B. *et al.* (1986) Atrial size, atrial fibrillation, and stroke. *Ann. Neurol.*, **19**, 158–61.
78. Abdon, N-J., Zettervall, O., Carlson, J. *et al.* (1982) Is occult atrial

disorder a frequent cause of non-hemorrhagic stroke? Long-term ECG in 86 patients. *Stroke*, 13, 832–7.

79. Francis, D.A., Heron, J.R. and Clarke, M. (1984) Ambulatory electrocardiographic monitoring in patients with transient focal cerebral ischaemia. *J. Neurol. Neurosurg. Psychiatry*, 47, 256–9.

80. Powers, W.J., Siegel, B.A., Davis II, H.H. *et al.* (1982) Indium-III platelet scintigraphy in cerebrovascular disease. *Neurology*, 32, 938–43.

81. Powers, W.J. and Raichle, M.E. (1985) Positron emission tomography and its application to the study of cerebrovascular disease in man. *Stroke*, 16, 361–76.

82. Bousser, M-G., Chiras, J., Bories, J. and Castaigne, P. (1985) Cerebral venous thrombosis – A review of 38 cases. *Stroke*, 16, 199–213.

83. Brant-Zawadzki, M., Chang, G.Y. and McCarty, G.E. (1982) Computed tomography in dural sinus thrombosis. *Neurology*, 39, 446–7.

84. Clifford Jones, R.E., Ellis, C.J.K., Stevens, J.M. and Turner, A. (1982) Cavernous sinus thrombosis. *J. Neurol. Neurosurg. Psychiatry*, 45, 1092–7.

85. Savino, P.J., Grossman, R.I., Schatz, N.J. *et al.* (1986) High-field magnetic resonance imaging in the diagnosis of cavernous sinus thrombosis. *Arch. Neurol.*, 43, 1081–2.

86. Rumbaugh, C.L. and Potts, D.G. (1966) Skull changes associated with intracranial arteriovenous malformations. *Am. J. Roentgenol.*, 98, 525–34.

87. Handa, J., Handa, H., Torizuka, K. *et al.* (1972) Radioisotopic study of arteriovenous anomalies. *Am. J. Roentgenol.*, 115, 751–9.

88. Goree, J.A. and Dukes, H.T. (1963) The angiographic differential diagnosis between the vascularized malignant glioma and the intracranial arteriovenous malformation. *Am. J. Roentgenol.*, 90, 512–21.

89. Kamrin, R.B. and Buchsbaum, H.W. (1965) Large vascular malformations of the brain not visualized by serial angiography. *Arch. Neurol.*, 13, 413–20.

90. Vlaikidis, N.D. and Kazis, A. (1984) CT in the diagnosis of cerebral vascular malformations. *J. Neurol.*, 231, 188–93.

4

Dementia
Epilepsy

4.1 DEMENTIA

A recent review suggested that dementia of severe degree affected between 3 and 5% of the population over the age of 65 years, with a similar percentage having milder disease[1]. All studies agree that Alzheimer's disease (including senile dementia of Alzheimer type) together with multi-infarct dementia account for at least three-quarters of cases[1]. Attempts have been made to define specific criteria for the diagnosis of Alzheimer's disease, influenced no doubt by the knowledge that some 20% of cases, diagnosed in life, are found to have other conditions at autopsy[2]. The clinical diagnosis of multi-infarct dementia is facilitated by the use of a system which scores a number of factors thought to be associated with an underlying ischaemic pathogenesis. The system has been verified by autopsy study[3]. Clinical features of particular importance in the diagnosis of multi-infarct dementia include abrupt onset of disability, a stepwise deterioration, a history of stroke and focal signs or symptoms. Patients with subcortical arteriosclerotic encephalopathy have a similar history and findings, though often with a more slowly evolving history[4]. Neither Alzheimer's disease nor multi-infarct dementia are reversible. Perhaps as a consequence, much has been written of the other disorders which either reproduce the features of dementia, but are triggered by psychopathological mechanisms, or are, at least theoretically, amenable to surgical or medical intervention. Reversibility is a subjective concept, and whilst authors have suggested that up to 30% of patients fall into this category[5], their appraisal and, critically, the quality of their follow-up require close scrutiny. A frequently quoted study analysed the results of the investigation of 106 patients admitted with a putative diagnosis of pre-senile dementia[6]. The diagnosis remained uncertain in seven, was confirmed in 84, and was excluded in 15 patients. The last group contained patients with depression, hysteria, mania and drug toxicity. No metabolic causes were discovered among the 84 confirmed cases, but eight proved to have mass lesions, and five normal-pressure hydrocephalus. None of the patients with normal-pressure hydrocephalus benefited from surgery, whilst only two of the mass lesions were benign. If the term reversibility is applied rigorously, therefore, 2.4% of the 84 cases benefited from therapeutic intervention. A divide between the theoretical and practical limits of reversibility is only too apparent from a study of the literature. At times, the discovery of hypothyroidism, drug intoxication or subdural haematoma has led to the assumption that the sole basis for the patient's dementia has been discovered with the expectation that the condition can be eliminated by appropriate treatment. In a careful study of 107 patients with a presumptive diagnosis of dementia, 15 were thought to have reversible factors[7]. In practice, three recovered. Of patients identified as having hypothyroidism, drug intoxication or subdural haematoma, three-quarters, two-thirds and half respectively showed a subsequent progressive mental deterioration suggesting the presence of Alzheimer's disease[7]. The same study, incidentally, emphasized that treatment of concomitant disorders, for example cardiac failure, might improve the mental status of individuals despite the fact that the underlying pathology of their dementia was thought to be Alzheimer's disease. It has been suggested that those patients with a potentially reversible dementia are more likely to have a shorter history, be less severely affected, to have had exposure to more drugs and more often give a history of sudden deterioration than those with Alzheimer's disease[7].

The term pseudo-dementia has been used to describe patients with a presentation suggesting dementia in whom psychiatric disease is thought to be the main triggering factor. Conditions responsible for this presentation include schizophrenia, the affective disorders, and a personality disorder. Where the pseudo-dementia is merely a caricature of the real condition, often associated with strenuous complaints of cognitive dysfunction incompatible with observed behaviour, an underlying hysterical conversion reaction is likely[8]. Depressive pseudo-dementia tends to occur in older individuals often with a past history of psychiatric illness. In these cases, pseudo-dementia can be indistinguishable from an organic mental disorder prompting some observers to suggest that an organic syndrome is indeed present, but based on neurochemical rather than

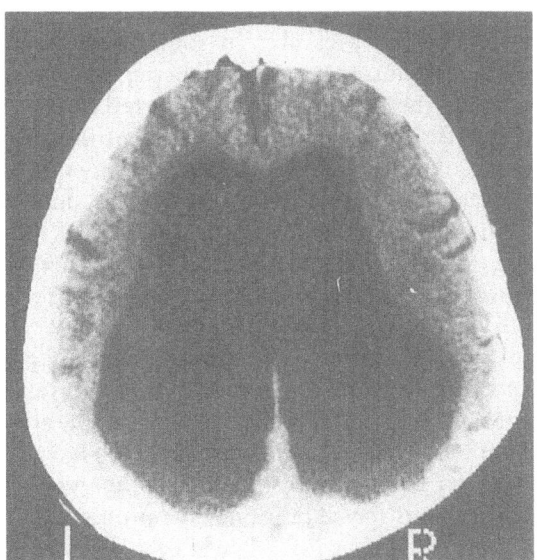

Fig. 4.1 CT scan showing gross hydrocephalus. The patient had presented with dementia accompanied by a gait disorder

irreversible structural change. Such cases may respond dramatically to appropriate therapy. Pseudo-dementia was encountered, among populations deemed to be demented at initial appraisal in 9.4, 14, 1.7 and 10% respectively in four separate series[6,7,9,10].

Subcortical dementia is considered a specific entity by some authors. Disorders of higher cortical function, for example aphasia and agnosia are lacking. A defect of fluency in the absence of aphasia is thought typical of the syndrome[11], which has been described in conditions such as Parkinson's and Huntington's disease.

Normal-pressure hydrocephalus (NPH) was found to account for 4.4% of 502 cases of dementia collected from five separate studies[12] (Fig. 4.1). The dementia associated with NPH is less likely to show aphasia, agnosia or apraxia than that due to Alzheimer's disease[13]. A clinical triad of dementia, incontinence and gait disorder is associated with radiological evidence of hydrocephalus. Some patients, with similar radiological findings, have dementia alone. Whereas early studies suggested a correlation between delayed emptying of radioisotope from the lateral ventricles after cisternal injection and response to shunting[14], this has not been the subsequent experience [15]. Demonstration of intermittently raised intradural pressures in some patients with normal-pressure hydrocephalus may allow a better prediction of shunt responders [16]. In three studies already referred to [6,9,10], 20 cases of normal-pressure hydrocephalus were identified. Response occurred in 42.1% of those shunted, with a mortality rate of 5.3%. In a survey of 73 patients with NPH, early response to shunting occurred in 45.2% falling to 37% during a longer period of follow-up [15]. The mortality rate was 6.9%. Of more relevance is the likely response, estimated at 20%, in patients who present with dementia alone.

The logic behind the intensive investigation of patients with dementia rests therefore on the knowledge that a certain proportion will be found to have triggering factors which are potentially treatable. Although some patients with dementia have evidence of a metabolic disorder or a mass lesion, critical analysis suggests that many of these patients have additional symptoms and signs incompatible with the diagnosis of Alzheimer's disease. A dementia syndrome is described in association with B_{12} deficiency, though in two of three cases in one, often quoted, study spontaneous remissions and relapses of the mental disorder had occurred [17]. A case of hypoparathyroidism associated with dementia is similarly used as a justification for calcium studies in dementia. At the time of diagnosis, neurological findings included nystagmus and bilateral extensor plantar responses [18]. Amongst 850 patients admitted for diagnostic investigation to a 'cerebral surgery and research unit', 41 proved to have tumours and 14 subdural haematomas [19]. In the latter group, eight had long tract signs and six were admitted in coma. The paper fails to indicate how many of the patients with mass lesions had a pure dementia syndrome. Adult-onset metachromatic leucodystrophy can present with dementia though, in one case report, extrapyramidal features accompanied the altered mental state [20]. Two patients with a dementia syndrome and idiopathic haemochromatosis improved after phlebotomy. Both patients were ataxic and one had limb rigidity [21]. The cases were considered to be similar to a group with non-Wilsonian hepatocerebral degeneration described previously. A condition with a superficial resemblance to Huntington's disease, neuronal intranuclear hyaline inclusion disease, generally presents in childhood and displays autosomal recessive inheritance. Cases with adult-onset have been described with, in one family, a pattern suggesting dominant inheritance[22]. A patient with improving cognition after treatment of a phaeochromocytoma has been described, despite a history of stroke-like events and the finding of multiple infarction on CT scanning[23]. Myxoedema may be found presenting with dementia but no other features[9,10], though there must be a suspicion, from subsequent events, that in some patients, a chance association between hypothyroidism and Alzheimer's disease has been discovered[7].

4.1.1 Investigation

The initial phase in the investigation of a patient suspected of dementia is a psychometric evaluation. Some authors have suggested that the findings in patients with depression are indistinguishable from those with an organic dementia[8], but others believe that distinguishing factors operate. In some instances the dementia is so florid that formal evaluation becomes redundant and, indeed, impossible. Debate continues as to the most valid testing scheme for distinguishing patients with dementia from the normal population. Any assessment method is likely to include appraisal of orientation, memory, language function, praxis, attention, visual perception, problem solving capacity and overall social function[2]. An analysis of individual tests concluded that, using four sub-tests alone, correct classification of dementia or no dementia was achieved in 82 of 84 patients and all 24 controls[24]. The tests used were the Wechsler Memory Scale, mental control and logical memory, word fluency and Trailmaking A (part of the Halstead–Reitan neuropsychological battery). The tests could be administered in 10 minutes. It has been suggested that a combination of CT scanning and psychometric assessment is more powerful in discriminating normals from dementia patients then either investigation alone[25].

(a) Electrophysiological investigation

In one study, a significant slowing of the dominant occipital rhythm of the EEG correctly identified 86% of patients with Alzheimer's disease[26] (Fig. 4.2). The view that the EEG is more normal in patients with pseudo-dementia has been challenged[8]. Prominent slowing of the EEG is a feature of subcortical arteriosclerotic encephalopathy[4]. In Pick's disease, on the other hand, the EEG is relatively normal[27]. Long latency, event-related components of the auditory and other evoked potentials are abnormal in Alzheimer's disease. In a group of 25 patients, significant delay of the P_3

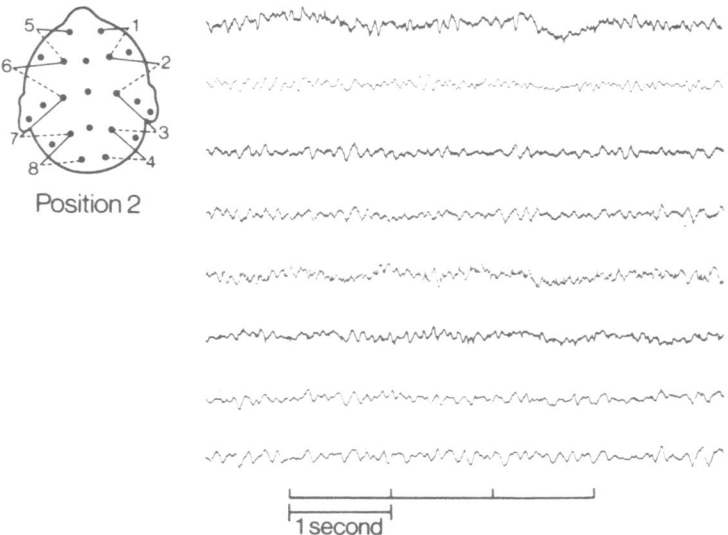

Position 2

Fig. 4.2 EEG showing diffuse increase in theta activity in a patient with dementia

wave was detected in 20, producing a correct classification, on electrophysiological criteria, in 80% [28].

(b) CSF abnormalities

The recognition of the neurotransmitter changes occurring in Alzheimer's disease has stimulated a search for transmitter activity, particularly relating to choline, in the CSF. A reduced level of cholinesterase activity has been reported in Alzheimer's disease [2,9,30]. Whilst some authors have found the level to correlate with the severity of the dementia [29], others have not [30]. Somatostatin-like immunoreactivity is similarly depressed in Alzheimer's disease [29,31] and in multi-infarct dementia [31]. However, peripheral acetylcholinesterase activity, (as measured in plasma and red cells), is unchanged and cannot, therefore, be used as a screening test for depletion of cerebral cholinergic activity [32]. Other transmitter systems have been assessed. CSF homovanillic acid levels have either been reported to be reduced overall in Alzheimer's disease [33], or only in more severely demented cases [34]. Levels of tetrahydrobiopterin, a cofactor in the hydroxylation of phenylalanine, tyrosine and tryptophan, correlate with CSF homovanillic acid concentrations, and are reduced in Alzheimer's disease[35]. Levels of the glycolytic enzyme enolase, localized to neurones and neuroendocrine cells, are similarly depressed[36]. Although the findings of these and other investigations of enzyme and transmitter systems in the CSF are of some interest in terms of the pathogenesis of the disease, overlap between patients and controls is substantial, and none of the investigations to date have been sufficiently specific to allow their use as a screening test for Alzheimer's disease.

The role of the conventional tests on the CSF in the investigation of dementia has been supported with varying levels of enthusiasm. Some have suggested that the examination is mandatory[5]. Others have indicated its potential role for the exclusion of conditions such as cryptococcosis and syphilis[2]. In one study of dementia syphilis accounted for a single case out of a total of 60. Rather than masquerading as Alzheimer's disease, the patient's condition was associated with a history of syphilis and findings on examination typical of tertiary syphilis, with Argyll Robertson pupils. Moreover, serology was positive in the blood as well as the CSF[9]. An evaluation of the role of CSF examination in the diagnosis of the pathogenesis of dementia[12] showed that among 80 patients reviewed retrospectively, 42 had had a lumbar puncture as part of their assessment. It says much about the role of the investigation that the authors were unable to elicit why it had been performed in some patients, but not in others. They found a non-specific elevation of the protein concentration in eleven patients, and concluded that 'no diagnoses were made with the information obtained from 42 LPs, despite a cost of approximately 16,000 dollars'.

(c) Radiological investigation
Many studies have been published in the last 10 years on the role of CT scanning in the investigation of suspected dementia. Two main aspects have been discussed. First, the value of scanning in the detection of unsuspected pathology, for example tumour, or sub-dural haematoma, and secondly, the relationship between various radiological markers of atrophy and the presence of dementia. Among 502 cases, collected from five studies, mass lesions were found in 3% [12]. In an analysis of the necessity for CT scanning as a screening procedure in dementia, it was concluded that if, for patients with severe dementia, and a history exceeding three years, or those without a history of sudden deterioration, no scan had been

performed, no potentially reversible structural lesion would have been missed [7].

The results of CT scanning among 500 consecutive patients with a presumed diagnosis of dementia have been published [37]. Atrophy was found in 38.4%, infarction in 34.8% and tumour in 8.4%. Of the 42 tumours, 38 were malignant. Despite this, the tumour cases were included among the treatable cases. Among the patients with dementia but no other symptoms or signs, 5% were said to have a treatable structural lesion though no indication is given as to how many of these were malignant. The authors found that the presence of headache, speech disturbance, focal signs and papilloedema discriminated in favour of patients with a treatable lesion.

Correlations have been made between dementia and radiological criteria of cerebral atrophy with varying degrees of success. In an early paper, it was concluded that the degree of intellectual impairment correlated with mean ventricular area but not with para-ventricular density, nor with the width of the widest sulcus [38]. Whereas a further study again failed to find a relationship between tissue density adjacent to the lateral ventricle and clinical evidence of dementia [39], a more recent analysis did find a positive relationship which, when combined with measures of the third and lateral ventricles, allowed a correct classification of demented patients in 97% [40]. Measurements of sulcal width have proved disappointing as a discriminant between demented patients and age-matched controls. Though some have found a significant difference [41] others have not [42], nor, when differences have been found, have they shown a correlation with the degree of dementia [41].

Measurement of ventricular size has proved more valuable though disagreement has been expressed regarding the most valuable index. Measurement of third ventricular size alone correctly classified 84% of demented patients [26]. Measurement of frontal horn size, the ratio of lateral ventricular width at the level of the cella media to the width of the outer skull table, the width of the third ventricle and the size of the temporal horn all produced significant differences between patients with senile dementia and controls, and between patients with multi-infarct dementia and controls [41]. For Alzheimer's disease, the ventricular area increased with increasing degree of intellectual impairment [41]. Measurement of lateral ventricular size combined with the width of the interhemispheric fissure correctly classified 84% of patients and control subjects [42].

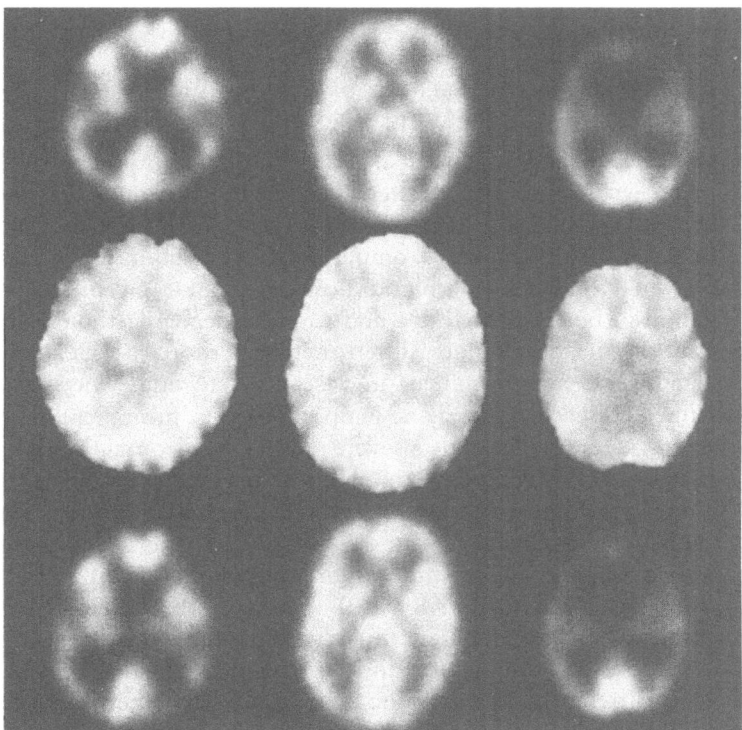

Fig. 4.3 Positron emission tomography in multi-infarct dementia (left), Alzheimer's disease (right) and control subject (centre). The top row shows cerebral blood flow, the centre the oxygen extraction ratio and the bottom row regional cerebral oxygen utilization. In the multi-infarct case there are matching patchy defects in blood flow and metabolism whereas in the Alzheimer patient there is depression of flow and metabolism more generally, maximally in the frontal cortex

A computed estimation of lateral ventricular volume discriminates dementia subjects more successfully than a simple measurement of width, particularly for those under the age of 65[43]. Whilst measurements of sulcal width have proved of limited value, a computed system measuring cortical surface area produced values that were significantly reduced in demented subjects[44]. Both CT and, in particular, MRI display a much higher incidence of white matter change in multi-infarct dementia than in Alzheimer's disease[45]. In Pick's disease, CT may display frontal rather than generalized atrophy, the changes sometimes preceding clinical declaration of the disease [27].

(d) Blood flow and positron emission tomography

Cerebral blood flow, measured by the xenon inhalation technique, shows bilateral and symmetrical reduction in grey matter which correlates with the severity of the dementia [46]. For milder degrees of dementia, however, there is an overlap with age-matched controls. Positron emission tomography has established a correlation between cerebral blood flow levels and mean oxygen utilization in both degenerative and vascular dementia though the distribution of the changes differs between the two (Fig. 4.3). Parietal defects are prominent in vascular dementia, whereas in Alzheimer's disease, parietal and temporal defects, prominent in the earlier stages, are replaced by a severe reduction in frontal flow with progression [47]. Metabolic activity has been assessed by the use of [^{18}F]fluorodeoxyglucose scanning, with the finding of diffuse hypometabolism in Alzheimer's disease but asymmetric cortical and subcortical suppression in multi-infarct dementia [48]. A relative reduction of metabolic activity in the parietal lobes compared to other cortical areas is apparent in the earliest stages of Alzheimer's disease, antedating radiological and electrophysiological abnormalities [49]. Differences in metabolic activity also exist between Alzheimer's disease and normal pressure hydrocephalus, the latter showing depression in all regions [50].

4.1.2 Recommendation (see flow chart A)

In patients with advanced dementia, formal psychometry is unnecessary. For other patients, a restricted analysis, using four discriminants, allows an accurate diagnosis in the majority. If psychometry fails to exclude a pseudo-dementia confidently, a trial of antidepressant therapy can be of value.

The degree of investigation required to exclude metabolic factors in dementia is debatable (see flow chart A). A full blood count, biochemical analysis and thyroid function tests are appropriate. A progressive dementia, without focal signs, must be a rare manifestation of vitamin B$_{12}$ deficiency or neurosyphilis. There is no justification for examining the CSF in dementia unless there are signs suggesting the diagnosis of neurosyphilis.

Neurophysiological tests are of some value as screening

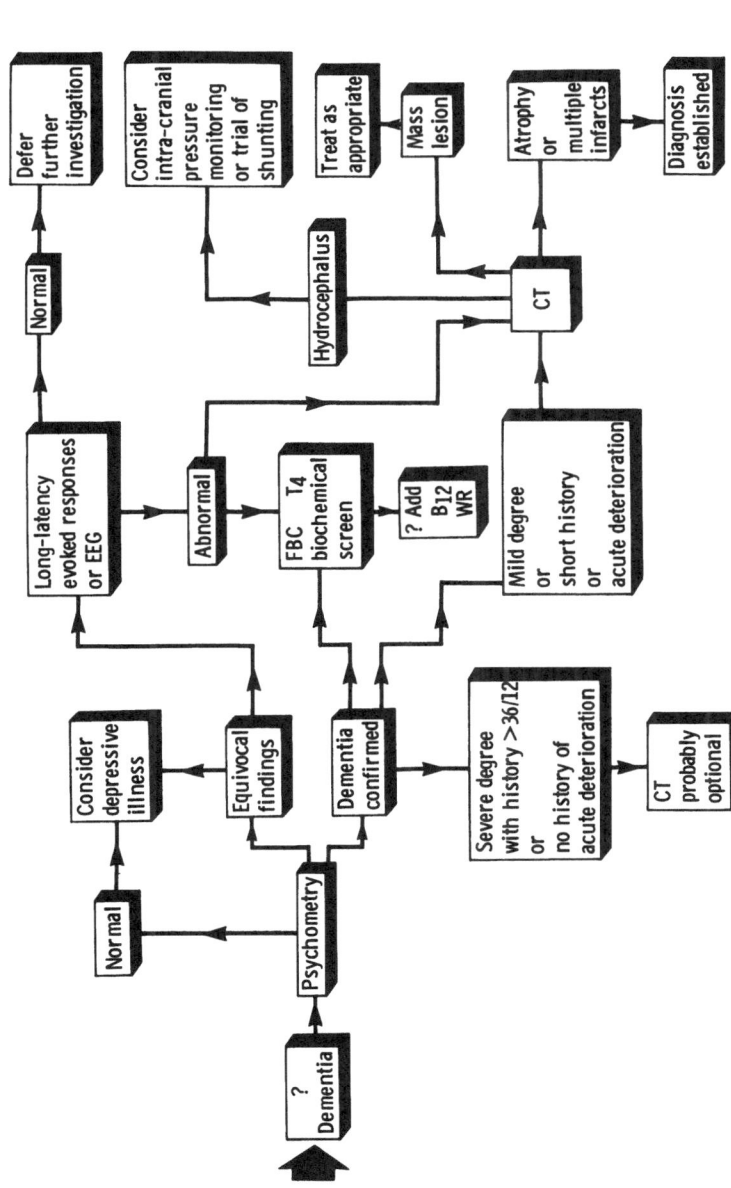

Flow chart A

procedures. Measurement of either long-latency components of the evoked responses, or performance of an EEG will identify 80% or more of cases of Alzheimer's disease.

A small proportion of patients with dementia alone will be found to have a structural lesion. Many tumours presenting in this way are malignant and barely amenable to therapy. Though normal pressure hydrocephalus is theoretically reversible, this is achieved in a minority when presentation has been with dementia alone. In patients with a severe dementia and a protracted history or with no history of a sudden deterioration, scanning is highly unlikely to reveal a space-occupying lesion or normal-pressure hydrocephalus.

4.2 EPILEPSY

The development of the EEG, and more recently, the capacity to record electrical brain activity over a prolonged period, combined with video recording of epileptic events, has resulted in an increasingly sophisticated scheme of seizure classification. One relevance of better classification lies in the realization that certain seizure types are much more likely to be related to structural brain pathology than are others. Absence seizures, when carefully defined, are very rarely associated with structural changes on CT scanning. On the other hand, an early study of CT scanning in patients with simple or complex partial seizures established abnormalities in nearly two-thirds[51]. There are other motives prompting the investigation of epilepsy, or episodes of altered awareness. A certain proportion of events, amounting to 20% in one report[52], initially considered to be epileptic, prove to have a cardiogenic basis. Equally important is the need to identify those patients whose seizures are the manifestation of conversion hysteria[53]. Further considerations worthy of attention include the role of particular investigations in the correct identification of those patients whose intractable, focal, seizures are likely to respond to surgical intervention[54], and the role of the EEG and estimation of serum anticonvulsant levels in the evaluation of treatment response.

In one large survey of epilepsy[55], amounting to 689 patients, 274 proved to have tonic–clonic convulsions. Less common forms included focal motor seizures (46) and complex partial seizures (54). The analysis had excluded patients known to have symptomatic epilepsy. With increasing age at onset, structural abnormalities are more likely to be identified. In an analysis of 80 patients developing epilepsy beyond the age of 50, 29 proved to have a cerebral tumour, whereas 20 were thought to have an arteriosclerotic basis[56]. Of the cerebral tumours, 21 were malignant. An appraisal of patients with angiographically proven carotid or middle cerebral occlusions indicated that 17.3% of the former, and 10.8% of the latter had seizures[57]. Some of these coincided with the acute stroke, others appeared later. The recurrence rate after a single seizure has been reported to lie between 21 and 71%[58]. The risk of recurrence begins to fall sharply once two years have elapsed from the initial attack[59].

4.2.1 Investigation

Many metabolic disorders can trigger epileptic activity, though usually this represents only part of their symptomatology. Nevertheless, biochemical screening is appropriate for patients with epilepsy with particular reference to sodium, calcium and glucose levels. Certain metabolic consequences of seizure activity have been advocated as a means for distinguishing geniune from hysterical seizures. Although creatine kinase levels remained normal after psychogenic seizures in six patients, they rose at 18–96 hours after 15% of tonic–clonic convulsions[60]. Other authors have found a higher incidence of abnormal values after organic seizure activity. Some increase in prolactin levels is almost inevitable immediately after tonic–clonic convulsions, returning to base-line levels at 60 min. Changes after simple partial seizures are less striking and often lacking[61].

Interpretation of CSF abnormalities in patients being investigated for epilepsy must take account of changes consequent to the seizure itself. Following 98 seizures in 91 patients, two examples of pleocytosis were recorded and seven of an elevated protein concentration. Pleocytosis seems only likely to appear after prolonged or repeated fits[62].

Skull radiography is irrelevant in the investigation of epilepsy. Among 200 consecutive patients with epilepsy presenting after the age of 15, none of whom had neurological signs, 158 had had skull X-rays performed. All but two were normal, the exceptions showing old skull fractures[63]. When 100 patients, of whom 83 had had skull X-rays, were followed, six subsequently developed evidence of an intracranial tumour. None of these had had an abnormal skull X-ray initially.

(a) Electroencephalography

No uniform opinion is available regarding the incidence of EEG abnormalities in epilepsy. Variables to be considered include whether there have been single or multiple seizures, and the type of epileptic event. In a review of 689 patients, where symptomatic cases had been excluded, 56% had borderline or abnormal EEGs[55]. An interesting observation in this study was that one-third of individuals with non-convulsive 'attacks' had borderline or abnormal records. Where a frequency of abnormal records is quoted, some care is needed when appraising how representative a sample of the epileptic population has been chosen. An early report found that 95% of EEG recordings in a group of 494 patients with epilepsy were abnormal. Perusal of the paper reveals, however, that some selection of patients with focal epilepsy was evident and that nearly half the patients had been admitted for intensive study with a view to possible surgery[64]. The role of the electroencephalogram in the diagnosis of epilepsy has been critically appraised[65]. There is general agreement that abnormalities are often found in focal epilepsy (Fig. 4.4). Gastaut[66] found abnormalities in 90% of his patients with temporal lobe epilepsy, though it is likely that this was achieved, in some instances, only after repeated recordings or after activation procedures. Video analysis of temporal lobe epilepsy has led to the differentiation of seizure types with individual EEG characteristics[67]. Whereas classical complex partial seizures are likely to have a temporal lobe focus[68], certain additional features, for example tonic adversive head or eye movements, suggest an initial focus elsewhere, for example the frontal lobe or the supplementary motor gyrus[69]. Certain activation procedures enhance the diagnostic value of the EEG. Recordings performed during sleep are more likely to be abnormal, especially when demonstrating spike foci in the temporal lobe. A comparison between sleep and metrazol-activated recordings indicates that the latter is more likely to demonstrate a focus in patients with temporal lobe epilepsy[70]. Among a group of patients with severe temporal lobe epilepsy, focal seizure activity on the EEG would have been missed if waking records alone had been taken[71]. In a comparison of sphenoidal and nasopharyngeal electrodes, EEG confirmation of epilepsy could invariably be made by using the latter without recourse to the former[72]. Moreover, when lateralizing epileptic foci are recorded in temporal lobe epilepsy, they always show their highest amplitude in nasopharyngeal electrodes[67].

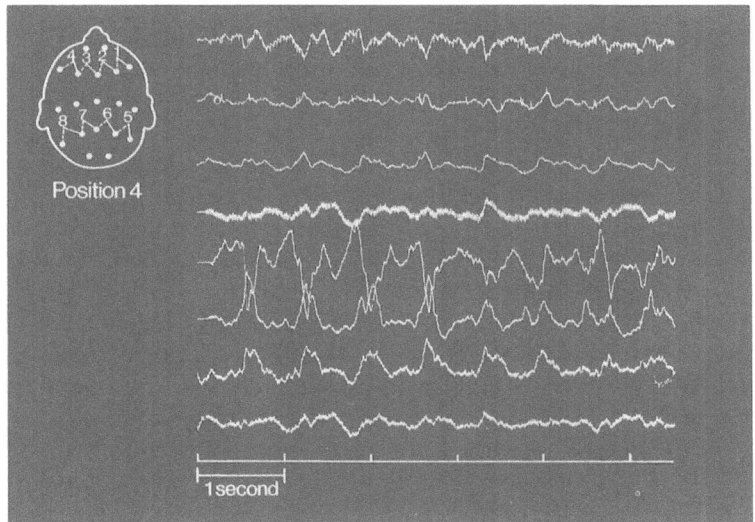

Fig. 4.4 EEG showing right posterior temporal sharp delta activity in a patient with a microglioma

A major advance in the diagnostic yield of EEG recording has stemmed from the introduction of prolonged monitoring, with or without video analysis. In one report of the role of continuous EEG monitoring, interictal changes had been recorded after the first 24 hours in two-thirds, rising to three-quarters of patients if recording was continued for 72 hours. Montages were used to preferentially detect anterior temporal and frontal discharges [73]. A comparison of 8-channel cable telemetry EEG with 3-channel ambulatory EEG indicated that the latter technique detected 79% of the focal and 100% of the generalized interictal abnormalities detected by the former [74]. Indeed the main limiting factor of either technique was the ability of the observer to identify epileptiform transients during video review. It has been suggested that if patients' attacks are occurring at monthly intervals or less, ambulatory recordings are not likely to be more successful than routine recordings in the detection of epileptic activity [75].

Depth electroencephalography assumes importance in those patients whose epilepsy may be amenable to surgical intervention. It has been estimated that 30% of the epileptic population, two-thirds of whom have focal attacks, have poor seizure control and that, if a well-defined epileptic focus can be established, its resection results in complete or near complete seizure relief in about two-thirds. Depth electrodes are positioned stereotactically at sites determined by clinical and surface EEG criteria. Complication of the procedure, including infection and haemorrhage, are said to be infrequent [76]. Depth recordings may show foci not apparent on surface recordings, may better localize foci demonstrated by surface recordings, and may display multiple foci [54]. It has been estimated that if patients with localized foci, as defined by surface EEG, have depth studies, and operation is restricted to those in whom the results of surface recordings had been confirmed, the percentage of patients with a successful outcome rises by 20% [54]. When a localized focus on scalp EEG can not be confirmed by depth studies, outcome from surgery is poor [77]. Anterior temporal foci on scalp recordings may be found, by depth electrodes, to emanate from posterior temporal, frontal or multiple foci [77]. It is apparent that sphenoidal or nasopharyngeal electrodes cannot achieve the localizing accuracy of depth recordings. It has been estimated, however, that a full evaluation of epilepsy, including depth recording can result in an average cost of 36 000 dollars [54].

(b) CT scanning

Some authors have recommended the performance of a CT scan in every patient with a seizure, but others have adopted a more selective approach. In one survey of 220 patients, 31 of whom had had a single seizure, 52 abnormal CT scans were encountered [78] (Fig. 4.5). Of the 15 patients considered to have potentially treatable lesions, all had either focal signs, or focal epilepsy, or localizing EEG changes. Another study, comparing similar groups, has reported a considerably higher incidence of CT abnormality in all the categories considered [72]. Among 62 adults with a single seizure, 64% had an abnormal EEG and 47% an abnormal CT. For those patients with abnormal neurological findings, the comparable figures were 78 and 71% [80]. Only 12% of patients with a normal examination and EEG had an abnormal CT; all were over 30 years of age, and all had diffuse atrophy. It was concluded that CT scanning was unnecessary in patients under the age of 30 who had had a single generalized seizure and whose neurological examination was normal. Whilst CT scanning might show abnormalities in similar patients over the age of 30, management would not necessarily be altered as a consequence. A survey of the findings on CT scanning in 148 patients with

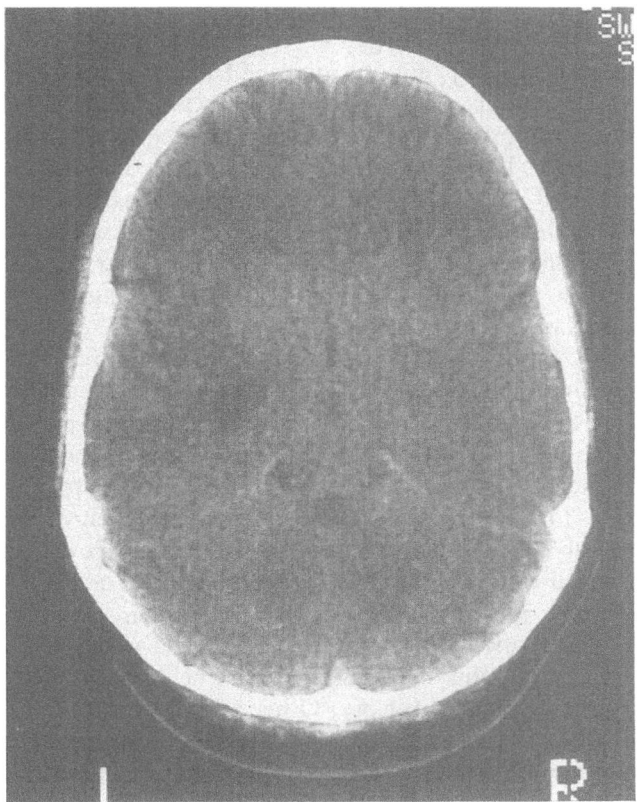

Fig. 4.5 CT showing low-density area deep in the left temporal lobe in a patient with complex partial seizures

seizures has been performed. Of these 53 had had two or more sei-zures within a 48 hour period amounting to status in 20 of them. The remainder had had a single fit. Similar conclusions were reached in terms of the screening role of the neurological examination [79]. Of 78 patients with a normal examination, only 12 had an abnormal scan (excluding atrophy and hydrocephalus). All the 15% of patients with a normal neurological examination but a structural lesion on CT, had an abnormal EEG. Among structural lesions there were nine patients with tumour (6%) but, of these, eight were gliomas and one metastatic. A metabolic basis for the seizures was discovered in 16 patients (11%), over half of whom had focal attacks. The impor-tance of structural, and certain metabolic factors in the causation of late-onset epilepsy has been frequently confirmed. Among 221 patients whose seizures began beyond the age of 24, alcohol was thought to be a significant precipitating factor in 51 and tumours in 36 [81]. Of the tumour group, 88% had focal EEG changes. Vascular disease has previously been underestimated as a factor in late-onset epilepsy. Ischaemic lesions were the only identified basis for seizures in 18% of a group of 89 patients who had developed epilepsy after the age of 40 [82]. No features of the seizures allowed identification of the likelihood of underlying vascular disease. Whilst the concern to identify a tumour basis for late-onset epilepsy is clearly paramount in many published studies of CT scanning in epilepsy, that enthusiasm has to be tempered by the realization that many of the lesions thereby identified prove to be malignant. In a group of 162 patients with adult-onset epilepsy, the presence of a low-grade glioma, unsuspected on clinical grounds, was identified in two. Both patients improved, in terms of epilepsy control, after surgery [83]. In patients with intractable partial seizures being appraised for surgical intervention, a proportion prove to have a glioma, even with a seizure history extending over many years [84]. In one survey, the onset of refractory partial seizures after the age of 30 was almost always due to underlying neoplasm [85]. A changing neurological examination suggested the likelihood of a neoplastic basis for the patient's epilepsy. Other pathological entities can be identified by CT scanning. It has been claimed that herniation of the mesial temporal lobe over the tentorial edge is associated with the presence of mesial temporal sclerosis. Identification of the former, by metrizamide CT, has been confirmed at surgery and shown to correlate with the changes of mesial temporal sclerosis in resected specimens [86]. Interpretation of CT changes in patients with epilepsy must take account of reports of evanescent abnormalities, consisting of low attenuation areas, sometimes with enhancement, resolving over periods of several weeks [87].

(c) MRI and PET

Several studies have been made of the role of MRI in the management of epilepsy, particularly in relationship to patients with intractable focal seizures. In a group of 30 patients with complex partial seizures, 26% had focal abnormalities on CT, but 43% on MRI [88]. A close correlation existed between the lateralization of MRI abnormalities and the site of the EEG focus. Spin–echo (T_2 weighted) images were more successful in detecting anatomical change than

Fig. 4.6 Right temporal hypometabolism on PET scan with [¹⁸F] fluoro-deoxyglucose in patient with focal seizures

inversion–recovery. In a survey of four publications, dealing with 36 patients with complex partial seizures who had had normal CT scans, 12 proved to have abnormal MRI. Typically, the abnormality most commonly described is in the mesial temporal lobe but, despite this, some authors have failed to find any correlation between pathological changes in resected specimens and abnormalities on MRI [89].

Positron emission tomography has also allowed identification of focal brain abnormalities in patients with normal CT scans. Reduction of regional oxygen metabolism is found in the temporal lobe ipsilateral to EEG foci in patients with complex partial seizures, though, additionally, changes are found in the contralateral temporal cortex and both cerebellar hemispheres [90] (Fig. 4.6). The hypometabolic region is often more extensive than the apparent EEG focus, and fails to correlate with the duration of the seizure disorder or the tendency to secondary generalization [91]. The same study suggested a close correlation between PET findings and foci elicited by depth electrode studies, a conclusion not confirmed by others [92]. In other words, some patients with defined epileptic foci have normal scans whereas some patients with hypometabolic zones have non-specific EEG changes. On the other hand, hypometabolic areas, defined with [^{18}F]fluorodeoxyglucose studies, correlate excellently with non-epileptic foci on EEG, suggesting that the latter might reflect sites of structural change but not necessarily the zone from which epileptic discharges are initiated. The correlation between MRI and PET is poor in patients with intractable partial epilepsy [93]. In general, PET scanning is more likely to define abnormalities in refractory partial seizures than either MRI or CT scanning [94]. The zones of PET hypometabolism tend to be larger than those defined by MRI. Furthermore, the finding of increased signal intensity on spin–echo MR images are relatively non-specific, being a reflection of either infarction, haemorrhage, multiple sclerosis or tumour. It has been suggested that, at present, MRI should be regarded as a research tool in the appraisal of patients with complex partial seizures. Even more experimental, at the time of writing, is the use of the magnetoencephalogram to localize focal discharges by the disposition of the changes in extracranial magnetic fields which they generate [95].

4.2.2 Differential diagnosis

Techniques for ambulatory recording of EEG and ECG activity have established that some episodes of altered awareness, or feeling, are triggered by cardiogenic rather than epileptogenic activity. The separation of these aetiological factors can sometimes prove difficult since epileptic activity itself can induce secondary changes in cardiac rhythm. In patients with complex partial seizures, for example, ECG concomitants to seizure activity include tachycardia and abrupt rate changes [96]. In one case report, complicated by the presence of hysterical attacks, tonic–clonic convulsions were associated with a secondary cardiac rhythm disturbance which included episodes of sinus arrest and supraventricular tachycardia [97]. The identification of non-organic seizures can prove equally difficult. Intensive monitoring techniques has allowed a system of clinical differentiation which separates the majority of organic from non-organic attacks [53]. In one study, however, neurologists observing video recordings of attacks, without access to EEG correlates or clinical information correctly identified only 72% of non-organic attacks [98].

Hysterical seizures were found to account for 6% of patients admitted to one hospital with a seizure disorder during the period of the study [99]. Over three-quarters of the patients were female. Self-injury, incontinence and tongue biting were sometimes a part of the hysterical seizure. The patients identified in this survey had had a non-organic attack provoked by suggestion (the intravenous injection of saline). Of the 51, six were finally considered to have a mixture of organic and non-organic seizures, and a further three were considered to have had a history of organic attacks which had been supplanted by non-organic episodes.

4.2.3 Recommendation (see flow chart B)

Metabolic studies are appropriate in all patients with single or multiple seizures, even though the yield of abnormalities is low. Focal seizures are sometimes the consequence of metabolic rather than structural disturbances. An EEG is probably appropriate even where there has been an isolated seizure, since the finding of a spike or, particularly, a delta focus would alert the physician to the desirability of carrying out further investigations. If the EEG is normal, and there are no neurological findings on examination, CT scanning is not necessary in patients under the age of 30 unless the seizure has been focal. Patients presenting over the age of 30 with a single seizure even if non-focal, and unassociated with clinical or EEG changes merit CT scanning. It must be recognized, however, both by physician and patient, that many structural changes thereby identified are either immune to or only marginally influenced by surgical intervention. If seizures continue, with persistently normal routine EEG recordings, activation procedures (e.g. sleep or metrazol) or special electrode placements (e.g. nasopharyngeal) can usefully serve to identify focal epileptic discharges. Where diagnostic doubt remains, ambulatory EEG recording, followed if negative by prolonged EEG telemetry with video analysis, with concomitant ECG, is of value, both in identifying patients with primary cardiac dysrhythmias, and in further establishing a potential focal basis for the clinical event. Any remaining doubt regarding the organic nature of the patient's attack merits estimation of prolactin levels 20 minutes after an attack, particularly if they are tonic–clonic in quality. For patients with intractable complex partial seizures, immune to medical intervention,

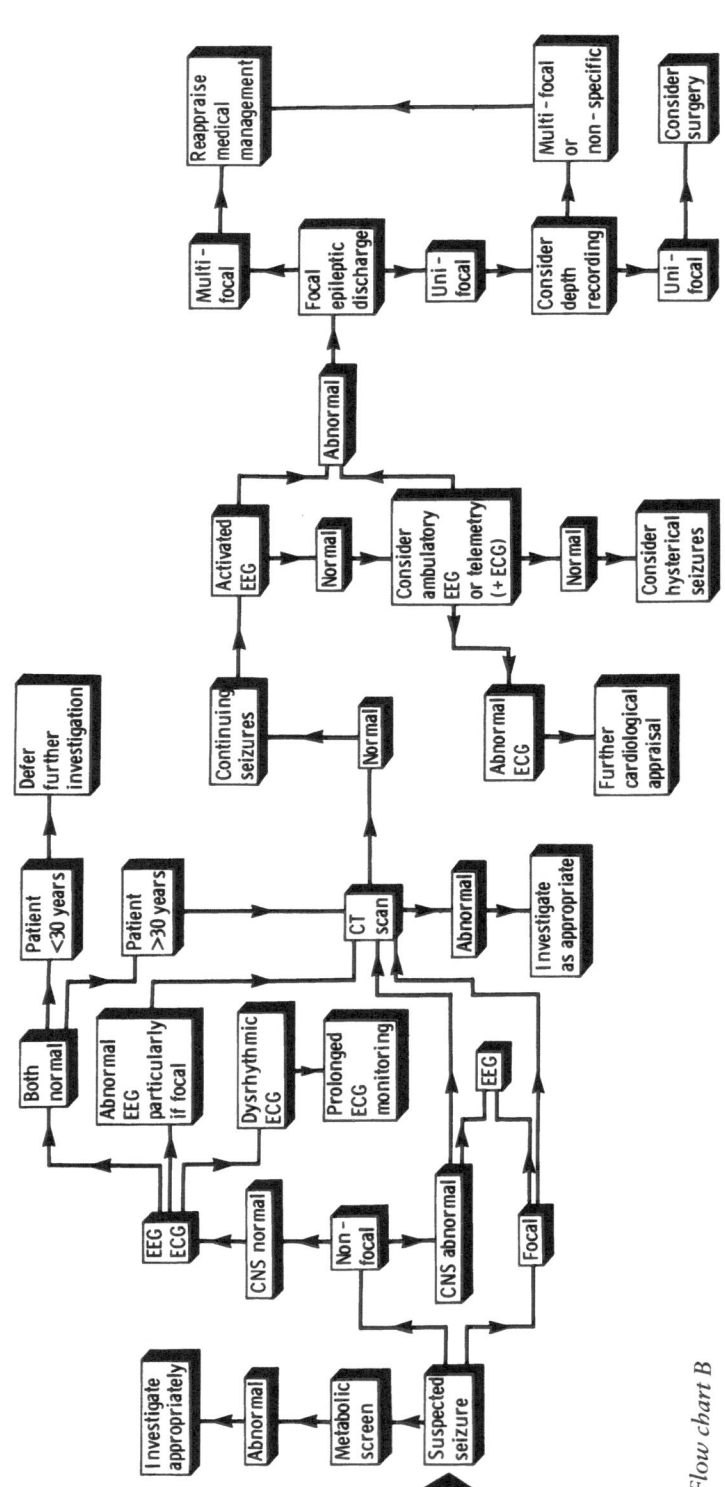

Flow chart B

further investigation is required to identify those who might benefit from surgery. Although MRI and PET are likely to identify focal temporal lobe changes in such patients, these do not necessarily correlate with the site of spike foci, removal of which would be critical to an attempt at seizure control. There is no doubt that the most accurate technique for the identification of the epileptic focus is the depth EEG recording. Use of this technique is expensive, and not without hazard. Without it, a reliance on localization from surface EEG recordings will diminish the success rate of surgery.

4.2.4 Other management problems

There is some evidence to suggest that an abnormal EEG, in a patient with a single fit, predicts a greater likelihood of seizure recurrence [59]. On the other hand, initial EEG findings do not predict which patients, with intractable epilepsy, are likely to benefit from video EEG monitoring, nor are serial EEG records helpful in monitoring seizure activity or identifying medication toxicity [100]. Differing opinions have been expressed regarding the value of the EEG in predicting the likelihood of a relapse following drug withdrawal. Some authors have found the EEG useful in this respect [101], others have not [102].

Monitoring drug levels is now well established as being of considerable value in the management of epilepsy. Brain concentrations of phenytoin, phenobarbitone and primidone correlate with plasma levels [103]. There is good evidence that seizure control with ethosuximide, phenytoin or carbamazepine is enhanced if drug levels are maintained within the therapeutic range [104]. There are, however, some patients who are controlled with sub-therapeutic levels, and others who appear to benefit, at least as far as phenytoin is concerned, from serum levels exceeding the therapeutic range.

REFERENCES

1. Mulley, G.P. (1986) Differential diagnosis of dementia. *Br. Med. J.*, **292**, 1416–18.
2. McKhann, G., Drachman, D., Folstein, M. *et al.* (1984) Clinical diagnosis of Alzheimer's disease: report of the NINCDS-ADRDA Work Group under the auspices of Department of Health and Human Services Task Force on Alzheimer's disease. *Neurology*, **34**, 939–44.
3. Rosen, W.G., Terry, R.D., Fuld, P.A. *et al.* (1980) Pathological verification of ischemic score in differentiation of dementias. *Ann. Neurol.*, **7**, 486–8.

4. Loizou, L.A., Kendall, B.E. and Marshall, J. (1981) Subcortical arteriosclerotic encephalopathy: a clinical and radiological investigation. *J. Neurol. Neurosurg. Psychiatry*, **44**, 294–304.
5. Ropper, A.H. (1979) A rational approach to dementia. *Can. Med. Assoc. J.*, **121**, 1175–90.
6. Marsden, C.D. and Harrison, M.J.G. (1972) Outcome of investigation of patients with presenile dementia. *Br. Med. J.* **2**, 249–52.
7. Larson, E.B., Reifler, B.V., Featherstone, H.J. and English, D.R. (1984) Dementia in elderly outpatients: A prospective study. *Ann. Intern. Med.*, **100**, 417–23.
8. McAllister, T.W. (1983) Overview: Pseudodementia. *Am. J. Psychiatry*, **140**, 528–33.
9. Freemon, F.R. (1976) Evaluation of patients with progressive intellectual deterioration. *Arch. Neurol.*, **33**, 658–9.
10. Smith, J.S. and Kiloh, L.G. (1981) The investigation of dementia: Results in 200 consecutive admissions. *Lancet*, i, 824–7.
11. Cummings, J.L. and Benson, F. (1984) Subcortical dementia. Review of an emerging concept. *Arch. Neurol.*, **41**, 874–9.
12. Hammerstrom, D.C. and Zimmer, B. (1985) The role of lumbar puncture in the evaluation of dementia: the University of Pittsburgh study. *J. Am. Geriatrics Soc.*, **33**, 397–400.
13. Gustafson, L. and Hagberg, B. (1978) Recovery in hydrocephalic dementia after shunt operation. *J. Neurol. Neurosurg. Psychiatry*, **41**, 940–7.
14. McCullough, D.C., Harbert, J.C., Di Chiro, G. and Ommaya, A.K. (1970) Prognostic criteria for cerebrospinal fluid shunting from isotope cisternography in communicating hydrocephalus. *Neurology*, **20**, 594–8.
15. Greenberg, J.O., Shenkin, H.A. and Adam, R. (1977) Idiopathic normal pressure hydrocephalus – A report of 73 patients. *J. Neurol. Neurosurg. Psychiatry*, **40**, 336–41.
16. Symon, L., Dorsch, N.W.C. and Stephens, R.J. (1972) Pressure waves in so-called low-pressure hydrocephalus. *Lancet*, ii, 1291–2.
17. Strachan, R.W. and Henderson, J.G. (1965) Psychiatric syndromes due to avitaminosis B_{12} with normal blood and marrow. *Quart. J. Med.*, **34**, 303–17.
18. Robinson, K.C., Kallberg, K.H. and Crowley, M.F. (1954) Idiopathic hypoparathyroidism presenting as dementia. *Br. Med. J.*, **2**, 1203–6.
19. Selecki, B.R. (1965) Intracranial space-occupying lesions among patients admitted to mental hospitals. *Med. J. Aust.*, **1**, 383–90.
20. Skomer, C., Stears, J. and Austin, J. (1983) Metachromatic leukodystrophy (MLD). XV. Adult MLD with focal lesions by computed tomography. *Arch. Neurol.*, **40**, 354–5.
21. Jones, H.R. Jr and Hedley-Whyte, E.T. (1983) Idiopathic hemochromatosis (IHC): Dementia and ataxia as presenting signs. *Neurology*, **33**, 1479–83.

22. Munoz-Garcia, D. and Ludwin, S.K. (1986) Adult-onset neuronal intranuclear hyaline inclusion disease. *Neurology*, 36, 785–90.
23. White, P.D., Lishman, W.A. and Wyke, M.A. (1986) Phaeochromocytoma as a cause of reversible dementia. *J. Neurol. Neurosurg. Psychiatry*, 49, 1449–51.
24. Storandt, M., Botwinick, J., Danziger, W.L. *et al.* (1984) Psychometric differentiation of mild senile dementia of the Alzheimer type. *Arch. Neurol.*, 41, 497–9.
25. Eslinger, P.J., Damasio, H., Graff-Radford, N. and Damasio, A.R. (1984) Examining the relationship between computed tomography and neuropsychological measures in normal and demented elderly. *J. Neurol. Neurosurg. Psychiatry*, 47, 1319–25.
26. Soininen, H., Partanen, J.V., Puranen, M. and Riekkinen, P.J. (1982) EEG and computed tomography in the investigation of patients with senile dementia. *J. Neurol. Neurosurg. Psychiatry*, 45, 711–14.
27. Groen, J.J. and Endtz, L.J. (1982) Hereditary Pick's disease. Second re-examination of a large family and discussion of other hereditary cases, with particular reference to electroencephalography and computerized tomography. *Brain*, 105, 443–59.
28. Goodin, D.S., Squires, K.C. and Starr, A. (1978) Long latency event-related components of the auditory evoked potential in dementia. *Brain*, 101, 635–48.
29. Soininen, H.S., Jolkkonen, J.T., Reinikainen, K.J. *et al.* (1984) Reduced choline esterase activity and somatostatin-like immunoreactivity in the cerebrospinal fluid of patients with dementia of the Alzheimer type. *J. Neurol. Sci.*, 63, 167–72.
30. Tune, L., Gucker, S., Folstein, M. *et al.* (1985) Cerebrospinal fluid acetylcholinesterase activity in senile dementia of the Alzheimer type. *Ann. Neurol.*, 17, 46–8.
31. Beal, M.F., Growdon, J.H., Mazurek, M.F. and Martin, J.B. (1986) CSF somatostatin-like immunoreactivity in dementia. *Neurology*, 36, 294–7.
32. St. Clair, D.M., Brock, D.J.H. and Barron, L. (1986) A monoclonal antibody assay technique for plasma and red cell acetylcholinesterase activity in Alzheimer's disease. *J. Neurol. Sci.*, 73, 169–76.
33. Bareggi, S.R., Franceschi, M., Bonini, L. *et al.* (1982) Decreased CSF concentrations of homovanillic acid and γ-aminobutyric acid in Alzheimer's disease. Age- or disease-related modifications? *Arch. Neurol.*, 39, 709–12.
34. Gibson, C.J., Logue, M. and Growdon, J.H. (1985) CSF monoamine metabolite levels in Alzheimer's and Parkinson's disease. *Arch. Neurol.*, 42, 489–92.
35. Kay, A.D., Milstien, S., Kaufman, S. *et al.* (1986) Cerebrospinal fluid biopterin is decreased in Alzheimer's disease. *Arch., Neurol.*, 43, 996–9.
36. Cutler, N.R., Kay, A.D., Marangos, P.J. and Burg, C. (1986)

104   Dementia. Epilepsy

Cerebrospinal fluid neuron-specific enolase is reduced in Alzheimer's disease. *Arch. Neurol.*, **43**, 153–4.
37. Bradshaw, J.R., Thomson, J.L.G. and Campbell, M.J. (1983) Computed tomography in the investigation of dementia. *Br. Med. J.,* **286**, 277–80.
38. Roberts, M.A. and Caird, F.I. (1976) Computerised tomography and intellectual impairment in the elderly. *J. Neurol. Neurosurg. Psychiatry*, **39**, 986–9.
39. Wilson, R.S., Fox, J.H., Huckman, M.S. *et al.* (1982) Computed tomography in dementia. *Neurology*, **32**, 1054–7.
40. Albert, M., Naeser, M.A., Levine, H.L. and Garvey, A.J. (1984) CT density numbers in patients with senile dementia of the Alzheimer's type. *Arch. Neurol.*, **41**, 1264–9.
41. Soininen, H., Puranen, M. and Riekkinen, P.J. (1982) Computed tomography findings in senile dementia and normal aging. *J. Neurol. Neurosurg. Psychiatry*, **45**, 50–4.
42. Damasio, H., Eslinger, P., Damasio, A.R. *et al.* (1983) Quantitative computed tomographic analysis in the diagnosis of dementia. *Arch. Neurol.*, **40**, 715–19.
43. Albert, M., Naeser, M.A., Levine, H.L. and Garvey, A.J. (1984) Ventricular size in patients with presenile dementia of the Alzheimer's type. *Arch. Neurol.*, **41**, 1258–63.
44. Turkheimer, E., Cullum, C.M., Hubler, D.W. *et al.* (1984) Quantifying cortical atrophy. *J. Neurol. Neurosurg. Psychiatry*, **47**, 1314–18.
45. Erkinjuntti, T., Ketonen, L., Sulkava, R. *et al.* (1987) Do white matter changes on MRI and CT differentiate vascular dementia from Alzheimer's disease? *J. Neurol. Neurosurg. Psychiatry*, **50**, 37–42.
46. Yamaguchi, F., Meyer, J.S., Yamamoto, M. *et al.* (1980) Noninvasive regional cerebral blood flow measurements in dementia. *Arch. Neurol.*, **37**, 410–18.
47. Frackowiak, R.S.J., Pozzilli, C., Legg, N.J. *et al.* (1981) Regional cerebral oxygen supply and utilization in dementia. A clinical and physiological study with oxygen-15 and positron tomography. *Brain*, **104**, 753–78.
48. Benson, D.F., Kuhl, D.E., Hawkins, R.A. *et al.* (1983) The fluoro-deoxyglucose ^{18}F scan in Alzheimer's disease and multi-infarct dementia. *Arch. Neurol.*, **40**, 711–14.
49. Duara, R., Grady, C., Haxby, J. *et al.* (1986) Positron emission tomography in Alzheimer's disease. *Neurology*, **36**, 879–87.
50. Jagust, W.J., Friedland, R.P. and Budinger, T.F. (1985) Positron emission tomography with [^{18}F]fluorodeoxyglucose differentiates normal pressure hydrocephalus from Alzheimer-type dementia. *J. Neurol. Neurosurg. Psychiatry*, **48**, 1091–6.
51. Gastaut, H. and Gastaut, J.L. (1976) Computerized transverse axial tomography in epilepsy. *Epilepsia*, **17**, 325–36.
52. Schott, G.D., McLeod, A.A. and Jewitt, D.E. (1977) Cardiac arrhythmias that masquerade as epilepsy. *Br. Med. J.*, **1**, 1454–7.

53. Desai, B.T., Porter, R.J. and Penry, J.K. (1982) Psychogenic seizures: A study of 42 attacks in six patients, with intensive monitoring. *Arch. Neurol.,* 39, 202–9.
54. Spencer, S.S. (1981) Depth electroencephalography in selection of refractory epilepsy for surgery. *Ann. Neurol.,* 9, 207–14.
55. Leibowitz, U. and Alter, M. (1968) Epilepsy in Jerusalem, Israel. *Epilepsia,* 9, 87–105.
56. Woodcock, S. and Cosgrove, J.B.R. (1964) Epilepsy after the age of 50. A five-year follow-up study. *Neurology,* 14, 34–40.
57. Cocito, L., Favale, E. and Reni, L. (1982) Epileptic seizures in cerebral arterial occlusive disease. *Stroke,* 13, 189–95.
58. Hart, R.G. and Easton, J.D. (1986) Seizure recurrence after a first, unprovoked seizure. *Arch. Neurol.,* 43, 1289–90.
59. Cleland, P.G., Mosquera, I., Steward, W.P. and Foster, J.B. (1981) Prognosis of isolated seizures in adult life. *Br. Med. J.,* 283, 1364.
60. Wyllie, E., Lueders, H., Pippenger, C. and Vanlente, F. (1985) Postictal serum creatine kinase in the diagnosis of seizure disorders. *Arch. Neurol.,* 42, 123–6.
61. Dana-Haeri, J., Trimble, M.R. and Oxley, J. (1983) Prolactin and gonadotrophin changes following generalised and partial seizures. *J. Neurol. Neurosurg. Psychiatry,* 46, 331–5.
62. Edwards, R., Schmidley, J.W. and Simon, R.P. (1983) How often does a CSF pleocytosis follow generalized convulsions? *Ann. Neurol.,* 13, 460–2.
63. Bull, J.W.D. and Zilkha, K.J. (1968) Rationalizing requests for X-ray films in neurology. *Br. Med. J.,* 4, 569–70.
64. Jasper, H. and Kershman, J. (1941) Electroencephalographic classification of the epilepsies. *Arch. Neurol. Psychiatry,* 45, 903–43.
65. Matthews, W.B. (1973) The clinical value of routine electroencephalography. *J. R. Coll. Physicians Lond.,* 7, 207–12.
66. Gastaut, H. (1953) So-called 'psychomotor' and 'temporal' epilepsy – A critical study. *Epilepsia,* 2, 59–76.
67. Escueta, A.V., Kunze, U., Waddell, G. *et al.* (1977) Lapse of consciousness and automatisms in temporal lobe epilepsy: A videotape analysis. *Neurology,* 27, 144–5.
68. Theodore, W.H., Porter, R.J. and Penry, J.K. (1983) Complex partial seizures: Clinical characteristics and differential diagnosis. *Neurology,* 33, 1115–21.
69. Delgado Escueta, A.V., Bacsal, Fe.E. and Treiman, D.M. (1982) Complex partial seizures on closed-circuit television and EEG: A study of 691 attacks in 79 patients. *Ann. Neurol.,* 11, 292–300.
70. Merlis, J.K., Grossman, C. and Henriksen, G.F. (1951) Comparative effectiveness of sleep and metrazol-activated electroencephalography. *Electroencephalogr. Clin. Neurophysiol.,* 3, 71–8.
71. Niedermeyer, E. and Rocca, U. (1972) The diagnostic significance of sleep electroencephalograms in temporal lobe epilepsy. A comparison of scalp and depth tracings. *Eur. Neurol.,* 7, 119–29.

72. Dejesus, P.V. Jr and Masland, W.S. (1970) The role of nasopharyngeal electrodes in clinical electroencephalography. *Neurology*, 20, 869–78.
73. Ebersole, J.S. and Leroy, R.F. (1983) An evaluation of ambulatory, cassette EEG monitoring: II. Detection of interictal abnormalities. *Neurology*, 33, 8–18.
74. Ebersole, J.S., Leroy, R.F. (1983) Evaluation of ambulatory cassette EEG monitoring: III. Diagnostic accuracy compared to intensive inpatient EEG monitoring. *Neurology*, 33, 853–60.
75. Cull, R.E. (1985) An assessment of 24-hour ambulatory EEG/ECG monitoring in a neurology clinic. *J. Neurol. Neurosurg. Psychiatry*, 48, 107–10.
76. Soloway, S.S., Williamson, P.D., Spencer, D.D. and Mattson, R.H. (1980) Surgery for epilepsy: Role of depth electroencephalography. *Conn. Med.*, 44, 70–5.
77. Spencer, S.S., Spencer, D.D., Williamson, P.D. and Mattson, R.H. (1982) The localizing value of depth electroencephalography in 32 patients with refractory epilepsy. *Ann. Neurol.*, 12, 248–53.
78. Young, A.C., Costanzi, J.B., Mohr, P.D. and Forbes, W. St. Clair (1982) Is routine computerised axial tomography in epilepsy worthwhile? *Lancet*, ii, 1446–7.
79. Ramirez-Lassepas, M., Cipolle, R.J., Morillo, L.R. and Gumnit, R.J. (1984) Value of computed tomographic scan in the evaluation of adult patients after their first seizure. *Ann. Neurol.*, 15, 536–43.
80. Russo, L.S. Jr. and Goldstein, K.H. (1983) The diagnostic assessment of single seizures. Is cranial computed tomography necessary? *Arch. Neurol.*, 40, 744–6.
81. Dam, A.M., Fuglsang-Frederiksen, A., Suarre-Olsen, V. and Dam, M. (1985) Late-onset epilepsy: Etiologies, types of seizure, and value of clinical investigation, EEG, and computerized tomography scan. *Epilepsia*, 26, 227–31.
82. Shorvon, S.D., Gilliatt, R.W., Cox, T.C.S. and Yu, Y.L. (1984) Evidence of vascular disease from CT scanning in late onset epilepsy. *J. Neurol. Neurosurg. Psychiatry*, 47, 225–30.
83. Jabbari, B., Huott, A.D., Di Chiro, G. *et al.* (1980) Surgically correctable lesions solely detected by CT scan in adult-onset chronic epilepsy. *Ann. Neurol.*, 7, 344–7.
84. Rich, K.M., Goldring, S. and Gado, M. (1985) Computed tomography in chronic seizure disorder caused by glioma. *Arch. Neurol.*, 42, 26–7.
85. Spencer, D.D., Spencer, S.S., Mattson, R.H. and Williamson, P.D. (1984) Intracerebral masses in patients with intractable partial epilepsy. *Neurology*, 34, 432–6.
86. Wyler, A.R. and Bolender, N.-Fr. (1983) Preoperative CT diagnosis of mesial temporal sclerosis for surgical treatment of epilepsy. *Ann. Neurol.*, 13, 59–64.
87. Sethi, P.K., Kumar, B.R., Madan, V.S. and Mohan, V. (1985) Appearing and disappearing CT scan abnormalities and seizures. *J. Neurol. Neurosurg. Psychiatry*, 48, 866–9.

88. Jabbari, B., Gunderson, C.H., Wippold, F. *et al.* (1986) Magnetic resonance imaging in partial complex epilepsy. *Arch. Neurol.*, 43, 869–72.

89. Lesser, R.P., Modic, M.T., Weinstein, M.A. *et al.* (1986) Magnetic resonance imaging (1.5 tesla) in patients with intractable focal seizures. *Arch. Neurol.*, 43,367–71.

90. Bernardi, S., Trimble, M.R., Frackowiak, R.S.J. *et al.* (1983) An interictal study of partial epilepsy using positron emission tomography and the oxygen-15 inhalation technique. *J. Neurol. Neurosurg. Psychiatry*, 46, 473–7.

91. Theodore, W.H., Newmark, M.E., Sato, S. *et al.* (1983) [^{18}F]Fluorodeoxyglucose positron emission tomography in refractory complex partial seizures. *Ann. Neurol.*, 14, 429–37.

92. Engel, J. Jr, Kuhl, D.E., Phelps, M.E. and Crandall, P.H. (1982) Comparative localization of epileptic foci in partial epilepsy by PCT and EEG. *Ann. Neurol.*, 12, 529–37.

93. Sperling, M.R., Wilson, G., Engel, J. Jr. *et al.* (1986) Magnetic resonance imaging in intractable partial epilepsy: Correlative studies. *Ann. Neurol.*, 20, 57–62.

94. Theodore, W.H., Dorwart, R., Holmes, M. *et al.* (1986) Neuroimaging in refractory partial seizures: Comparison of PET, CT, and MRI. *Neurology*, 36, 750–9.

95. Barth, D.S., Sutherling, W., Engel, J. Jr and Beatty, J. (1982) Neuromagnetic localization of epileptiform spike activity in the human brain. *Science*, 218, 891–4.

96. Blumhardt, L.D., Smith, P.E.M. and Owen, L. (1986) Electrocardiographic accompaniments of temporal lobe epileptic seizures. *Lancet*, i, 1051–6.

97. Gilchrist, J.M. (1985) Arrhythmogenic seizures: Diagnosis by simultaneous EEG/ECG recording. *Neurology*, 35, 1503–6.

98. King, D.W., Gallagher, B.B., Muruin, A.J. *et al.* (1982) Pseudoseizures: Diagnostic evaluation. *Neurology*, 32, 18–23.

99. Cohen, R.J. and Suter, C. (1982) Hysterical seizures: Suggestion as a provocative EEG test. *Ann. Neurol.*, 11, 391–5.

100. Theodore, W.H., Sato, S. and Porter, R.J. (1984) Serial EEG in intractable epilepsy. *Neurology*, 34, 863–7.

101. Emerson, R., D'Souza, B.J., Vining, E.P. *et al.* (1981) Stopping medication in children with epilepsy. Predictors of outcome. *N. Engl. J. Med.*, 304, 1125–9.

102. Thurston, J.H., Thurston, D.L., Hixon, B.B. and Keller, A.J. (1982) Prognosis in childhood epilepsy. Additional follow-up of 148 children 15 to 23 years after withdrawal of anticonvulsant therapy. *N. Engl. J. Med.*, 306, 831–6.

103. Houghton, G.W., Richens, A., Toseland, P.A. *et al.* (1975) Brain concentrations of phenytoin, phenobarbitone and primidone in epileptic patients. *Eur. J. Clin. Pharmacol.*, 9, 73–8.

104. Reynolds, E.H. (1978) Drug treatment of epilepsy. *Lancet*, ii, 721–5.

5

Extra-pyramidal disease

5.1 PARKINSON'S DISEASE

The clinical triad of bradykinesia, tremor and rigidity is felt to be sufficient to diagnose idiopathic Parkinson's disease, the assumption being made that the underlying pathology is centred on the zona compacta of the substantia nigra. That assumption is probably correct in the majority of patients with this clinical picture, though it is likely that other neuropathological disorders, generally undiagnosable in life, can present with a similar pattern of disability. Drug-induced Parkinsonism may be indistinguishable from the idiopathic form, though tremor is less conspicuous. The clinical spectrum of post-encephalitic Parkinsonism is broader, whilst extrapyramidal features are only a part of the disorder accruing from multi-infarction. The frequency with which dementia occurs in Parkinson's disease, and its severity, remains a matter of debate. One reviewer has suggested that one third of Parkinsonian patients become demented in the later stages of the disease [1], based on a study which recorded moderate to marked dementia in 32% of 520 patients [2]. Included among these patients, however, were some with atypical features (wasting, cerebellar tremor, dystonia or pyramidal signs), though, even in these, the parkinsonian features predominated. Though the authors claimed that dementia was as likely in the typical as in the atypical cases, another paper, including 93 patients, came to the opposite conclusion. There, an organic mental syndrome (principally dementia) was found in 15% of typical but in 68% of atypical cases [3].

5.1.1 Investigation

Clinical investigative techniques have proved of little value in the diagnosis of Parkinson's disease, largely because abnormal findings are often shared by other extra-pyramidal disorders. Abnormalities of ocular saccadic velocities are common to a number of extrapyramidal syndromes, whereas electrical measurement of the blink reflex simply confirms the clinical finding of depressed habituation [4]. Though some early studies suggested that visual evoked responses were delayed in Parkinson's disease, the degree of delay corresponding to the severity of the disease [5,6], a recent paper has refuted both conclusions [7].

Routine CSF studies are unproductive. Though one report described oligoclonal banding in two post-encephalitic patients [8], neither was typical nor has the finding been confirmed by others [9]. Knowledge of the underlying neurochemical changes of Parkinson's disease suggested that levels of homovanillic acid, dopamine's major metabolite, would be depressed in the CSF. That prediction has been verified, but the degree of overlap with normal individuals limits the diagnostic value of the investigation [10]. Other biochemical abnormalities have been detected in the parkinsonian brain. Markers reflecting GABA neuronal activity are depressed in the substantia nigra and changes in levels of met-enkephalin and substance P have been recorded. Despite this, CSF GABA levels in untreated patients do not differ significantly from controls [11], nor are there detectable alterations in the level of substance P [12].

The role of radiological investigation is similarly limited. A study of air encephalography revealed cortical atrophy in 46.7% and ventricular dilatation in 77.8% of patients, though no correlation existed between the degree of radiological abnormality and the severity of symptoms [13]. In a group of 93 parkinsonian patients, 22 of whom were atypical, 40% had evidence of generalized atrophy on CT scanning. The parkinsonian patients had significantly larger ventricles and cortical sulci than age-matched controls, the changes being more evident in atypical cases [3].

A discrepancy in the reported incidence of dementia in Parkinsonian patients has already been referred to. It has been suggested that, in Parkinson's disease, the dementia is of subcortical type, displaying changes in mood, cognition and memory but without dysphasia or apraxia [14].

No consistent abnormality has been reported for regional glucose metabolism, studied by positron emission tomography, in patients with bilateral parkinsonian symptoms. Where the Parkinson's is predominantly unilateral, relative increased regional blood flow and oxygen metabolism have been found in the contralateral basal ganglia [15]. Studies with 6-fluoro-L-Dopa, in patients with a pure unilateral syndrome, have shown impaired putamenal activity in the contralateral hemisphere [16].

5.1.2 Recommendation

Investigation is unnecessary for the majority of patients with a clinical diagnosis of Parkinson's disease. A substantial dementia is an accepted part of the condition in a proportion of individuals. If the dementia has cortical features, or if there are signs incompatible with the diagnosis of Parkinson's disease (for example, nystagmus, myoclonus or pyramidal signs) then CT scanning is indicated.

5.2 HUNTINGTON'S DISEASE

The clinical spectrum of Huntington's disease includes involuntary movements, choreiform in type, associated with alteration of personality and progressive dementia. The condition is inherited as an autosomal dominant, though new mutations undoubtedly occur and are thought to account for those cases genuinely lacking a family history of the disease. Where the family history is known, the diagnosis is usually only too obvious but confusion can occur if the presentation is atypical. Sometimes the abnormal movements are subtle, and easily overlooked. There probably exists a familial form of chorea in which dementia is lacking. Cases beginning before the age of 20 often display prominent rigidity, suggesting a diagnosis of Parkinson's disease. Investigations are sometimes necessary in these atypical cases, but undoubtedly a more pressing concern is whether certain investigative techniques allow diagnosis in pre-symptomatic individuals.

5.2.1 Investigation

Sophisticated methods for analysis of movement abnormalities have been devised to detect the earliest changes of the condition. A defect of saccadic eye movements, detected either clinically or by measurement of saccadic velocities, is of a type seen in other extrapyramidal disorders [17]. The EEG tends to be of low voltage, sometimes even relatively early in the course of the disease [18]. The latency of flash-evoked visual potentials does not differ from that of normal individuals though the amplitude tends to be lower [19]. Psychometric assessment reveals a deterioration in intelligence, more marked for performance than verbal function, associated with a disturbance of memory in which long-term memory is particularly affected. Aphasia, apraxia and agnosia are usually absent until the dementia has advanced substantially [20]. The finding of depressed γ-aminobutyric acid (GABA) and glutamic acid decarboxylase (GAD) levels in the brains of patients with Huntington's disease has prompted a study of CSF changes. GABA levels are significantly depressed compared to controls though without showing a correlation with duration of disease or the severity of the choreiform movements [21]. Although the caudate has a high concentration of somatostatin, and substance P levels are depressed in the substantia nigra in Huntington's disease, only levels of the former are significantly depressed in the CSF [22]. Radiological abnormalities described in Huntington's disease include cortical atrophy and an alteration of the configuration of the frontal horns of the lateral ventricles, consequent to caudate atrophy. Measurement of the intercaudate span and its ratio to the frontal horn span differentiates, though not completely, patients with Huntington's disease from those with dementia of Alzheimer type [23].

PET studies have shown a reduction in caudate glucose metabolism in patients in the early stages of the disease with little or no evidence of caudate atrophy on CT scanning [24]. Similar changes are reported in benign hereditary chorea.

5.2.2 Recommendation

Where the clinical pattern is characteristic, and the family history supportive, there is little indication to investigate patients with suspected Huntington's disease. In the absence of a family history, or where there are atypical features, support for the diagnosis is obtained through certain radiological abnormalities detectable on CT scanning and by the particular pattern of dementia revealed by psychometry.

5.2.3 Predictive tests

Much has been written on which investigations might allow a confident diagnosis to be established at a stage when the individual is asymptomatic. The value of such prediction does not lie in the availability of preventative treatment, but in the desire to give genetic counselling at a time when it is still relevant. Often, however, enthusiasm for the role of a particular investigation has not been borne out in practice, as the experience with EEG analysis clearly demonstrates. An EEG study of the offspring of Huntington's disease patients was reported in 1948 [25]. The EEG was abnormal in 26 (73.1%) with bilateral paroxysmal bursts in eight of them. All but two of those at-risk individuals were traced, and reported on 18 years later [26]. No correlation was found between the degree of EEG abnormality in 1948 and the subsequent development of the disease. Other electrophysiological tests have fared no better. Abnormal blink reflexes have been recorded electrically in 7 of 17 offspring, in some of them only after a L-Dopa load, but without evidence that this identifies the at-risk group [27]. The amplitude and latency of flash-evoked visual potentials in offspring do not differ from control subjects [19]. Similarly, CSF levels of GABA are unchanged [21); though somatostatin levels have been reported as low in seven offspring, of these, one had reported restlessness, and several had abnormalities of saccadic velocities or the presence of involuntary jerks during pursuit movements [22]. It is clear that CT scanning does not identify patients with Huntington's disease before the onset of symptoms [28].

The ethical aspects of attempting to predict the eventual development of the disease were particularly triggered when a group of workers reported, in 1972, that when 28 patients at risk for Huntington's disease were given L-Dopa, 10 developed choreiform movements [29]. By 1980, 30 patients had been entered in the study. Of 10 subjects who developed movements with L-Dopa, five had, by 1980, developed the disease, whereas of the 20 who did not develop movements, only one has developed the disease. The difference was significant [30].

Similar ethical dilemmas are encountered if PET scanning is used for predictive purposes. Caudate hypometabolism, based on regional glucose studies, was found in six of fifteen asymptomatic individuals at risk for Huntington's disease. Over the next two years, three of the six had developed signs of the disease. A more recent study, using the same technique, failed to identify significant changes in caudate metabolism in any of 29 individuals at risk for Huntington's disease [31].

5.2.4 Genetic studies

Linkage analysis has established the presence of a particular allele on the G8 locus of chromosome 4 which co-inherits with the Huntington gene 96% of the time [32]. At present, attempts are being made to identify markers closer to, and on both sides of, the Huntington gene to facilitate genetic counselling and establish the practicality of ante-natal diagnosis.

5.2.5 Recommendation

No electrophysiological, radiological or biochemical test has convincingly allowed an accurate prediction of the disease in the offspring of patients. Provocation of movements by L-Dopa does allow some certainty in prediction, though identification of the at-risk group is not absolute. The ethical dilemma involved in the use of this test is clear, and the group originally reporting its use have not enrolled new patients since 1980.

5.3 PROGRESSIVE SUPRANUCLEAR PALSY

In this condition, there is a combination of supranuclear ophthalmoplegia, limb and neck rigidity, pseudobulbar palsy and dementia[33]. With increasing experience of the condition, other features have been described, and variants recognized. Pyramidal and cerebellar signs can occur, whilst the ophthalmoplegia may incorporate an internuclear element. As in Parkinson's and Huntington's disease, the dementia is sub-cortical in quality[34], but exceptions occur, some patients displaying cortical features, for example dysphasia[35]. The main difficulty in establishing the diagnosis occurs when the ophthalmoplegia appears either late in the clinical course[36], or not at all.

5.3.1 Investigation

No specific CSF changes have been described. CT scanning demonstrates atrophic changes in the cerebrum, brain stem and cerebellum[37]. PET scanning, using [¹¹C]bromospiperone, reflects the pathological evidence of a reduction of striatal D-2 receptors[38].

5.3.2 Recommendation

Neuro-otological appraisal is sensible in suspected progressive supranuclear palsy even if the clinical findings are suggestive. Electrophysiological and radiological investigation are of limited value.

5.4 WILSON'S DISEASE

Wilson's disease is seldom seen in neurological practice. In one study, of 40 patients, the mean age at onset of symptoms was 16.3 years [39]. It is rare for the disease to present beyond the age of 30. Clinical features relate to deposition of copper in the liver, kidney and brain. Neurological manifestations include tremor, dysarthria and dystonia. Patients who have neurological findings are generally, but not inevitably, found to have Kayser–Fleischer rings [40].

5.4.1 Investigations

An abnormal prothrombin time is the most commonly detected abnormal liver function test. Serum caeruloplasmin levels are almost always depressed in Wilson's disease. Copper levels are more variable. Abnormal evoked responses have been rarely reported [41]. CT scanning demonstrates ventricular dilatation and cortical atrophy together with areas of reduced density in the basal ganglia [41,42]. A higher yield of abnormal findings is obtained with magnetic resonance imaging [43].

5.4.3 Recommendation

Serum copper and caeruloplasmin levels should be measured in any patient suspected of having Wilson's disease. The absence of Kayser–Fleischer rings in a patient with neurological disease makes the diagnosis of Wilson's disease highly unlikely, but not impossible. The diagnosis is strongly supported by the finding, on CT or MRI scanning, of lucencies in the basal ganglia.

5.5 DYSTONIA

In dystonia, sustained muscular contraction leads to the adoption of an abnormal posture of the limbs, trunk, or both. Where the contractions are only briefly sustained, rapidly changing movements (dyskinesias) result. Some authors use the term athetosis to describe such dyskinetic movements affecting the periphery of the limb. It has been suggested that the term torsion dystonia should be employed to include all types of movement disorder characterized by sustained muscle contraction irrespective of its distribution [44].

Generalized torsion dystonia in adult life is rarely the consequence of an identifiable structural brain abnormality. Investigation is more relevant where there are additional neurological signs, or where the dystonia is unilateral. Causes of hemidystonia, presenting in adult life, include trauma, cerebrovascular disease, basal ganglia tumour and arteriovenous malformation. CT scanning indicates that the responsible lesion lies in the thalamus, caudate or lentiform nucleus [45].

Dystonia was reported as the presenting feature of ataxia–telangiectasia in a child of 10 [46], whereas dystonic manifestations occur in a syndrome resembling Niemann–Pick disease, embracing vertical supranuclear ophthalmoplegia, dementia, seizures and ataxia [47]. Rarely, this syndrome can appear in adult life [48]. Whatever the age of presentation, the neurological features are likely to be accompanied by hepatosplenomegaly. In a review of 40 cases of Hallervorden–Spatz disease, three were found who had developed the disease in adult life (at 30, 57 and 64 years old respectively). Typically such patients display, in addition to dystonia, visual impairment and dementia [49]. Leigh's disease presents in early childhood or, rarely, in juveniles. Clinical findings include, besides extra-pyramidal features, retardation, ataxia, and spasticity. CT scanning demonstrates low attenuation areas distributed symmetrically in the basal ganglia [50]. A similar CT appearance has been recently described in a familial disorder sometimes presenting with dystonia alone but later accompanied by visual failure. All cases, however, appeared by the age of 14 [51]. Some patients with acanthocytes, with or without abnormal lipoprotein levels, have a neurological syndrome including choreiform movements or dystonia [52].

A familial disorder, inherited as an autosomal dominant, has been described which combines intellectual impairment and dystonia with evidence of intracranial calcification in the absence of disordered calcium metabolism. Onset was sometimes delayed until the age of 20 [53]. Amongst the extensive array of other disorders associated with dystonia [54], few need to be considered if the condition has commenced in adult life. Metachromatic leucodystrophy resulting in pure dystonia has been recorded, though in the single case in the literature, onset was at the age of 8 [55]. An adult form of G_{M1}-gangliosidosis is described with extra-pyramidal features including dystonia. In two siblings of one case, minimal dystonia triggered by voluntary movement was the sole clinical manifestation of the disease. Diagnosis is established by finding depressed β-galactosidase activity in leucocytes [56]. Hartnup disease produces a combination of dementia, optic atrophy and ataxia, sometimes combined with dystonic posturing. Many patients show early, childhood, evidence of intellectual and motor retardation, but sudden progression of disability may emerge as late as the seventeenth year of life [57].

5.5.1 Recommendation

In adults with hemidystonia, focal structural lesions should be excluded by CT scanning. In all adult onset cases of dystonia, whether or not there are accompanying signs, Wilson's disease requires exclusion by the measurement of serum and 24 hour urinary copper levels, and serum caeruloplasmin. If the dystonia is generalized, and unaccompanied by other physical signs, further investigation is unlikely to be rewarding, though a history of drug intake, particularly the neuroleptics, should be sought. Measurement of leucocyte or fibroblastic arylsulphatase A activity is indicated, however, together with measurement of leucocyte β-galactosidase activity to exclude the remote possibilities of adult-onset metachromatic leucodystrophy and G_{M1}-gangliosidosis respectively. If a supranuclear ophthalmoplegia is present, then bone marrow examination is required, searching for foamy storage cells ('sea-blue histiocytes'). The presence of visual failure and dementia suggests Hallervorden–Spatz disease (though this diagnosis is difficult to establish in life). The combination of dystonia with visual failure requires CT scanning looking, particularly, for the presence of striatal lucencies. An atypical dystonia, with prominent choreiform movements and particularly if accompanied by neuropathic features requires estimation of serum lipoprotein levels and examination of a wet blood film for spiny erythrocytes (acanthocytes). Dystonia combined with dementia, optic atrophy and ataxia merits exclusion of Hartnup disease by urinary amino acid analysis.

5.6 THE FOCAL DYSTONIAS

A number of clinical disorders, once relegated to the province of psychiatry, are now considered to be examples of a focal dystonia. They include blepharospasm, oro-mandibular dystonia, spasmodic torticollis and writer's cramp. The exact pathogenesis of these disorders remains unsettled, but they are not the manifestation of an underlying structural or biochemical disorder and investigations, apart from, perhaps, those designed to exclude Wilson's disease, are not warranted.

5.7 CHOREA

There are a number of disorders, besides Huntington's disease, in which choreiform movements are prominent. Choreo-athetoid movements are more likely than dystonia in patients with ataxia–telangiectasia. In abeta lipoproteinaemia (Bassen–Kornzweig syndrome) choreiform movements sometimes appear, though more prominent is a progressive cerebellar syndrome with pyramidal signs and proprioceptive loss [58]. Chorea combined with seizures, dysarthria, areflexia and pes cavus has been described as a familial disorder. Laboratory abnormalities include normal lipoprotein levels, but acanthocytosis and elevated CPK levels [59]. Choreiform movements may occur in thyrotoxicosis, in pregnancy, in phenytoin intoxication, and in association with systemic lupus erythematosus and polycythaemia. In one review of the causes of chorea, over 40 conditions or disorders were found with which it had been associated [60]. Added to that list are cases, sometimes strikingly asymmetrical, triggered by the oral contraceptive.

5.7.1 Recommendation

In adults with chorea, Huntington's disease and familial senile chorea require exclusion. Drug history analysis should concentrate on exposure to phenytoin or the oral contraceptive. Appropriate investigations are required to exclude polycythaemia, thyrotoxicosis and systemic lupus erythematosus. Serum lipoproteins should be measured and a wet blood film examined for acanthocytes. Many of the conditions producing a dystonic syndrome may sometimes be associated with choreiform movements.

5.8 OTHER DISORDERS

Essential tremor is a familial disorder displaying a postural tremor of the hands (and sometimes of the head or voice) at a frequency around 6 Hz. The pathological substrate of this disorder has not been identified, and investigation is unwarranted. In Gilles de la Tourette's syndrome investigation seldom reveals any specific abnormalities. The EEG shows an excess of slow wave activity in a minority of patients [61], but the CT scan is almost always normal [62]. Evoked responses show no significant deviation from normal controls [61]. Though CT scan abnormalities have been described in some patients with tardive dyskinesia, measurement of ventricular size did not differ from controls [63].

REFERENCES

1. Marsden, C.D. (1982) Basal ganglia disease. *Lancet*, ii, 1141–7.
2. Lieberman, A, Dziatolowski, M., Kupersmith, M. *et al.* (1979) Dementia in Parkinson disease. *Ann. Neurol.*, 6, 355–9.
3. Sroka, H., Elizan, T.S., Yahr, M.D. *et al.* (1981) Organic mental syndrome and confusional states in Parkinson's disease. *Arch. Neurol.*, 38, 339–42.
4. Esteban, A. and Giménez-Roldán, S. (1975) Blink reflex in Huntington's chorea and Parkinson's disease. *Acta Neurol. Scand.*, 52, 145–57.
5. Gawel, M.J., Das, P., Vincent, S. and Rose, F.C. (1981) Visual and auditory evoked responses in patients with Parkinson's disease. *J. Neurol. Neurosurg. Psychiatry*, 44, 227–32.
6. Kupersmith, M.J., Shakin, E., Siegel, I.M. and Lieberman, A. (1982) Visual system abnormalities in patients with Parkinson's disease. *Arch. Neurol.*, 39, 284–6.
7. Dinner, D.S., Lüders, H., Hanson, M. *et al.* (1985) Pattern evoked potentials (PEPs) in Parkinson's disease. *Neurology*, 35, 610–13.
8. Williams, A., Houff, S., Lees, A. and Calne, D.B. (1979) Oligoclonal banding in the cerebrospinal fluid of patients with postencephalitic Parkinsonism. *J. Neurol. Neurosurg. Psychiatry*, 42, 790–2.
9. Behan, P.O., Thomas, A.M. and Behan, W.M.H. (1981) Cerebrospinal fluid immunoglobulin profiles in Parkinson's disease. in *Research Progress in Parkinson's Disease* (ed. F.C. Rose and R. Capildeo), Pitman Medical, London, pp. 181–5.
10. Johansson, B. and Roos, B-E. (1967) 5-Hydroxyindoleacetic and homovanillic acid levels in the cerebrospinal fluid of healthy volunteers and patients with Parkinson's syndrome. *Life Sci.*, 6, 1449–54.
11. Abbott, R.J., Pye, I.F. and Nahorski, S.R. (1982) CSF and plasma GABA levels in Parkinson's disease. *J. Neurol. Neurosurg. Psychiatry*, 45, 253–6.
12. Nutt, J.G., Mroz, E.A., Leeman, S.E. *et al.* (1980) Substance P in human cerebrospinal fluid: Reductions in peripheral neuropathy and autonomic dysfunction. *Neurology*, 30, 1280–5.
13. Gath, I., Jörgensen, A., Sjaastad, O. and Berstad, J. (1975) Pneumoencephalographic findings in Parkinsonism. *Arch. Neurol.*, 32, 769–73.
14. Mayeux, R., Stern, Y., Rosen, J. and Benson, D.F. (1981) Subcortical dementia: A recognizable clinical entity. *Ann. Neurol.*, 10, 100–1.
15. Wolfson, L.I., Leenders, K.L., Brown, L.L. and Jones, T. (1985) Alterations of regional cerebral blood flow and oxygen metabolism in

Parkinson's disease. *Neurology*, 35, 1399–405.

16. Nahmias, C., Garnett, E.S., Firnau, G. and Lang, A. (1985) Striatal dopamine distribution in Parkinsonian patients during life. *J. Neurol. Sci.*, 69, 223–30.

17. Starr, A. (1967) A disorder of rapid eye movements in Huntington's chorea. *Brain*, 90, 545–64.

18. Scott, D.F., Heathfield, K.W.G., Toone, B. and Margerison, J.H. (1972) The EEG in Huntington's chorea: a clinical and neuropathological study. *J. Neurol. Neurosurg. Psychiatry*, 35, 97–102.

19. Ellenberger, C. Jr, Petro, D.J. and Ziegler, S.B. (1978) The visually evoked potential in Huntington's disease. *Neurology*, 28, 95–7.

20. Wilson, R.S. and Garron, D.C. (1979) Cognitive and affective aspects of Huntington's disease. In *Advances in Neurology*, Vol. 23 (ed. T.N. Chase, N.S. Wexler and A. Barbeau), Raven Press, New York, pp. 193–201.

21. Bala Manyam, N.V., Hare, T.A. and Katz, L. (1979) Cerebrospinal fluid GABA levels in Huntington's disease, 'at risk' for Huntington's disease and normal controls. in *Advances in Neurology*, Vol. 23 (ed. T.N. Chase, N.S. Wexler and A. Barbeau), Raven Press, New York, pp. 547–56.

22. Cramer, H., Kohler, J., Oepen, G. *et al.* (1981) Huntington's chorea – measurements of somatostatin, substance P and cyclic nucleotides in the cerebrospinal fluid. *J. Neurol.*, 225, 183–7.

23. Barr, A.N., Heinze, W.J., Dobben, G.D. *et al.* (1978) Bicaudate index in computerized tomography of Huntington's disease and cerebral atrophy. *Neurology*, 28, 1196–200.

24. Martin, W.R.W., Hayden, M.R., Suchowersky, O. *et al.* (1984) Striatal metabolism in Huntington's disease and in benign hereditary chorea. *Ann. Neurol.*, 16, 126.

25. Patterson, R.M., Bagchi, B.K. and Test, A. (1948) The prediction of Huntington's chorea. An electroencephalographic and genetic study. *Am. J. Psychiatry*, 104, 786–97.

26. Chandler, J.H. (1966) EEG in prediction of Huntington's chorea. An eighteen year follow-up. *Electroencephalogr. Clin. Neurophysiol.*, 21, 79–80.

27. Esteban, A., Mateo, D. and Giménez-Roldán, S. (1981) Early detection of Huntington's disease. Blink reflex and levodopa load in presymptomatic and incipient subjects. *J. Neurol. Neurosurg. Psychiatry*, 44, 43–8.

28. Oepen, G. and Ostertag, Ch. (1981) Diagnostic value of CT in patients with Huntington's chorea and their offspring. *J. Neurol.*, 225, 189–96.

29. Klawans, H.L. Jr, Paulson, G.W., Ringel, S.P. and Barbeau, A. (1972) Use of L-dopa in the detection of presymptomatic Huntington's chorea. *N. Engl. J. Med.*, 286, 1332–4.

30. Klawans, H.L., Goetz, C.G., Paulson, G.W. and Barbeau, A. (1980) Levodopa and presymptomatic detection of Huntington's disease – eight-year follow-up. *N. Engl. J. Med.*, 302, 1090.

31. Young, A.B., Penney, J.B., Starosta-Rubinstein, S. *et al.* (1987) Normal caudate glucose metabolism in persons at risk for Huntington's disease. *Arch. Neurol.*, **44**, 254–7.

32. Gusella, J.F., Wexler, N.S., Conneally, P.M. *et al.* (1983) A polymorphic DNA marker genetically linked to Huntington's disease. *Nature,* **306**, 234–8.

33. Richardson, J.C., Steele, J. and Olszewski, J. (1963) Supranuclear ophthalmoplegia, pseudobulbar palsy, nuchal dystonia and dementia. *Trans. Am. Neurol. Assoc.*, **88**, 25–7.

34. Albert, M.L., Feldman, R.G., and Willis, A.L. (1974) The 'subcortical dementia' of progressive supranuclear palsy. *J. Neurol. Neurosurg. Psychiatry*, **37**, 121–30.

35. Perkin, G.D., Lees, A.J., Stern, G.M. and Kocen, R.S. (1978) Problems in the diagnosis of progressive supranuclear palsy (Steele–Richardson–Olszewski syndrome). *Can. J. Neurol. Sci.*, **5**, 167–73.

36. Pfaffenbach, D.D., Layton, D.D. and Kearns, T.P. (1972) Ocular manifestations in progressive supranuclear palsy. *Am. J. Ophthalmol.*, **74**, 1179–84.

37. Haldeman, S., Goldman, J.W., Hyde, J. and Pribram, H.F.W. (1981) Progressive supranuclear palsy, computed tomography and response to antiparkinsonian drugs. *Neurology*, **31**, 442–5.

38. Baron, J.C., Maziere, B., Loch, C. *et al.* (1985) Progressive supranuclear palsy: loss of striatal dopamine receptors demonstrated *in vivo* by positron tomography. *Lancet*, **i**, 1163–4.

39. Strickland, G.T. and Leu, M-L. (1975) Wilson's disease. Clinical and laboratory manifestations in 40 patients. *Medicine (Baltimore)*, **54**, 113–37.

40. Ross, M.E., Jacobson, I.M., Dienstag, J.L. and Martin, J.B. (1985) Late-onset Wilson's disease with neurological involvement in the absence of Kayser–Fleischer rings. *Ann. Neurol.*, **17**, 411–13.

41. Roach, E.S., Ford, C.S., Spudis, E.V. *et al.* (1985) Wilson's disease: evoked potentials and computed tomography. *J. Neurol.*, **232**, 20–3.

42. Williams, F.J.B. and Walshe, J.M. (1981) Wilson's disease. An analysis of the cranial computerized tomographic appearances found in 60 patients and the changes in response to treatment with chelating agents. *Brain*, **104**, 735–52.

43. Lawler, G.A., Pennock, J.M., Steiner, R.E. *et al.* (1983) Nuclear magnetic resonance (NMR) imaging in Wilson's disease. *J. Comput. Assist. Tomogr.*, **7**, 1–8.

44. Marsden, C.D. (1976) Dystonia: the spectrum of the disease. in *The Basal Ganglia* (ed. M.D. Yahr), Raven Press, New York, pp. 351–67.

45. Marsden, C.D., Obeso, J.A., Zarranz, J.J. and Lang, A.E. (1985) The anatomical basis of symptomatic hemidystonia. *Brain*, **108**, 463–83.

46. Bodensteiner, J.B., Goldblum, R.M. and Goldman, A.S. (1980) Progressive dystonia masking ataxia in ataxia–telangiectasia. *Arch. Neurol.*, **37**, 464–5.

47. Neville, B.G.R., Lake, B.D., Stephens, R. and Sanders, M.D. (1973) A

neurovisceral storage disease with vertical supranuclear ophthalmoplegia, and its relationship to Niemann–Pick disease. A report of nine patients. *Brain*, **96**, 97–120.
48. Longstreth, W.T. Jr, Farrell, D.F., Bolen, J.W. *et al.* (1982) Adult dystonic lipidosis: clinical, histologic, and biochemical findings of a neurovisceral storage disease. *Neurology*, **32**(2), A141.
49. Dooling, E.C., Schoene, W.C. and Richardson, E.P. Jr (1974) Hallervorden–Spatz syndrome. *Arch. Neurol.*, **30**, 70–83.
50. Hall, K. and Gardner-Medwin, D. (1978) CT scan appearances in Leigh's disease (subacute necrotizing encephalomyelopathy). *Neuroradiology*, **16**, 48–50.
51. Marsden, C.D., Lang, A.E., Quinn, N.P. *et al.* (1986) Familial dystonia and visual failure with striatal CT lucencies. *J. Neurol. Neurosurg. Psychiatry*, **49**, 500–9.
52. Aminoff, M.J. (1972) Acanthocytosis and neurological disease. *Brain*, **95**, 749–60.
53. Larsen, T.A., Dunn, H.G., Jan, J.E. and Calne, D.B. (1985) Dystonia and calcification of the basal ganglia. *Neurology*, **35**, 533–7.
54. Fahn, S., Marsden, C.D. and Calne, D.B. (1987) Classification and investigation of dystonia. in *Movement Disorders*, 2 (ed. C.D. Marsden and S. Fahn), Butterworths, London, pp. 332–58.
55. Lang, A.E., Clarke, J.T.R., Resch, L. *et al.* (1985) Progressive longstanding 'pure' dystonia: a new phenotype of juvenile metachromatic leukodystrophy (MLD). *Neurology*, **35**, (Suppl. 1), 194.
56. Nakano, T., Ikeda, S.-I., Kondo, K. *et al.* (1985) Adult G$_{M1}$-gangliosidosis: clinical patterns and rectal biopsy. *Neurology*, **35**, 875–80.
57. Tahmoush, A.J., Alpers, D.H., Feigin, R.D. *et al.* (1976) Hartnup disease. Clinical, pathological and biochemical observations. *Arch. Neurol.*, **33**, 797–807.
58. Schwartz, J.F., Rowland, L.P., Eder, H. *et al.* (1963) Bassen–Kornzweig syndrome: deficiency of serum β-lipoprotein. *Arch. Neurol.*, **8**, 438–54.
59. Gross, K.B., Skrivanek, J.A., Carlson, K.C. and Kaufman, D.M. (1985) Familial amyotrophic chorea with acanthocytosis. New clinical and laboratory investigations. *Arch. Neurol.*, **42**, 753–6.
60. Greenhouse, A.H. (1966) On chorea, lupus erythematosus, and cerebral arteritis. *Arch. Intern. Med.*, **117**, 389–93.
61. Krumholz, A., Singer, H.S., Niedermeyer, E. *et al.* (1983) Electrophysiological studies in Tourette's syndrome. *Ann. Neurol.*, **14**, 638–41.
62. Lees, A.J., Robertson, M., Trimble, M.R. and Murray, N.M.F. (1984) A clinical study of Gilles de la Tourette syndrome in the United Kingdom. *J. Neurol. Neurosurg. Psychiatry*, **47**, 1–8.
63. Brainin, M., Reisner, Th. and Zeitlhofer, J. (1983) Tardive dyskinesia: clinical correlation with computed tomography in patients aged less than 60 years. *J. Neurol. Neurosurg. Psychiatry*, **46**, 1037–40.

6

Multiple sclerosis
CNS infection

6.1 MULTIPLE SCLEROSIS

For many patients, the diagnosis of multiple sclerosis is evident from their clinical characteristics. A remitting and relapsing illness in a young adult with signs reflecting scattered white matter dysfunction, hardly requires investigation, though the picture so defined is not unique to multiple sclerosis. Greater uncertainty occurs in the early course of the illness before a remitting and relapsing pattern has been established, or where the disability is progressive from the outset. Previous classifications of the disease allowed for such uncertainties by designating definite, probable or possible categories [1] or definite, early probable/latent and progressive probable/possible cases [2]. The latter criteria include data based on electrophysiological studies. More recently, a classification incorporating CSF data has been introduced [3]. There are no tests which infallibly identify patients with multiple sclerosis. Certainly CSF changes, for example oligoclonal IgG, and abnormalities of central conduction time are seen in other neurological disorders. Even the demonstration of paraventricular pathology by magnetic resonance imagery does not allow a certain diagnosis, since identical appearances are encountered in some patients with cerebrovascular disease [4].

6.1.1 Immunological studies

A vast literature has accumulated detailing evidence of an altered immunological status in patients with MS including the demonstration of antibodies in serum and CSF to various CNS components. Although these studies have been of some value in exploring possible pathogenetic mechanisms, they do not provide diagnostic information in patients with suspected MS. Antibodies to oligodendrocytes are found in both MS and other neurological diseases [5]. Antibrain antibodies are more common in MS than in other neurological disorders, higher titres correlating with a more malignant course of the disease [6].

Whilst antibodies to myelin basic protein are found in the CSF of MS patients, they occur in diverse neurological diseases, including sub-acute sclerosing panencephalitis [7], Guillain–Barré syndrome and cerebrovascular disease [8]. The antibodies belong to the IgG_1 or IgG_3 subclass [9]. Levels of bound or free forms of the antibody in the CSF are elevated in patients with clinically active disease, falling as a remission appears. In patients with chronic progressive disease, titres of bound antibody tend to exceed those of the free form [10].

Immune complexes have been detected in the serum and CSF of patients with MS [11]. Plasma levels of the terminal complement component (C9) are not altered, but are depressed in the CSF. Overlap with control subjects is, however, considerable [12]. Antinuclear antibodies have been found in MS subjects but in low titres and in a differing pattern from that described in patients with neurological involvement from systemic lupus erythematosus. [13].

Depression of suppressor T cells in the blood in acute exacerbations of the disease has not been found consistently nor is its significance certain. Indeed much of the data relating to immunological dysfunction in MS remains contradictory. Cytotoxic activity in CNS cultures from experimental animals has been demonstrated using T cells derived from MS patients in relapse [14].

Studies of viral antibodies in serum and CSF have consistently demonstrated elevated levels against measles, rubella and vaccinia [15]. However, measles-specific IgG antibody represents less than 5% of total CSF IgG in MS patients, compared to 30–60% of total IgG in subacute sclerosing panencephalitis [16]. Analysis of antibody levels to the measles-related canine distemper virus has failed to demonstrate significant specific elevations in MS [17].

Examination of histocompatibility status has identified an association of certain HLA antigens with MS, though the pattern varies according to the racial origins of the patient. In Northern Europe, associations are described with A3, B7, Dw2 and DR2, being strongest for the last of these [18]. The correlation fails to apply to residents of the Orkneys, whilst differing HLA antigens predominate in non-European populations with MS. None of the studies discussed in this section can be used in a diagnostic sense in patients suspected of having MS, and they will not be considered in further detail.

6.1.2 CSF changes

In an early review of CSF changes in MS, an elevated protein concentration was found in 15–75% of cases, and a pleocytosis in 30–70% [19]. A more recent study suggested figures of 25% for each [20]. The cell count rarely exceeds $50/mm^3$. Whereas the cell count tends to rise after an acute exacerbation, the protein concentration remains stable. The protein concentration is of no value when attempting to predict the further course of the disease. The cell count tends to be lower in more severely disabled patients, and in those with a longer history.

6.1.3 IgG

Elevated concentrations of IgG have been found in 70–80% of patients with MS [22]. The sensitivity of the estimation is increased by calculating the ratio of IgG to albumin, or by comparing that ratio in the CSF with the same ratio in the serum (IgG index) [23]. Despite this, the number of clinical lesions and degree of disability appear to correlate better with IgG levels than with the above ratios [24]. IgG levels tend to rise in acute exacerbations and to be higher in those with severe disability. The proportion of patients with abnormal IgG ratios increases with increasing diagnostic certainty [25]. Among 34 patients with MS, an abnormal IgG, IgG/albumin ratio, IgG index or IgG synthesis rate was found in 33 [23]. The specificity of the IgG ratios has been variously reported. An abnormal IgG index was found in 27% of patients with other neurological diseases in one study [23], the figure in another control group was 7.3% [25].

6.1.4 Electrophoresis

In most hands, CSF electrophoresis for the demonstration of oligoclonal bands has proved a more sensitive technique for the diagnosis of multiple sclerosis than measurement of IgG ratios (Fig. 6.1). Exceptionally, calculation of the IgG index has been found preferable to electrophoresis [25,26]. Variability in the frequency with which oligoclonal banding can be demonstrated in MS clearly relates to methodology. Electrophoresis has been performed on both

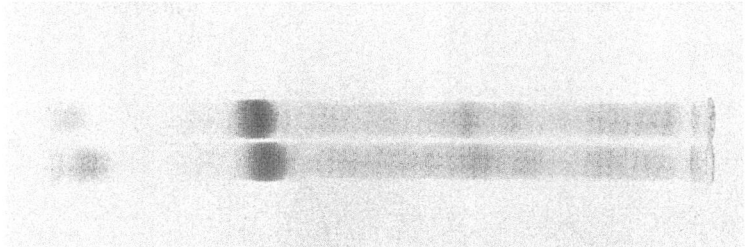

Fig. 6.1 Oligoclonal bands in the CSF of an MS patient

unconcentrated and concentrated CSF, and on a number of media, including agar, agarose and polyacrylamide gel. The use of unconcentrated fluid has the advantages of requiring a smaller volume of CSF and of being freer of artefacts [27]. In one review, oligoclonal IgG had been reported in between 85 and 95% of definite MS cases, in 40% of CNS inflammatory diseases and in 2–10% of other CNS diseases [20]. The use of isoelectric focusing has allowed a more sensitive separation of IgG fractions in the CSF. It has been suggested that separate colonies of lymphocytes are activated intrathecally in MS, one synthesizing oligoclonal, the other polyclonal IgG. Polyclonal, but not oligoclonal, IgG is found in some normal individuals. In MS patients, oligoclonal IgG can also be detected in the serum but in lower concentrations and in fewer bands [28]. The oligoclonal pattern does not necessarily remain constant during the course of the disease, some bands appearing, others fading [29]. Irrespective of the mode of onset of MS, an oligoclonal pattern at that stage anticipates a greater likelihood of further activity [30]. In a study confined to patients with sensory symptoms alone, all those developing evidence of MS during a mean follow up exceeding five years had had oligoclonal IgG originally [31]. A similar trend, in terms of the anticipation of further neurological events, applies to abnormal IgG ratios [32]. IgA oligoclonal bands occur in MS, rarely in the absence of IgG bands [33].

An increased ratio of kappa to lambda light chains in the IgG of the CSF has been reported in 53% of MS patients, and appears a more selective investigation than either IgG ratios or electrophoresis [22]. A correlation between the presence of free kappa light chains and silent brain lesions on MRI has been reported in eight patients with isolated optic neuritis [34].

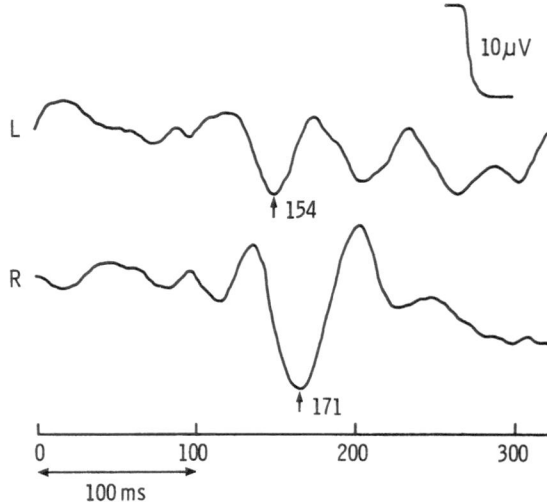

Fig. 6.2 VEP demonstrating bilateral delay

6.1.5 Electrophysiology

Whilst visual evoked potentials (VEP) have proved of supreme value in the detection of subclinical optic nerve involvement, careful visual field analysis can detect abnormalities in two-thirds of patients with no history of visual disturbance [35] (Fig. 6.2). Since many of these defects are found at 15–30° from fixation, whereas the VER, using standard techniques, is generated by a central retinal area of about 12°, the two methods of examination are complementary [36]. In an early report of the use of pattern evoked potentials in MS, abnormalities were found in over 90% of definite cases, but in a smaller proportion of patients with lesser evidence of the disease [37]. The pattern-onset VER is generally better defined, and larger than the pattern-reversal VER, and more often abnormal in suspected MS [38]. Foveal, rather than central, field stimulation produces a higher yield of abnormal results in all categories of MS [39], particularly if the check size is limited to a subtended angle of 30′ or less [40]. The fact that some patients with MS, despite preserving their ability to see fine detail, have lost their capacity to see coarser detail has been appraised by testing contrast sensitivity using a grating of bright and dim bars of varying contrast and spatial frequency [41]. In a comparison of contrast sensitivity with visual-evoked potentials in patients with normal visual acuity, abnormalities of the former were found in 78% and of the latter in 67% [42]. The number of abnormal findings from VER studies can be increased if differing stimulus orientations are used [43]. Psychophysical methods for testing visual function depend on excellent patient cooperation.

Abnormal VER latencies are not unique to MS. They occur in many other conditions, including glaucoma, optic nerve compression, vitamin B_{12} deficiency and Friedreich's ataxia. The use of abnormal VER latencies as the sole criterion for the diagnosis of MS in patients with spinal cord disease will result in a false positive diagnosis in 10%. If oligoclonal IgG is added to the diagnostic criteria, the false positive rate falls to zero [44].

The fact that a rise in body temperature exacerbates symptoms in some patients with MS has been used in a number of tests in which the effect of an artificial elevation of body temperature on various parameters of optic nerve function is assessed [45]. Fatiguing of optic nerve pathways by artificial means, for example by superimposing upon a VER stimulus either flicker or a moving pattern can cause alteration of the VER amplitude. The phenomenon, however, is not unique to MS [46].

Brain-stem auditory evoked responses (BAER) have proved of less value than visual evoked responses in demonstrating occult CNS lesions in early MS. Most studies have concentrated on the amplitude or latency of the NV potential, the one most reliably present in normal individuals. An early study reported abnormalities of NV (either latency or amplitude) in 71, 20 and 41% of definite, probable and possible MS cases who had no clinical evidence of brain stem disease [47]. Another group, using the same diagnostic categories, and using, as abnormal criteria, altered interwave latencies between I, III and V, or an altered amplitude ratio between I and V, reported abnormal results in 19, 21 and 24% respectively, again excluding those with symptoms or signs of brain stem disease [48]. Whereas the amplitude of the NV wave increases by about two-thirds in normal individuals when unilateral is switched to simultaneous bilateral stimulation, this enhancement fails to materialize in MS patients [49]. A comparison of the relative values of BAER and the blink reflex in MS concluded that the former was a more sensitive technique for detecting brain stem lesions [50]. A pontine lesion tends to affect the II–III or III–V interwave latency ipsilaterally. A comparison bewteen BAER and the acoustic stapedius reflex found more abnormalities with the former but concluded that the two methods of examination were complementary. A surprisingly high yield of abnormal findings for BAER was found in the study, amounting to 72, 64 and 50% of definite, probable and possible cases respectively [51]. In a study of 54 patients, comparison was made between the jaw jerk, blink and corneal reflex latencies. The blink reflex has an early ipsilateral response, mediated via the pons, and a delayed bilateral response which is mediated via pons, spinal trigeminal tract and medulla. The latter pathway is similar to that involved in the corneal response. The corneal reflex latency revealed the highest and the jaw jerk the lowest frequency of abnormalities [52]. All reflex latencies were normal in 26% of patients, including five with definite MS, all of whom had brain stem signs. The authors concluded that none of the tests replaced clinical examination in the appraisal of brain stem involvement.

Somatosensory potentials, elicited usually by stimulation of the median or tibial nerves, can be recorded over the cervical spine and parietal cortex. Measurement of peak latency is a more sensitive test than amplitude for detection of abnormalities in MS [53]. Comparison of visual, auditory and somatosensory responses has been made. In general, the yield of abnormalities from testing of somatosensory responses falls below that obtained from visual but above that from auditory responses [54]. Not surprisingly, the frequency of abnormal findings increases during the course of the disease, mirroring a progression of disability [55]. In a small number of patients, normal evoked potentials become prolonged during artificial elevation of body temperature [56].

The most recent development in the assessment of central conduction in MS has been measurement of motor velocities. Delayed latencies have been reported following either scalp [57] or spinal stimulation [58] in patients with clinical signs of pyramidal dysfunction (Fig. 6.3). A magnetic stimulator, effecting discharge from the motor cortex via a fluctuating magnetic field is more acceptable to the patient than a conventional electric stimulator. Abnormal central motor slowing has been demonstrated in some MS patients though, surprisingly, showing no correlation with clinical signs of upper motor-neurone involvement except for pathological finger jerks [59].

Where a combination of electrophysiological techniques was used to measure function in patients with isolated optic neuritis, abnormalities, outside the optic pathway, were found in 50% [60].

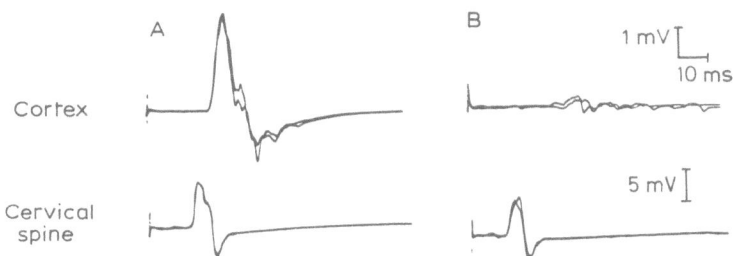

Fig. 6.3 Consecutive thenar muscle responses to single magnetic stimuli applied over the cortex and cervical spine. A, Normal subject. B, MS patient. The responses in the patient are delayed, dispersed, of low amplitude and variable morphology following cortical stimulation.

6.1.6 Radiological investigation and MRI

Although air encephalography demonstrates cortical atrophy and ventricular dilatation in some MS patients, the investigation now has no place in the investigation of suspected MS. In an early discussion of CT scanning, of 80 focal lesions diagnosed clinically in MS patients, 31 were detected radiologically. The majority of foci not detected were localized to the brain stem or cerebellum [61]. Using a second generation scanner, evidence of cerebral atrophy was detected in 44% of 202 patients, 81 of whom had definite evidence of the disease. White matter lucencies were seen in 35, and periventricular lucencies in 10 [62]. The degree of atrophy correlated with disease duration and severity. In a recent review of high-resolution scanning in definite, probable and possible cases, abnormalities were detected in 85, 39 and 51% respectively. The changes found included low density areas, enlarged CSF spaces and areas of abnormal enhancement. Indeed in 47% of patients with CT abnormalities, these only materialized following contrast injection [63]. Enhancement is particularly found in patients with recent acute exacerbations. It is more readily detected by the use of high dose contrast, and diminishes during corticosteroid therapy [64].

MRI has demonstrated the remarkable discrepancy in some patients between clinical declaration of the disease and the extent of its pathological distribution. In one analysis of 10 patients, MRI detected between 9 and 22 lesions in each, with a total of 112 more lesions than had been detected by CT [65]. Generally spin–echo sequences have proved of greater value than inversion–recovery [66]. In two studies, both of patients with definite disease,

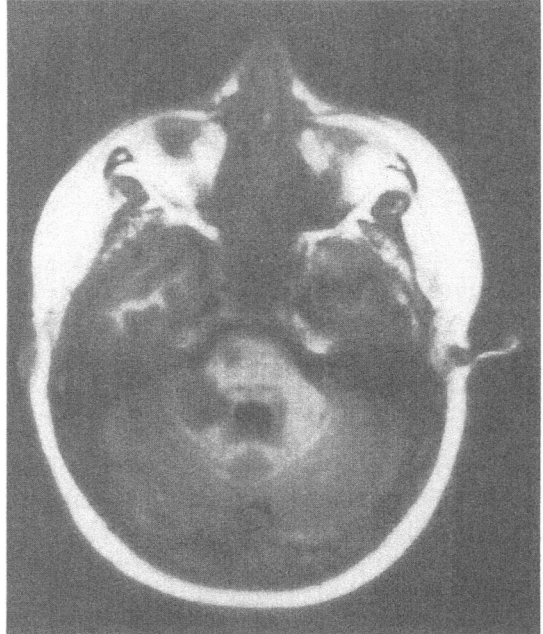

Fig. 6.4 MRI scan in MS patient. Inversion–recovery sequence demonstrating brain-stem and cerebellar lesions.

abnormalities were reported in 83 [67] and 78% [68] of patients (Fig. 6.4). Others, however, have reported periventricular changes in all definite cases [69]. These predominate posteriorly and appear white on spin–echo sequences. The spin characteristics of lesions found in any one patient are not necessarily uniform, requiring imaging with a range of sequences if their full extent is to be determined. Imaging of the posterior fossa has proved particularly valuable for the demonstration of brain-stem and cerebellar demyelination.

Data are accumulating on the extent of MRI changes in patients with clinically unifocal disease. In acute optic neuritis, changes in the optic nerve are found in the majority, best demonstrated by inversion–recovery sequences with a short inversion time [70]. Silent brain lesions in optic neuritis have been found in 50 [71] and 70% [72] of cases in two recent publications. The lesions predominated in the periventricular regions, and were of a type seen in patients with established MS. Although in one of the studies, further neurological events (in two patients) were confined to those with MRI changes, in the other a patient with abnormal MRI at the onset of optic neuritis failed to develop clinical signs of dissemination over a follow-up period of 7 years. No consistent correlation has been demonstrated between MRI abnormalities and CSF changes in optic neuritis [71]. An MRI investigation of patients with isolated brainstem lesions has produced similar findings. Among 27 patients, clinically silent lesions were detected elsewhere in 20 [73].

Numerous studies have appeared comparing the sensitivity of CT, MRI, evoked responses and CSF examination in the diagnosis of MS. MRI has, almost always, proved the superior method of investigation.

6.1.7 Recommendation (flow chart)

The requirement for laboratory based data to supplement a clinical diagnosis of MS is reinforced when patients who fulfil clinical criteria for the diagnosis are found to have other neurological diseases [74]. Features considered to cast doubt on the diagnosis include an absence of optic nerve or oculomotor involvement, absence of remission in younger patients, disease localized to one area, absence of sensory findings or bladder disturbance and normal CSF findings.

In patients with a history of remitting and relapsing disease, with signs of lesions at two or more sites, the diagnosis of MS is very likely. In such cases, CSF analysis alone is probably sufficient. If the CSF is normal, electrophysiological investigation of clinically unaffected sites is appropriate. Negative findings suggest the need for MRI, if available. For individuals with slowly progressive, unifocal disease, more extensive investigation will probably be necessary. Combined electrophysiological and CSF investigation is needed. Abnormalities of both make the diagnosis almost certain. If one or other is normal, then CT or, preferably, MRI should be considered in an attempt to exclude other pathologies whilst establishing evidence of multi-focal demyelinating disease. More vexing is the extent to which patients with isolated episodes of a type known to occur in established MS should be investigated. Certain CSF abnormalities in these patients increase the likelihood of progression of the disease, though the fact is hardly likely to be of great consolation to the patient in the absence of an effective treatment. Despite the fact that MRI will establish disseminated lesions in over 50% of patients with

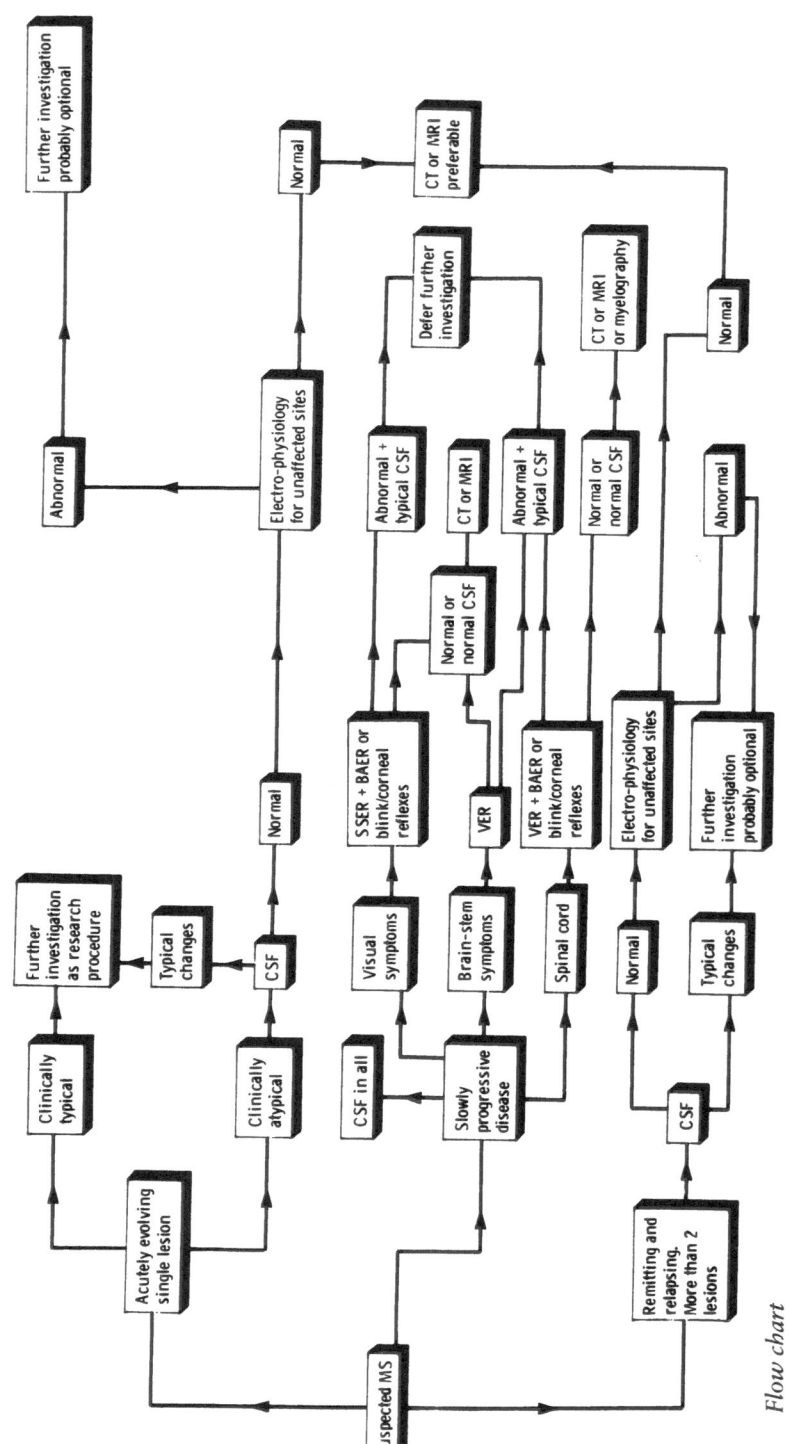

Flow chart

isolated optic nerve or brain stem disease, experience indicates that, in at least some of these individuals, clinical progression fails to appear over a follow-up period lasting several years. At the present time, MRI and, perhaps, CSF analysis should be regarded as research procedures in patients with monosymptomatic disease unless doubt exists as to the underlying pathological mechanism.

6.2 CNS INFECTION

6.2.1 Cerebral abscess

With the advent of CT scanning, the capacity for early diagnosis of cerebritis and cerebral abscess has been enhanced. Delay in diagnosis still occurs, either from failure to appreciate the need for scanning, or from misinterpretation of the findings. Multiple enhancing masses on CT are most likely the consequence of metastatic malignancy, but a similar appearance occurs in some patients with disseminated sepsis. Increasingly frequently, patients with abscess fail to show signs of an infective process, and are diagnosed initially as having a space-occupying lesion, an experience encountered in 45% of patients in one series [75].

(a) Investigation

Measurement of ESR and white cell count is of limited value, since many patients have normal values. In one series, of 400 cases, 70% had an elevated white cell count in peripheral blood [76]. Blood cultures, although mandatory in patients with suspected intracranial sepsis, will be negative in otogenic cases. Sterile cultures from the abscess itself were reported in 23% of cases in one study [75].

(b) CSF findings

The majority of patients with cerebral abscess have an elevated cell count in the CSF. Culture of the fluid is likely to yield the causative organism where rupture of the abscess has occurred into the ventricular system but the hazards of the procedure far outweigh its diagnostic value. A significant deterioration of the conscious level within 48 hours of lumbar puncture occurred in 29% of cases in one series, with a corresponding increase in mortality rate over those individuals whose conscious state remained stable [77]. The same hazard and lack of specific diagnostic information, applies to the use of the procedure in cases of subdural empyema [78].

(c) Technetium scanning

Although the role of isotope scanning has been supplanted by CT, its use is worth considering where immediate access to CT is not available. In one series, of 50 cases, scanning had been performed in 16 patients, and was abnormal in all of them. One review has suggested a yield of between 80 and 100% from the procedure [76]. The resolution capacity of scanning is limited, however. In one patient, with a single abscess detected by technetium scanning, autopsy revealed numerous smaller abscesses between 0.3 and 0.7 cm in diameter [79].

(d) EEG

The EEG is abnormal in the majority of patients with abscess, abnormal findings being recorded in up to 90% of cases [80]. A focal delta wave discharge is highly suggestive of the diagnosis but more often, the EEG merely suggests the likely localization of the underlying disorder. The sensitivity of echo encephalography does not allow its use as a screening procedure.

(e) Radiology

Skull X-rays are often performed in patients with suspected intra-cranial sepsis and, by demonstrating focal sinus disease, can suggest the site of the abscess. Both ventriculography and angiography achieve localization in the majority of cases but the former is never, and the latter seldom, now performed.

CT scanning will detect all symptomatic intracerebral abscesses. In an early study, the appearances of cerebritis and abscess were summarized [81]. The former, on pre-contrast films, appears as a non-homogeneous mass with irregular margins, with diffuse enhancement following contrast injection. The pre-contrast appearance of abscess is similar. Following contrast, ring enhancement appears around a low-density core. Less commonly, dense, homo-geneous enhancement is seen. Periventricular or intraventricular enhancement may be found. It was noted that the same pattern of ring enhancement might be seen in other processes, including neoplasm and infarction. A thin ring of uniform enhancement is highly suggestive of abscess but 40–50% of cases do not show this pattern [82] (Fig. 6.5). Other findings suggestive of abscess include multi-loculation, localization at the cortico-medullary junction and

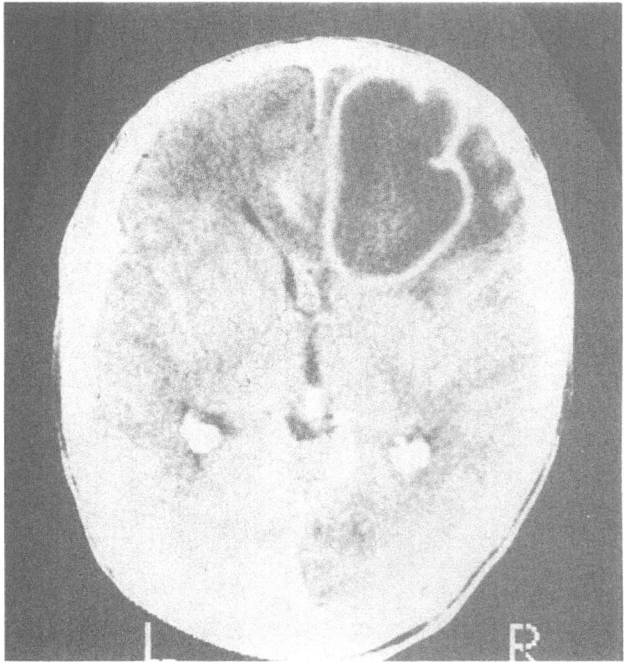

Fig. 6.5 CT with contrast showing uniform ring enhancement in a right frontal abscess

ependymal enhancement. Differing patterns of enhancement have been used to differentiate abscess from cerebritis. With the latter, a ring-pattern of enhancement may be seen, which remains stable at rescanning after 60 minutes but shows a tendency to diffuse into the central core. With the formation of abscess, the ring pattern of enchancement diminishes after 60 minutes, and no central penetration occurs [82]. The use of corticosteroids tends to inhibit enhancement, particularly at the cerebritis stage.

Serial scanning has proved of considerable value in the assessment of treatment response. Contrast enhancement fades rapidly after aspiration. Repeat aspiration is indicated if the size of the cavity fails to diminish after the initial procedure. Where patients are managed without surgery, weekly scanning is advisable. In one study, a mean of 2.4 weeks elapsed before abscess size reduced and 10 weeks before mass effect and contrast enhancement resolved [82].

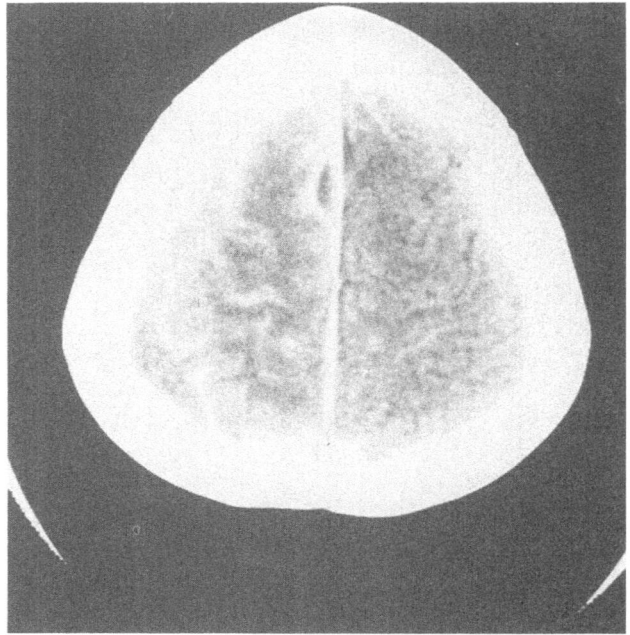

Fig. 6.6 CT with contrast – subdural abscess overlying left hemisphere with separate loculus in interhemispheric fissure

6.2.2 Subdural and epidural abscess

Carotid angiography is abnormal in the majority of cases of subdural abscess [78]. In the review already referred to, CT was considered to be entirely reliable in the diagnosis of subdural abscess (empyema), demonstrating a non-homogeneous lenticular or semi-lunar extracerebral lesion with mass effect [81] (Fig. 6.6). Further experience has indicated that initially negative scans can be obtained in proven cases [83]. The value of EEG in the diagnosis of subdural empyema has been stressed [84]. In one series, of nine cases, focal delta waves lasting up to 2 s, and extensive unilateral depression of cortical activity, were universal [84]. Focal abnormalities corresponded to the area of subdural pus. The authors suggested that the absence of focal EEG changes in a patient with a meningo-encephalitic syndrome made cerebral abscess or subdural empyema very unlikely.

Epidural abscess is detected by carotid angiography in over 90%

of cases [85]. CT demonstrates a homogeneous, low-density lenticular mass sometimes appearing contiguous with bone [81].

6.2.3 Brucellosis

The neurological manifestations of brucellosis include radiculitis, myelitis, meningitis and encephalitis [86]. CSF changes are inevitable. In a series of 91 patients, the mean protein concentration was 1.77 g/l. A lymphocytic pleocytosis is virtually always present. IgG ratios are abnormal, and oligoclonal IgG is described [87]. An enzyme-linked immunosorbent assay (ELISA) for brucella specific IgG, IgM and IgA was positive in 11 out of 11 cases and a tube agglutination test for brucella (in serum) exceeded 1:320 in all [87]. Myelography is negative in the myelitic cases, apart from occasionally demonstrating arachnoiditis. CT scanning simply demonstrates cerebral oedema in the meningo-encephalitic group [87].

6.2.4 Syphilis

In an extensive survey, details of CSF changes in the various types of neurosyphilis were reviewed [88]. Acute syphilitic meningitis, encountered within two years of primary infection was always associated with positive blood and CSF serology. CSF is always abnormal in meningovascular syphilis, where angiography demonstrates concentric narrowing of large vessels with focal dilatation and constriction of smaller vessels. In tabes dorsalis, the CSF is sometimes normal, with, individually, normal protein concentrations and cell counts in about 50%. Positive blood serology is estimated to occur in 88% of cases, compared to probably 100% in patients with general paralysis of the insane. Positive CSF serology was estimated to occur in some three-quarters of cases of tabes, but was considered to be inevitable in general paralysis.

A confusing array of serological tests is now available. The serum VDRL test is relatively non-specific and may become non-reactive in up to 25% of late cases. The serum FTA-ABS is more specific than the VDRL. It remains active indefinitely, despite treatment, and is reported positive in over 95% of patients with late syphilis. In a recent study, the serum MHA:TP (microhaemagglutination assay for *Treponema pallidum* antibodies) – a variant of the TPHA – was positive in all the cases of neurosyphilis in whom it was tested [89]. The serum TPI always remains positive following treatment.

The sensitivity of CSF-VDRL ranges from 10 to 89% according to the type of presentation [90]. False positive CSF-VDRL tests are rare. The CSF FTA-ABS has a higher sensitivity than CSF-VDRL but false positive results have also been recorded [88]. All patients with a positive CSF-FTA-ABS have a positive serum FTA-ABS [88]. The same probably applies to MHA:TP.

Following institution of treatment, the CSF cell count falls. An adequate response at six months after completion of therapy is considered likely if the cell count has returned to normal and if the protein concentration (if previously raised) has fallen. Repeat examination at six monthly intervals for two years is recommended, during which the cell count should remain normal and the protein concentration fall further. The VDRL titre in the CSF falls but may not become unreactive.

Atypical clinical presentations of neurosyphilis have been described, including transverse myelitis [91]. Other investigations are of limited value in diagnosis. Abnormal visual-evoked potentials occur in about 20% of cases of neurosyphilis, with latencies less prolonged than those found in MS [92].

(a) Recommendation

Patients with suspected neurosyphilis should have serum FTA-ABS, MHA:TP or TPHA measured. If these are negative, CSF examination is not worthwhile. If positive, CSF should be examined. Reactivity is judged by the presence of an increased protein concentration and cell count and a positive CSF VDRL. Response to treatment is judged by normalization of cell count, a fall in protein concentration, and a fall in VDRL titre.

6.2.5 Subacute sclerosing panencephalitis (SSPE)

SSPE appears as a late sequelae of measles infection. The EEG shows a characteristic pattern, in which periodic burst potentials discharge repetitively, sometimes coinciding with myoclonic jerking of the limbs [93]. The CSF protein and cell count may be slightly elevated. Abnormal IgG ratios are present, together with oligoclonal IgG. Measles antibody accounts for up to 60% of the latter [16]. CSF and serum titres of complement-fixation and haemagglutination inhibition measles antibody are elevated. CT findings include dilated ventricles, cortical atrophy, brain-stem atrophy and areas of parenchymal attenuation [94].

6.2.6 Cytomegalovirus

Whilst congenital cytomegalovirus infection is well recognized, and associated neurological conditions described, acquired cytomegalovirus infection only rarely results in CNS involvement. A meningo-encephalitic syndrome has been described usually in hosts with evidence of immunoparesis. Serological evidence of recent cytomegalovirus infection has been reported in 11 and 33% of patients with Guillain–Barré syndrome in two series. The diagnosis of cytomegalovirus infection depends on recovery of virus material, most readily achieved from urine, saliva or the buffy coat of leucocytes. Alternatively, demonstration of a fourfold rise in antibody titres (most commonly complement fixing) is used to support the diagnosis [95].

6.2.7 Progressive multifocal leucoencephalopathy

In this condition, CNS oligodendroglia are infected by papovavirus resulting in patchy necrosis and demyelination. The CSF and EEG changes are slight, and non-specific. CT reveals patchy attenuation in white matter. More extensive abnormalities appear on MRI [96]. Brain biopsy is definitive.

6.2.8 Creutzfeldt–Jakob disease

A purely clinical diagnosis of Creutzfeldt–Jakob disease is prone to error. More protracted cases (some 9% produce an illness of more than two years' duration) may be mistaken for cases of Alzheimer's disease with myoclonus. Familial involvement has been reported in 5–15% of cases of Creutzfeldt–Jakob disease, producing a clinical picture similar to familial myoclonic dementia [97]. Whereas the identification of a transmissible agent, by the development of the disease in an inoculated primate, provides definitive evidence for the disease, the diagnosis, of necessity, is usually based on laboratory criteria, aided, in some cases, by ante-mortem brain biopsy material.

(a) Investigation
CSF findings are normal in the majority of patients. About 10% have a moderate increase in protein concentration [98]. The EEG can provide powerful support for the diagnosis. Regularly recurring, diffuse, high-voltage sharp waves appear, often at about 2 Hz [99].

This periodic activity is almost inevitable in the fully developed case, but is less conspicuous in the prodromal and terminal phases [100]. Rarely, the EEG remains normal [98]. CT scanning has proved of little value in diagnosis. In many, it remains normal even in the latter stages of the disease. The changes that are found, including ventricular dilatation and cortical atrophy, are not specific [101].

With increasing knowledge of the disease's pathogenesis, further methods of diagnosis have been developed. Various abnormal proteins have been detected in the CSF by electrophoresis. Two, with specified relative molecular masses, and isoelectric points, were found in all 21 cases tested, in 5 of 10 cases of herpes simplex encephalitis, but in no other neurological condition [102]. The detection of status spongiosus, on light microscopy of brain material remains the most definitive diagnostic aid [103]. A unique fibrillary structure has been found in brain tissue. Antibody, prepared against an antigen from hamster brain inoculated with scrapie, can be used to identify a marker protein in human brain tissue. The test was positive in 25 of 31 cases; no false-positive tests occurred amongst cases of Alzheimer's disease, dementia with myoclonus and dementia with amyotrophic lateral sclerosis. The test is positive in the majority of patients with the Gerstmann–Straussler–Scheinker syndrome, in which a progressive cerebellar syndrome coincides with dementia and spinal tract signs, some cases of which are caused by a spongiform encephalopathy agent [104].

6.2.9 Aspergillosis

CNS aspergillosis appears in patients with immunological incompetence, or disabling medical conditions. Granulomatous masses are found intracranially or within the spinal cord. Invasion of blood vessels results in arterial occlusion or mycotic aneurysm. The CSF cell count and protein concentration are usually elevated [105]. The CT changes are non-specific, consisting of low-density areas sometimes with enhancement [106]. In some patients, the organism can be detected by culture during life. Pulmonary infiltration is frequent in patients with neurological involvement and is detectable on chest X-ray.

6.2.10 Cryptococcosis

Cryptococcal meningitis has been discussed elsewhere (Section 11.4). It has been suggested that the discovery of hypodense grey matter lesions on CT in patients with minimal or no focal deficits, but clinical and laboratory evidence of a sub-acute meningitis, is highly suggestive of cryptococcal infection [107].

6.2.11 Schistosomiasis

Schistosomiasis rarely affects the central nervous system. Involvement is more likely with *S. mansoni* than *S. haematobium*. Granulomata are found in the cerebrum and in the spinal cord, most often in the region of the conus [108]. Eosinophilia in the peripheral blood is common but not inevitable. The CSF usually shows a cellular reaction, occasionally including eosinophils. Myelography, in cases of cord involvement, shows partial or complete block with cord swelling, typically at the T12–L1 level. CT detects cord swelling and can demonstrate intracerebral granulomata.

Serological tests are of limited specificity. An enzyme-linked immunosorbent assay (ELISA) confirms response to schistosoma though false negative results occur. A greater antibody response in CSF compared to serum is suggestive of CNS involvement [108].

6.2.12 Cysticercosis

Seizures represent the initial manifestation of neurocysticercosis in nearly half the cases and continue as the only manifestation in a third [109]. The other major presenting symptoms reflect an increased intracranial pressure. The CSF changes are non-specific, incorporating an elevated cell count, seldom exceeding $100/mm^3$ and predominantly polymorphonuclear, together with a mild increase in protein concentration [110]. Occasionally an eosinophilic pleocytosis is detected in the CSF [109]. Less than a third of patients have ova or proglottides of *Taenia solium* in the stool. An abnormal titre of indirect haemagglutination (IH) antibodies ($\geq 1/128$) has been reported in the serum in up to 92% of patients. A technique for detection of antibodies to larval antigen bound to radioactive iodine labelled staphylococcal protein was always positive in patients with ventricular cysts or meningitis, using either serum or CSF [111]. An enzyme-linked immunosorbent assay (ELISA) detects anti-larval IgG antibodies or larval antigen in the CSF in all patients with histologically confirmed neurocysticercosis [112]. The technique proved more sensitive than an IH assay.

CT changes in neurocysticercosis include calcification and the presence of cysts, appearing as areas of low attenuation with or

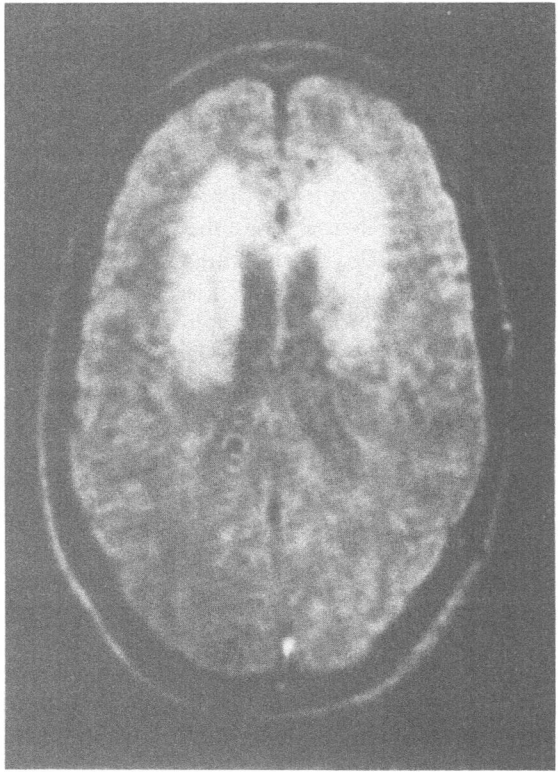

Fig. 6.7 MRI scan in patient with AIDS. Biopsy of the periventricular zone revealed evidence of both lymphoma and toxoplasmosis

without slight enhancement [113]. Acutely evolving, diffuse lesions are associated with oedema and more florid enhancement. The oedema is responsive to corticosteroid therapy. Acute lesions may calcify within a two year period.

6.2.13 Acquired immune deficiency syndrome

A slowly progressing encephalopathic syndrome in AIDS patients, once loosely ascribed to cytomegalovirus infection, is now considered the consequence of direct CNS invasion by the virus. Opportunistic infections occurring in AIDS patients include candidiasis, cryptococcal meningitis, progressive multi-focal leucoencephalopathy and toxoplasmosis [114]. Cerebral toxoplasmosis is the commonest cause of focal brain lesions in AIDS patients [115] (Fig. 6.7).

The clinical features of toxoplasmic encephalitis are not particularly specific. The majority of patients have an illness evolving over one to two weeks in which focal neurological findings are prominent from the outset. Evidence of raised intracranial pressure is common. At some point, many patients display a global reduction in cognitive function, with retained arousal, indistinguishable from the AIDS-related encephalopathy [115].

The CSF findings are of little value in diagnosis, revealing, at most, a mild increase in cell count and protein concentration with a normal, or slightly depressed, glucose level [116]. At times, the CSF is normal [117]. CT is the most useful radiological procedure. Single or multiple rounded hypodense areas are found, sometimes with enhancement, usually ring in type [115,118].

In patients with normal immune systems, primary toxoplasmic infection produces an IgM antibody response, peaking after a few weeks, together with a slower more sustained rise in IgG antibody levels [117]. For such patients, a fourfold rise of IgM or IgG immunofluorescent antibody titres, or a single marked rise in IgM titre (> 1/160) has been considered sufficient to establish the diagnosis [116]. The majority of AIDS patients, however, fail to develop an antibody response indicative of acute infection with *Toxoplasma gondii* [118]. Among 37 cases, none had positive titres for IgM-IFA, and only one had positive titres for DS-IgM-ELISA [118]. IgG antibody titres, however, are of greater value. In the same series, all 37 patients had a positive dye test and IgG-IFA in the serum. However, only 20 had titres of 1/256 or more, and four had titres of 1/32 or less [118]. In another study of 27 patients, three had titres of 1/16 or less [115]. Comparison of an agglutination (AGG) technique for antibody detection, with the dye test (DT), suggests that a serum AGG/DT ratio exceeding five indicates toxoplasmic encephalitis in an AIDS patient [118].

Definitive diagnosis rests on the results of brain biopsy, though a note of caution is required regarding histological techniques. In one analysis, over 50% of cases that had had toxoplasma organisms or antigens detected by the peroxidase–antiperoxidase technique had negative findings from conventional histology of brain biopsy sections [118]. Clinical and CT response to anti-toxoplasmic therapy is rapid, usually within two weeks of initiating treatment, and has prompted some observers to use a therapeutic trial as a diagnostic procedure in the place of brain biopsy [115].

Recommendation

Development of neurological deficit in an AIDS patient should prompt CT scanning. If the scan is normal, or shows atrophy alone, the CSF should be examined. Specific changes in the CSF will suggest the diagnosis of meningitis or meningeal lymphoma. Normal CSF indicates the probable diagnosis of an AIDS-related dementia, providing metabolic derangement has been excluded. A CT demonstrating non-enhancing, white matter lesions is compatible with a diagnosis of PMLE. Confirmation should be sought by biopsy. Enhancing white matter lesions, or lesions confined to grey matter, are highly suggestive of toxoplasma encephalitis. Serological investigations are necessary. If DT, IgG-IFA or AGG in the serum are negative, the diagnosis of toxoplasma encephalitis is virtually excluded. If titres are positive, some authors then use a therapeutic trial, typically of pyrimethamine, to confirm the diagnosis, reserving biopsy for those patients failing to respond. Others advocate biopsy of any accessible lesions to exclude diagnoses such as lymphoma or fungal infection.

REFERENCES

1. McAlpine, D., Lumsden, C.E. and Acheson, E.D. (1972) *Multiple Sclerosis. A Reappraisal.* 2nd edn, Churchill Livingstone, Edinburgh, London.
2. McDonald, W.I. and Halliday, A.M. (1977) Diagnosis and classification of multiple sclerosis. *Br. Med. Bull.*, 33, 4–8.
3. Poser, C.M., Paty, D.M., Scheinberg, L. *et al.* (1983) New diagnostic criteria for multiple sclerosis: guidelines for research proposals. *Ann. Neurol.*, 13, 227–31.
4. Ormerod, I.E.C., Roberts, R.C., du Boulay, E.P.G.H. *et al.* (1984) NMR in multiple sclerosis and cerebral vascular disease. *Lancet*, ii, 1334–5.
5. Traugott, U. and Raine, C.S. (1981) Antioligodendrocyte antibodies in cerebrospinal fluid of multiple sclerosis and other neurologic diseases. *Neurology*, 31, 695–700.
6. Ryberg, B. (1982) Antibrain antibodies in multiple sclerosis. Relation to clinical variables. *J. Neurol. Sci.*, 54, 239–61.
7. Panitch, H.S., Hooper, C.J. and Johnson, K.P. (1980) CSF antibody to myelin basic protein. Measurement in patients with multiple sclerosis and subacute sclerosing panencephalitis. *Arch. Neurol.*, 37, 206–9.

8. Biber, A., Englert, D., Dommasch, D. and Hempel, K. (1981) Myelin basic protein in cerebrospinal fluid of patients with multiple sclerosis and other neurological diseases. *J. Neurol.,* **225**, 231–6.

9. Garcia-Merino, A., Persson, M.A.A., Ernerudh, J. *et al.* (1986) Serum and cerebrospinal fluid antibodies against myelin basic protein and their IgG subclass distribution in multiple sclerosis. *J. Neurol. Neurosurg. Psychiatry,* **49**, 1066–70.

10. Warren, K.G. and Catz, I. (1986) Diagnostic value of cerebrospinal fluid anti-myelin basic protein in patients with multiple sclerosis. *Ann. Neurol.* **20**, 20–5.

11. Tachousky, T.G., Lisak, R.P., Koprowski, H. *et al.* (1976) Circulating immune complexes in multiple sclerosis and other neurological diseases. *Lancet,* **ii**, 997–9.

12. Compston, D.A.S., Morgan, B.P., Oleesky, D. *et al.* (1986) Cerebrospinal fluid C9 in demyelinating disease. *Neurology,* **36**, 1503–5.

13. Dore-Duffy, P., Donaldson, J.O., Rothman, B.L. and Zurier, R.B. (1982) Antinuclear antibodies in multiple sclerosis. *Arch. Neurol.,* **39**, 504–6.

14. Selmaj, K., Alam, R., Perkin, G.D. and Clifford Rose, F. (1987) T lymphocyte-derived demyelinating activity in multiple sclerosis patients in acute relapse. *J. Neurol. Neurosurg. Psychiatry,* **50**, 532–7.

15. Cremer, N.E., Johnson, K.P., Fein, G. and Likosky, W.H. (1980) Analysis of serum and CSF antibodies by standard serologic methods. *Arch. Neurol,* **37**, 610–15.

16. Mehta, P.D., Thormar, H. and Wisniewski, H.M. (1980) Quantitation of measles-specific IgG. Its presence in CSF and brain extracts of patients with multiple sclerosis. *Arch. Neurol.,* **37**, 607–9.

17. Appel, M.J., Glickman, L.T., Raine, C.S. and Tourtellotte, W.W. (1981) Canine viruses and multiple sclerosis. *Neurology,* **31**, 944–9.

18. Batchelor, J.R., Compston, A. and McDonald, W.I. (1978) The significance of the association between HLA and multiple sclerosis. *Br. Med. Bull.,* **34**, 279–84.

19. Müller, R. (1951) The correlation between the state of the cerebrospinal fluid and the clinical picture in disseminated sclerosis. *Acta Med. Scand.,* **139**, 153–63.

20. Hart, R.G. and Sherman, D.G. (1982) The diagnosis of multiple sclerosis. *J. Am. Med. Assoc.,* **247**, 498–503.

21. Johnson, K.P. (1980) Cerebrospinal fluid and blood assays of diagnostic usefulness in multiple sclerosis. *Neurology,* **30**, 106–9.

22. Link, H. and Müller, R. (1971) Immunoglobulins in multiple sclerosis and infections of the nervous system. *Arch. Neurol.,* **25**, 326–44.

23. Caroscio, J.T., Kochwa, S., Sacks, H. *et al.* (1983) Quantitative CSF IgG measurements in multiple sclerosis and other neurologic diseases. An update. *Arch. Neurol.,* **40**, 409–13.

24. Caroscio, J.T., Kochwa, S., Sacks, H. *et al.* (1986) Quantitative cerebrospinal fluid IgG measurements as a marker of disease activity in multiple sclerosis. *Arch. Neurol.,* **43**, 1129–31.

25. Perkin, G.D., Sethi, K. and Muller, B.R. (1983) IgG ratios and oligoclonal IgG in multiple sclerosis and other neurological disorders. *J. Neurol. Sci.*, 60, 325–36.
26. Kolar, O.J., Rice, P.H., Jones, F.H. *et al.* (1980) Cerebrospinal fluid immunoelectrophoresis in multiple sclerosis. *J. Neurol. Sci.*, 47, 221–30.
27. Kostulas, V.K. and Link, H. (1982) Agarose isoelectric focusing of unconcentrated CSF and radioimmunofixation for detection of oligoclonal bands in patients with multiple sclerosis and other neurological diseases. *J. Neurol. Sci.*, 54, 117–27.
28. Laurenzi, M.A., Mavra, M., Kam-Hansen, S. and Link, H. (1980) Oligoclonal IgG and free light chains in multiple sclerosis demonstrated by thin-layer polyacrylamide gel isoelectric focusing and immunofixation. *Ann. Neurol.*, 8, 241–7.
29. Thompson, E.J., Kaufmann, P. and Rudge, P. (1983) Sequential changes in oligoclonal patterns during the course of multiple sclerosis. *J. Neurol. Neurosurg. Psychiatry*, 46, 115–18.
30. Easmark, B. and Sidén, Å. (1984) Isoelectric focusing of CSF proteins and the future evolution of multiple sclerosis: a clinical follow-up. *J. Neurol.*, 231, 117–21.
31. Kostulas, V.K., Henriksson, A. and Link, H. (1986) Monosymptomatic sensory symptoms and cerebrospinal fluid immunoglobulin levels in relation to multiple sclerosis. *Arch. Neurol.*, 43, 447–51.
32. Perkin, G.D. and Muller, B.K. (1987) The influence of abnormal IgG ratios in the CSF on further development of the disease in single lesion multiple sclerosis in *Multiple Sclerosis. Immunological, diagnostic and therapeutic aspects*. Eds F.C. Rose and R. Jones. John Libbey, London, Paris pp 115–119.
33. Grimaldi, L.M.E., Roos, R.P., Nalefski, E.A. and Arnason, B.G.W. (1985) Oligoclonal IgA bands in multiple sclerosis and subacute sclerosing panencephalitis. *Neurology*, 35, 813–17.
34. Rudick, R.A., Jacobs, L., Kinkel, P.R. and Kinkel, W.R. (1986) Isolated idiopathic optic neuritis. Analysis of free κ-light chains in cerebrospinal fluid and correlation with nuclear magnetic resonance findings. *Arch. Neurol.*, 43, 456–8.
35. Patterson, V.H. and Heron, J.R. (1980) Visual field abnormalities in multiple sclerosis. *J. Neurol. Neurosurg. Psychiatry*, 43, 205–8.
36. Meienberg, O., Flammer, J. and Ludin, H.-P. (1982) Subclinical visual field defects in multiple sclerosis. Demonstration and quantification with automated perimetry and comparison with visual evoked potentials. *J. Neurol.*, 227, 125–33.
37. Halliday, A.M., McDonald, W.I. and Mushin, J. (1973) Visual evoked response in diagnosis of multiple sclerosis. *Br. Med. J.*, 4, 661–4.
38. Aminoff, M.J. and Ochs, A.L. (1981) Pattern-onset visual evoked potentials in suspected multiple sclerosis. *J. Neurol. Neurosurg. Psychiatry*, 44, 608–14.
39. Hennerici, M., Wenzel, D. and Freund, H.-J. (1977) The comparison

of small-sized rectangle and checkerboard stimulation for the evaluation of delayed visual evoked responses in patients suspected of multiple sclerosis. *Brain*, **100**, 119–36.

40. Hammond, S.R. and Yiannikas, C. (1986) Contribution of pattern reversal foveal and half-field stimulation to analysis of VEP abnormalities in multiple sclerosis. *Electroencephalogr. Clin. Neurophysiol.*, **64**, 101–18.

41. Regan, D., Bartol, S., Murray, T.J. and Beverley, K.I. (1982) Spatial frequency discrimination in normal vision and in patients with multiple sclerosis. *Brain*, **105**, 735–54.

42. Kupersmith, M.J., Nelson, J.I., Seiple, W.H. *et al.* (1983) The 20/20 eye in multiple sclerosis. *Neurology*, **33**, 1015–20.

43. Camisa, J., Mylin, L.H. and Bodis-Wollner, I. (1981) The effect of stimulus orientation on the visual evoked potential in multiple sclerosis. *Ann. Neurology*, **10**, 532–9.

44. Kempster, P.A., Iansek, R., Balla, J.I. *et al.* (1987) Value of visual evoked response and oligoclonal bands in cerebrospinal fluid in diagnosis of spinal multiple sclerosis. *Lancet*, **i**, 769–71.

45. Perkin, G.D. and Rose, F.C. (1979) *Optic Neuritis and its Differential Diagnosis.* Oxford University Press, Oxford.

46. Regan, D. and Neima, D. (1984) Visual fatigue and visual evoked potentials in multiple sclerosis, glaucoma, ocular hypertension and Parkinson's disease. *J. Neurol. Sci.*, **47**, 673–8.

47. Robinson, K. and Rudge, P. (1980) The use of the auditory evoked potential in the diagnosis of multiple sclerosis. *J. Neurol. Sci.*, **45**, 235–44.

48. Chiappa, K.H., Harrison, J.L., Brooks, E.B. and Young, R.R. (1980) Brainstem auditory evoked responses in 200 patients with multiple sclerosis. *Ann. Neurol.*, **17**, 135–43.

49. Prasher, D.K., Sainz, M. and Gibson, W.P.R. (1982) Binaural voltage summation of brain stem auditory evoked potentials: an adjunct to the diagnostic criteria for multiple sclerosis. *Ann. Neurol.*, **11**, 86–91.

50. Kayamori, R., Dickins, Q.S., Yamada, T. and Kimura, J. (1984) Brainstem auditory evoked potential and blink reflex in multiple sclerosis. *Neurol.*, **34**, 1318–23.

51. Kofler, B., Oberascher, G. and Pommer, B. (1984) Brain-stem involvement in multiple sclerosis: a comparison between brain-stem auditory evoked potentials and the acoustic stapedius reflex. *J. Neurol.*, **231**, 145–7.

52. Sanders, E.A.C.M., Ongerboer de Visser, B.W., Barendswaard, E.C. and Arts, R.J.H.M. (1985) Jaw, blink and corneal reflex latencies in multiple sclerosis. *J. Neurol. Neurosurg. Psychiatry*, **48**, 1284–9.

53. Abbruzzese, G., Cocito, L., Ratto, S. *et al.* (1981) A reassessment of sensory evoked potential parameters in multiple sclerosis: a discriminant analysis approach. *J. Neurol. Neurosurg. Psychiatry*, **44**, 133–9.

54. Chiappa, K.H. (1980) Pattern shift visual, brainstem auditory, and

short-latency somatosensory evoked potentials in multiple sclerosis. *Neurology*, 30, 110–23.

55. Walsh, J.C., Garrick, R., Cameron, J. and McLeod, J.G. (1982) Evoked potential changes in clinically definite multiple sclerosis: a two year follow up study. *J. Neurol. Neurosurg. Psychiatry*, 45, 494–500.

56. Phillips, K.R., Potvin, A.R., Syndulko, K. *et al.* (1983) Multimodality evoked potentials and neurophysiological tests in multiple sclerosis. *Arch. Neurol.*, 40, 159–64.

57. Cowan, J.M.A., Rothwell, J.C., Dick, J.P.R. *et al.* (1984) Abnormalities in central motor pathway conduction in multiple sclerosis. *Lancet*, ii, 304–7.

58. Snooks, S.J. and Swash, M. (1985) Motor conduction velocity in the human spinal cord: slowed conduction in multiple sclerosis and radiation myelopathy. *J. Neurol. Neurosurg. Psychiatry.*, 48, 1135–9.

59. Hess, C.W., Mills, K.R. and Murray, N.M.F. (1986) Measurement of central motor conduction in multiple sclerosis by magnetic brain stimulation. *Lancet*, ii, 355–8.

60. Sanders, E.A.C.M., Reulen, J.P.H. and Hogenhuis, L.A.H. (1984) Central nervous system involvement in optic neuritis. *J. Neurol. Neurosurg. Psychiatry*, 47, 241–9.

61. Reisner, T. and Maida, E. (1980) Computerized tomography in multiple sclerosis. *Arch. Neurol.*, 37, 475–7.

62. Loizou, L.A., Rolfe, E.B. and Hewazy, H. (1982) Cranial computed tomography in the diagnosis of multiple sclerosis. *J. Neurol. Neurosurg. Psychiatry*, 45, 905–12.

63. Barrett, L., Drayer, B. and Shin, C. (1985) High-resolution computed tomography in multiple sclerosis. *Ann. Neurol.*, 17, 33–8.

64. Lodder, J., de Weerd, A.W., Koetsier, J.C. and van der Lugt, P.J.M. (1983) Computed tomography in acute cerebral multiple sclerosis. *Arch. Neurol.*, 40, 320–2.

65. Young, I.R., Hall, A.S., Pallis, C.A. *et al.* (1981) Nuclear magnetic resonance imaging of the brain in multiple sclerosis. *Lancet*, ii, 1063–6.

66. Lukes, S.A., Crooks, L.E., Aminoff, M.J. *et al.* (1983) Nuclear magnetic resonance imaging in multiple sclerosis. *Ann. Neurol.*, 13, 592–601.

67. Farlow, M.R., Markand, O.N., Edwards, M.K. *et al.* (1986) Multiple sclerosis: magnetic resonance imaging, evoked responses, and spinal fluid electrophoresis. *Neurology*, 36, 828–31.

68. Jacobs, L., Kinkel, W.R., Polachini, I. and Kinkel, R.P. (1986) Correlation of nuclear magnetic resonance imaging, computerized tomography, and clinical profiles in multiple sclerosis. *Neurology*, 36, 27–34.

69. Runge, V.M., Price, A.C., Kirschner, H.S. *et al.* (1984) Magnetic resonance imaging of multiple sclerosis: a study of pulse-technique efficiency. *Am. J. Roentgenol.*, 143, 1015–26.

70. Miller, D.H., Johnson, G., McDonald, W.I. *et al.* (1986) Detection of

optic nerve lesions in optic neuritis with magnetic resonance imaging. *Lancet*, i, 1490–1.

71. Jacobs, L., Kinkel, P.R. and Kinkel, W.R. (1986) Silent brain lesions in patients with isolated idiopathic optic neuritis. A clinical and nuclear magnetic resonance imaging study. *Arch. Neurol.*, 43, 452–5.

72. Johns, K., Lavin, P., Elliot, J.H. and Partain, L. (1986) Magnetic resonance imaging of the brain in isolated optic neuritis. *Arch. Ophthalmol.*, 104, 1486–8.

73. Ormerod, I.E.C., Bronstein, A., Rudge, P. et al. (1986) Magnetic resonance imaging in clinically isolated lesions of the brain stem. *J. Neurol. Neurosurg. Psychiatry*, 49, 737–43.

74. Rudick, R.A., Schiffer, R.B., Schwetz, K.M. and Herndon, R.M. (1986) Multiple sclerosis. The problem of incorrect diagnosis. *Arch. Neurol.*, 43, 578–83.

75. Beller, A.J., Sahar, A. and Praiss, I. (1973) Brain abscess. Review of 89 cases over a period of 30 years. *J. Neurol. Neurosurg. Psychiatry*, 36, 757–68.

76. Yang, S.-Y. (1981) Brain abscess: a review of 400 cases. *J. Neurosurg.*, 55, 794–9.

77. Garfield, J. (1969) Management of supratentorial intracranial abscess: a review of 200 cases. *Br. Med. J.*, 2, 7–11.

78. Bhandari, Y.S. and Sarkari, N.B.S. (1970) Subdural empyema. A review of 37 cases. *J. Neurosurg.*, 32, 35–9.

79. Davis, D.O. and Potchen, E.J. (1970) Brain scanning and intracranial inflammatory disease. *Radiology*, 95, 345–6.

80. Brewer, N.S., MacCarty, C.S. and Wellman, W.E. (1975) Brain abscess: a review of recent experience. *Ann. Intern. Med.*, 82, 571–6.

81. Weisberg, L.A. (1980) Cerebral computerized tomography in intracranial inflammatory disorders. *Arch. Neurol.*, 37, 137–42.

82. Britt, R.H. and Enzmann, D.R. (1983) Clinical stages of human brain abscesses on serial CT scans after contrast infusion. Computerized tomographic, neuropathological, and clinical correlations. *J. Neurosurg.*, 59, 972–89.

83. Dunker, R.O. and Khakoo, R.A. (1981) Failure of computed tomographic scanning to demonstrate subdural empyema. *J. Am. Med. Assoc.*, 246, 1116–18.

84. Mauser, H.W., van Huffelen, A.C. and Tulleken, C.A.F. (1986) The EEG in the diagnosis of subdural empyema. *Electroencephalogr. Clin. Neurophysiol.*, 64, 511–16.

85. Sharif, H.S. and Ibrahim, A. (1982) Intracranial epidural abscess. *Br. J. Radiol.*, 55, 81–4.

86. Bashir, R., Zuheir Al-Kawi, M. and Harder, E.J. (1985) Nervous system brucellosis: diagnosis and treatment. *Neurology*, 35, 1576–81.

87. Shakir, R.A., Al-Din, A.S.N., Araj, G.F. et al. (1987) Clinical categories of neurobrucellosis. A report on 19 cases. *Brain*, 110, 213–24.

88. Simon, R.P. (1985) Neurosyphilis. *Arch. Neurol.*, 42, 606–13.

89. Kinnunen, E. and Hillbom, M. (1986) The significance of cerebrospinal fluid routine screening for neurosyphilis. *J. Neurol. Sci.,* 75, 205–11.
90. Dans, P.E., Cafferty, L., Otter, S.E. and Johnson, R.J. (1986) Inappropriate use of the cerebrospinal fluid venereal disease research laboratory (VDRL) test to exclude neurosyphilis. *Ann. Intern. Med.,* 104, 86–9.
91. Harrigan, E.P., McLaughlin, T.J. and Feldman, R.G. (1984) Transverse myelitis due to meningovascular syphilis. *Arch. Neurol.,* 41, 337–8.
92. Conrad, B., Benecke, R., Müsers, H. *et al.* (1983) Visual evoked potentials in neurosyphilis. *J. Neurol. Neurosurg. Psychiatry,* 46, 23–7.
93. Cobb, W. and Hill, D. (1950) Electroencephalogram in subacute progressive encephalitis. *Brain,* 73, 392–404.
94. Krawiecki, N.S., Dyken, P.R., El Gammal, T. *et al.* (1984) Computed tomography of the brain in subacute sclerosing panencephalitis. *Ann. Neurol.,* 15, 489–93.
95. Bale, J.F. Jr (1984) Human cytomegalovirus infection and disorders of the nervous system. *Arch. Neurol.,* 41, 310–20.
96. Levy, J.D., Cottingham, K.L., Campbell, R.J. *et al.* (1986) Progressive multifocal leukoencephalopathy and magnetic resonance imaging. *Ann. Neurol.,* 19, 399–401.
97. Little, B.W., Brown, P.W., Rodgers-Johnson, P. *et al.* (1986) Familial myoclonic dementia masquerading as Creutzfeldt–Jakob disease. *Ann. Neurol.,* 20, 231–9.
98. May, W.W. (1968) Creutzfeldt–Jakob disease. *Acta Neurol. Scand.,* 44, 1–32.
99. Abbott, J. (1959) The EEG in Jakob–Creutzfeldt's disease. *Electroencephalogr. Clin. Neurophysiol.,* 11, 184–5.
100. Chiofalo, N., Fuentes, A. and Gálvez, S. (1980) Serial EEG findings in 27 cases of Creutzfeldt–Jakob disease. *Arch. Neurol.,* 37, 143–5.
101. Gálvez, S. and Cartier, L. (1984) Computed tomography findings in 15 cases of Creutzfeldt–Jakob disease with histological verification. *J. Neurol. Neurosurg. Psychiatry,* 47, 1244–6.
102. Harrington, M.G., Merril, C.R., Asher, D.M. and Gajdusek, D.C. (1986) Abnormal proteins in the cerebrospinal fluid of patients with Creutzfeldt–Jakob disease. *N. Engl. J. Med.,* 315, 279–82.
103. Brown, P., Rodgers-Johnson, P., Cathala, F. *et al.* (1984) Creutzfeldt–Jakob disease of long duration: clinico-pathological characteristics, transmissibility, and differential diagnosis. *Ann. Neurol.,* 16, 295–304.
104. Brown, P., Coker-Vann, M., Pomeroy, K. *et al.* (1986) Diagnosis of Creutzfeldt–Jakob disease by western blot identification of marker protein in human brain tissue. *N. Engl. J. Med.,* 314, 547–51.
105. Walsh, T.J., Hier, D.B. and Caplan, L..R. (1985) Aspergillosis of the central nervous system: clinico-pathological analysis of 17 patients. *Ann. Neurol.,* 18, 574–82.

106. Beal, M.F., O'Carroll, C.P., Kleinman, G.M. and Grossman, R.I. (1982) Aspergillosis of the nervous system. *Neurology*, 32, 473–9.
107. Garcia, C.A., Weisberg, L.A. and Lacorte, W.S.J. (1985) Cryptococcal intracerebral mass lesions: CT-pathologic considerations. *Neurology*, 35, 731–4.
108. Scrimgeour, E.M. and Gajdusek, D.C. (1985) Involvement of the central nervous system in *Schistosoma mansoni* and *S. haematobium* infection. A review. *Brain*, 108, 1023–38.
109. McCormick, G.F., Zee, C.-S. and Heiden, J. (1982) Cysticercosis cerebri. Review of 127 cases. *Arch. Neurol.*, 39, 534–9.
110. Torrealba, G., Villar, S.D., Tagle, P. *et al.* (1984) Cysticercosis of the central nervous system: clinical and therapeutic considerations. *J. Neurol. Neurosurg. Psychiatry*, 47, 784–90.
111. Miller, B., Goldberg, M.A., Heiner, D. *et al.* (1984) A new immunologic test for CNS cysticercosis. *Neurology*, 34, 695–7.
112. Estrada, J.J. and Kuhn, R.E. (1985) Immunochemical detection of antigens of larval *Taenia solium* and anti-larval antibodies in the cerebrospinal fluid of patients with neurocysticercosis. *J. Neurol. Sci.*, 71, 39–48.
113. Minguetti, G. and Ferreira, M.V.C. (1983) Computed tomography in neurocysticercosis. *J. Neurol. Neurosurg. Psychiatry*, 46, 936–42.
114. Snider, W.D., Simpson, D.M., Nielsen, S. *et al.* (1983) Neurological complications of acquired immune deficiency syndrome: analysis of 50 patients. *Ann. Neurol.*, 14, 403–18.
115. Navia, B.A., Petito, C.K., Gold, J.W.M. *et al.* (1986) Cerebral toxoplasmosis complicating the acquired immune deficiency syndrome: clinical and neuropathological findings in 27 patients. *Ann. Neurol.*, 19, 224–38.
116. Alonso, R., Heiman-Patterson, T. and Mancall, E.L. (1984) Cerebral toxoplasmosis in acquired immune deficiency syndrome. *Arch. Neurol.*, 41, 321–3.
117. Horowitz, S.L., Bentson, J.R., Benson, F. *et al.* (1983) CNS toxoplasmosis in acquired immunodeficiency syndrome. *Arch. Neurol.*, 40, 649–52.
118. Luft, B.J., Brooks, R.G., Conley, F.K. *et al.* (1984) Toxoplasmic encephalitis in patients with acquired immune deficiency syndrome. *J. Am. Med. Assoc.*, 252, 913–17.

7

Cerebral tumour
Syringomyelia

7.1 CEREBRAL TUMOUR

It is often difficult, on clinical grounds, to distinguish the underlying pathology in a patient suspected of having a space-occupying lesion. In general the symptomatology of primary and secondary malignant tumours of the brain is partly determined by focal effects related to their position, and partly the consequence of raised intracranial pressure. Some patients present with epilepsy. The headache associated with intracranial tumour is often mild and poorly localized, though, for supratentorial tumours, lateralization of the headache is a fairly accurate guide to the site of the tumour. At times sudden disability appears, in some the result of haemorrhage into the tumour, in others, however, post-mortem examination fails to establish the cause of the abrupt progression of disability.

The evaluation of a large series of proven tumours by computerized tomography gives some indication as to their relative frequency (Table 7.1)[1]. Non-malignant processes can, by acting as space-occupying lesions, mimic the effects of a malignancy. Abscesses can present in such a way that differentiation from malignancy is difficult even after recourse to investigation.

7.1.1 Investigation

Plain skull X-rays are now, rightly, only rarely performed in patients suspected of having a malignant brain tumour. Calcification, for example, was detected overall in 9.3% of cases in one series[2], the figure reaching nearly 50% for oligodendroglioma. Reliance on the procedure for diagnosis led to a false negative diagnosis in 66% of 374 cases[1]. Before the advent of the CT scanner, technetium scanning and electroencephalography were widely used as non-

Table 7.1 Distribution of 1071 tumours as
evaluated by computerized tomography [1]

Glioma	366
Metastasis	343
Meningioma	164
Acoustic neuroma	49
Pituitary adenoma	42
Lymphoma	18
Craniopharyngioma	12
Others	77

invasive procedures for the diagnosis of intracranial malignancy.
Technetium scanning produced a detection rate in 76 and 80.6% in
two series [1,3]. The yield is lowest in low-grade tumours, rising to
nearly 100% for glioblastoma multiforme and is higher for supratentorial than for infratentorial lesions [3]. It has been suggested that
technetium scanning is particularly successful in the detection of
convexity tumours [4]. The yield is related to the size of the tumour.
Supratentorial tumours exceeding 2.7 cm diameter can be detected
in over 95% of cases, the detection rate falling for infratentorial
tumours [5]. The value of electroencephalography in diagnosis is
largely determined by the site of the neoplasm. Cortical lesions
resulted in an abnormal EEG in 96% of 100 cases, with focal
abnormalities in 87% [6]. Experience with deep or subtentorial
tumours suggested that the typical EEG abnormality in such cases
was either localized or generalized bursts of bilate.al synchronous
delta, theta or alpha activity, an association being established
between these findings and the presence of raised intracranial
pressure [7,8]. Angiographic findings in glioma include the presence
of a mass, with abnormal vessels a prominent feature of the more
malignant tumours. In one study of 124 metastatic lesions, a
pathological circulation was detected in 56 [9] being particularly
common in those associated with renal carcinoma. Angiographic
differentiation of a primary from a secondary tumour is often
unsuccessful. In the National Cancer Institute study, angiography
led to a false negative diagnosis in 3% of cases [1].
   The advent of CT scanning revolutionized the investigation of
suspected cerebral malignancy. Increasingly, the diagnostic methods
already referred to have virtually ceased to be used. In an early
report [10], 100 histologically proven tumours had been assessed by

CT scanning. Most of the tumours showed a mixed density pattern with only a small number being either homogeneously hyper- or hypodense. Enhancement, performed in 77, was present in 74 and showed a whorl or ring pattern more often than patchy changes. A more extensive study was reported in 1977[11]. The predominance on the pre-enhancement scan of a mixed density pattern was confirmed, particularly for more malignant gliomas. Enhancement was found in 98% overall and was most commonly ring-shaped. A similar pattern of enhancement was seen in 32.6% of metastases, 73% of abscesses but in only 1.5% of meningiomas. Overall, the tumour was detected in 96.1% of cases on the pre-contrast scan. The initial radiological diagnosis was correct for virtually 70% of the glioblastomas, the diagnosis being considered in a further 12%. It was noted that an irregularity of the enhanced rim tended to exclude abscess. In general, therefore, low-grade tumours tend to be hypodense, with perhaps half exerting mass effect, and a similar proportion showing contrast enhancement. As the degree of malignancy increases, mixed-density patterns emerge, mass effect is the rule, and almost all highly malignant tumours show enhancement. It has been suggested that thickening and widening of the septum pellucidum on the enhanced scan is highly specific for an intra-axial neoplasm [12]. The exact volume of contrast and the time delay after injection most suited for the demonstration of enhancement remain subjects for debate. In one study, the use of delayed scanning 1.5 hours after high dose contrast increased the yield of demonstrable tumours by 11.5% compared to routine immediate post-contrast scanning[13].

Particular problems related to the role of CT scanning in the diagnosis of intracranial tumour are the sensitivity and specificity of the investigation. Negative scans in malignant tumours have been rarely reported[14,15], though with improving resolution, the possibility diminishes. A negative scan, therefore, cannot absolutely exclude a cerebral tumour. Radionuclide scanning in such cases is of dubious value[1]. More relevant is to perform serial scans in tumour suspects, particularly if there is a persistent slow-wave EEG focus[15]. Equally vexing are the cases where differentiation from metastatic disease, or from non-malignant lesions proves difficult.

Common primary sites responsible for CNS metastases include breast, bronchus, kidney, large bowel and skin (melanoma) (Fig. 7.1). Skull X-ray is of little value in diagnosis, whereas angiography achieves the same sensitivity of CT with or without contrast. In one

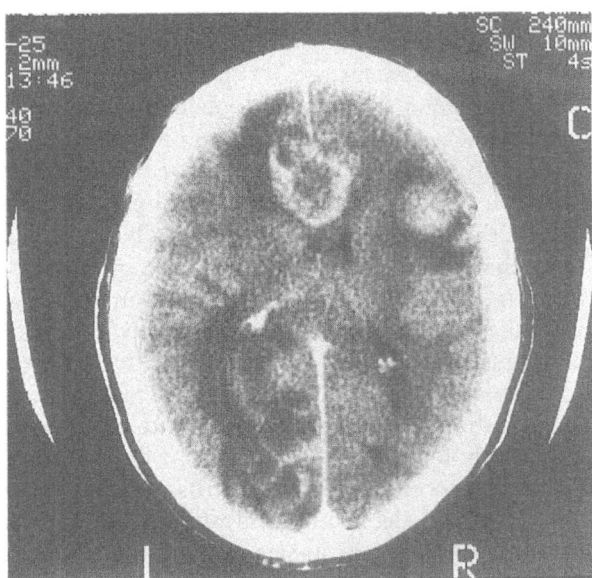

Fig. 7.1 CT scan. Multiple cerebral metastases from carcinoma of the bronchus

study of metastatic tumours, CT scanning failed to detect lesions in 8 of 225 cases. In one of these, technetium scanning was positive[16]. The CT patterns are not uniform. On pre-contrast scans there may be hypodense or hyperdense lesions, or isodense tumours which only visualize following contrast injection. Delayed scanning after high-dose contrast appears to increase the diagnostic yield[13]. Surrounding oedema tends to be prominent. Though multiple lesions are likely to be metastatic tumours, alternative diagnoses include multiple abscess, and multi-centric lymphoma. Lymphomas tend to be deeply sited, or sub-cortical often showing subependymal spread. In two series of lymphomas, multicentric tumours were present in 30% [17] and 50% of cases[18] respectively. The majority appear hyperdense and usually display homogeneous enhancement. They are commonly diagnosed as metastatic when multiple, and as meningiomas when single. CSF examination may be of value in differential diagnosis, since, in the majority of cases, there is an increase in protein concentration and cell count.

Infrequently, other pathological processes, for example infarction, can mimic malignant cerebral tumours. Generally there are clear differentiating features, including grey matter enhancement (far more common in infarction) and white matter oedema (far more common in gliomas or metastases)[19]. In one study, only four of 339 non-haemorrhagic infarcts had oedema confined to white matter pathways whereas 260 had oedema in both grey and white matter. Conversely tumours rarely result in oedema confined to grey matter[20]. Both cerebritis and abscess can mimic neoplasm. In the case of abscess, the ring enhancement is typically more uniform and thinner than that found in tumours, but exceptions to this rule occur[11]. It is evident that areas of radiation necrosis may be impossible to distinguish from tumour recurrence[21].

CT scanning is also of value in determining treatment response. Following remission of glioblastoma multiforme, the CT shows a discrete mass with little or no mass effect, and enhancement which corresponds, pathologically, to the most cellular regions of the lesion. With recurrence, mass effect returns with peritumoural low density composed of oedema and infiltrating neoplasm. Indeed it is clear that CT scanning, despite its sensitivity, fails to indicate the true extent of intracerebral malignancy. At the time of recurrence, post-mortem examination establishes the presence of microscopic islands of neoplasm in the contralateral hemisphere, and in the brain stem or cerebellum which have been undetected by scanning[22].

A number of studies have addressed themselves to the role of MR imaging in the diagnosis of intracranial tumour and its sensitivity compared to CT scanning. Early accounts suggested that MRI revealed a greater extent of glioma spread than was apparent from CT imaging[23,24] and was particularly successful in demonstrating tumours of the posterior fossa. In one study of 19 malignancies arising in the posterior fossa, all were seen by MRI (compared to 17 by CT scan), but more extensive changes were apparent on MRI in 12 out of 17, and better delineation of mass effect in 13[25]. Other series have come to the same conclusion[26,27]. Brain-stem gliomas are most readily detected by the spin–echo (T_2 weighted) technique, appearing then as a bright signal intensity lesion, compared to a dark, low signal, intensity on inversion–recovery (T_1 weighted)[27].

7.1.2 Recommendation

If intracerebral malignancy is suspected, then CT scanning should be carried out. The yield of abnormal findings is probably increased by performing delayed scans after high-dosage contrast injection.

Rarely an initial scan may be negative, but serial scanning, particularly appropriate if there is a persisting EEG slow-wave focus, will eventually reveal the underlying process. Differentiation from cerebrovascular disease is seldom difficult, but exclusion of an infective process may prove impossible, demanding then histological confirmation of the diagnosis. Multiple lesions are likely to be metastatic but a similar appearance may occur with infection or lymphoma. MR scanning defines the extent of the tumour more accurately but is probably not essential in the investigation of supratentorial malignancy. It is the investigation of choice in patients who are suspected of having a posterior fossa tumour.

7.2 MENINGIOMA

Meningiomas are said to constitute some 15% of all intracranial neoplasms. They tend to arise at certain sites, most commonly over the convexity and present either with focal effects from their particular distribution, or with epilepsy. In one study of 164 cases, 62 arose from the convexity or parasagittal region, and 37 from the sphenoid or the parasellar area[28].

A retrospective analysis of the value of plain skull films was performed in 133 proven cases of meningioma[29]. An abnormality strongly suggesting the diagnosis of meningioma was present in 63%. The most common finding was bone sclerosis (particularly with basal lesions) followed by bone destruction, increased vascularity (indicated by prominent and tortuous middle meningeal arterial grooves) and tumour calcification. An abnormality of any type was found in 73%. In the National Cancer Institute Study, technetium scanning was abnormal in 84% of cases, though in only 31% was it possible to make a specific diagnosis[28]. It has been suggested that the combination of an abnormal static image, and an abnormal dynamic scintigram, with increasing signal in the late arterial or capillary phase, persisting into the venous wash out phase is highly specific for meningioma[30].

Angiography is highly successful in detecting meningiomas, though demonstration of abnormal feeding vessels, or a tumour circulation, is by no means inevitable. In a study of 71 supratentorial meningiomas, an abnormal meningeal supply was detected in 42, and an abnormal tumour circulation in 34[31]. Selective external carotid angiography is not relevant for sub-frontal, sub-temporal and supra-sellar meningiomas, since most of these obtain their blood

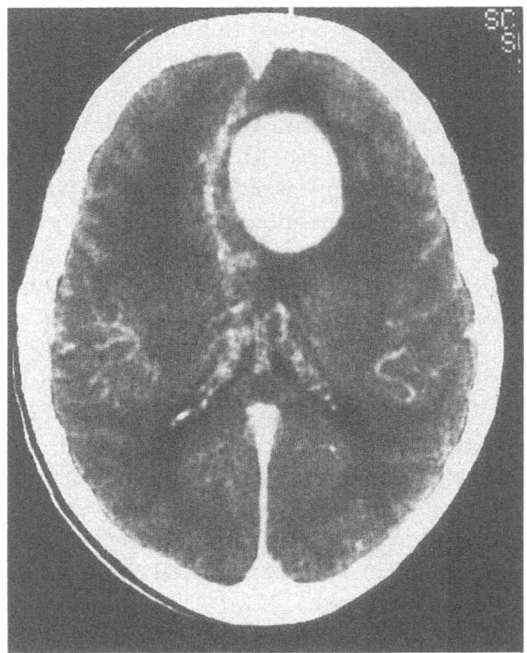

Fig. 7.2 CT scan after enhancement. Falx meningioma

supply from meningeal branches of the internal carotid artery. In the National Cancer Institute study, angiography was performed in 88% of cases. An intracranial mass was identified in 94–96% of cases with a certain or probable diagnosis of meningioma being possible in 83%. A comparative study of scintigraphy, angiography and encephalography has been attempted in 41 patients, though not all patients had all three investigations[32]. Scintigraphy and angiography were abnormal in all the cases. The specificity of diagnosis using scintigraphy for convexity tumours reached 90%, compared to a specific diagnosis following angiography in 73%. Encephalography was performed in only nine patients, and was abnormal in eight of them.

The unenhanced CT in meningioma generally reveals a slightly hyperdense tumour with fairly homogeneous enhancement (Fig. 7.2). Adjacent oedema is found in up to two-thirds of cases but bears little relationship to the size of the tumour[28]. Among 164 proven cases, CT detected some form of tumour in 84.5% of pre-contrast and in 96.3% of post-contrast studies. Combining pre- and post-contrast films, a specific diagnosis was achieved in 90.5% [28]. False-negative and false-positive diagnoses occurred with a frequency, in the series already quoted, of 6 and 1.9% respectively [28].

Some of the problems in diagnosis have been reviewed in a series of 347 proven meningiomas [33] of which 92.2% were correctly diagnosed on the initial scan. False negative diagnoses in the remainder included glioma, tumour of uncertain type, and a normal study. Angiography was performed in 22 of the 27 misdiagnosed cases. A definite abnormality was found in 21, but the correct diagnosis in only 10. Eventually, for 12 patients, the diagnosis was only established at operation. Among the 353 diagnoses of meningioma made by CT scan, 33 (9.3%) proved incorrect. Of these, 22 had some form of malignancy. Angiography, performed in 25 of the 33 cases produced diagnostic data in nine. A certain proportion of meningiomas recur, and some of these display malignant tendencies on histological examination. CT evidence suggesting this tendency includes extensive bone lysis, irregular or indistinct tumour margins, deeply penetrating fronds of tumour, extensive necrosis and absent or minimal calcification. It is suggested that malignancy is also indicated if a mushrooming pannus of tumour extends over the cerebral surface for a considerable distance from the globoid part of the tumour [34].

Meningiomas arising from particular sites can require other diagnostic procedures. Optic nerve sheath meningiomas are notoriously difficult to diagnose. It has been suggested that complex motion tomography of the optic canals can reveal abnormalities (canal enlargement, altered contour or atypical cortical bone) in all cases, even when CT has been negative [35]. Others have concluded that with the introduction of later generation CT, this has become the investigation of choice [36]. The features on scanning have been summarized as hyperostosis of the sphenoid, tumour calcification, marked enhancement, optic canal widening and a distinction of abnormal sheath from normal nerve. With optic nerve glioma, however, the sheath and tumour are indistinguishable [37]. Meningiomas arising from the CP angle tend to have a broad base aligned against the petrous bone, are eccentric in relationship to the internal auditory meatus and are more liable to show calcification but less likely to produce bone erosion compared to acoustic neuromas [28].

Experience with MRI scanning in meningioma has been recently published [38]. In 12 cases, definition was better by MRI in seven, better by CT scanning in two and equivalent in three. Two patterns of signal were encountered, one showing long T_1 and T_2, the other, long T_1 but normal or only slightly prolonged T_2. CT was found to be superior for demonstrating calcification, hyperostosis or bone erosion. MRI produced better imaging in the posterior fossa, at the base of the brain, at the skull apex and around the tentorium.

7.2.1 Recommendation

Though skull X-ray changes are common in meningioma, the investigation can be bypassed if CT scanning is available, with, perhaps, the exception of optic nerve sheath meningioma. The vast majority of meningiomas are diagnosed by CT. Uncertainties regarding the differential diagnosis can be partly resolved by the use of angiography. MR scanning is likely to be of value as an alternative and probably superior investigation for basal and posterior fossa growths.

7.3 PARA-SELLAR AND SELLAR TUMOURS

Microadenoma (< 10 mm diameter) of the pituitary may be insufficiently large to distort the pituitary fossa and certainly too small to extend above it. Their presentation, therefore, is almost always the result of an endocrinological disturbance. Adenoma, on the other hand, can spread beyond the confines of the pituitary fossa. Inferiorly, they invade the sphenoid sinus, laterally the cavernous sinus, and superiorly the supra-sellar cistern. At this site they are liable to encounter the visual pathway, most commonly in the region of the chiasm, with resulting visual failure. Headache can be prominent with pituitary tumour, though as a presenting complaint it figures in no more than 10% of patients. Lesions most commonly encountered in the region of the pituitary include pituitary adenoma, supra-sellar meningioma, craniopharyngioma and chiasmatic glioma. Less common pathologies include aneurysm, metastasis and chordoma.

The relative diagnostic value of plain X-rays, encephalography and angiography has been compared for parasellar masses [39]. For meningioma or pituitary adenoma, abnormalities of the sella were found in around 90%. The figure for craniopharyngioma was between 31 and 69%, depending on the criteria used. Patterns of calcification were unhelpful, as shell-like or cystic calcification was seen in pituitary adenoma and craniopharyngioma as well as in cases of aneurysm. Encephalography, performed via the ventricular or lumbar route, revealed all lesions, whereas angiography demonstrated all the aneurysm cases. Ballooning of the sella was found to be highly suggestive of pituitary adenoma, being found in only 10% of cases of craniopharyngioma and seldom in cases of meningioma where it was usually accompanied by enostosis. Technetium scanning has proved of limited value in cases of pituitary tumour. In one series, positive scans were found in 50%, correlating with evidence of supra-sellar extension [40]. Air encephalography, employing polytomographic sections, detects supra-sellar extension of a pituitary tumour in the vast majority of cases [41]. Angiography has often been considered a requisite in the investigation of para-sellar masses for fear of misdiagnosing an aneurysm, with potentially catastrophic consequences at surgery. Aneurysms are generally placed laterally, rather than occupying the sella. Though conventional angiography often fails to identify a tumour circulation in pituitary adenomas, a combined subtraction and magnification technique suggested that tumour vessels or tumour staining could be detected in all cases [42]. Despite this, prior to the introduction of CT, encephalography remained the investigation of choice for pituitary tumours. The value of CT scanning in the diagnosis of para-sellar masses is established. In an early report, pituitary tumour was detected in 86.2% of cases, a para-sellar mass in 97% of cases and normality of the fossa, or an empty sella, correctly identified in all cases [43]. The pituitary tumours were usually iso- or slightly hyperdense, showed calcification in a fifth and enhancement in four-fifths, usually in a homogeneous pattern (Fig. 7.3). Craniopharyngiomas were often indistinguishable from pituitary adenomas. CT appearance of secretory and non-secretory tumours are similar [44], though growth hormone-producing tumours tend to be more dense. Craniopharyngiomas generally arise from the supra-sellar cistern though some 20% originate in the pituitary fossa. Their supra-sellar site, and more posterior position result in a high incidence of obstruction of the foramina of Munro. Calcification has been reported in up to 77% of cases, more so in children. The margins of the tumours are usually well defined and the majority contain cystic components [45]. Enhancement may be lacking if the cystic component predominates. Para-sellar meningiomas have similar characteristics to meningiomas elsewhere. They are usually anterior and slightly lateral to the sella [12] (Fig. 7.4). Aneurysms arising from the internal

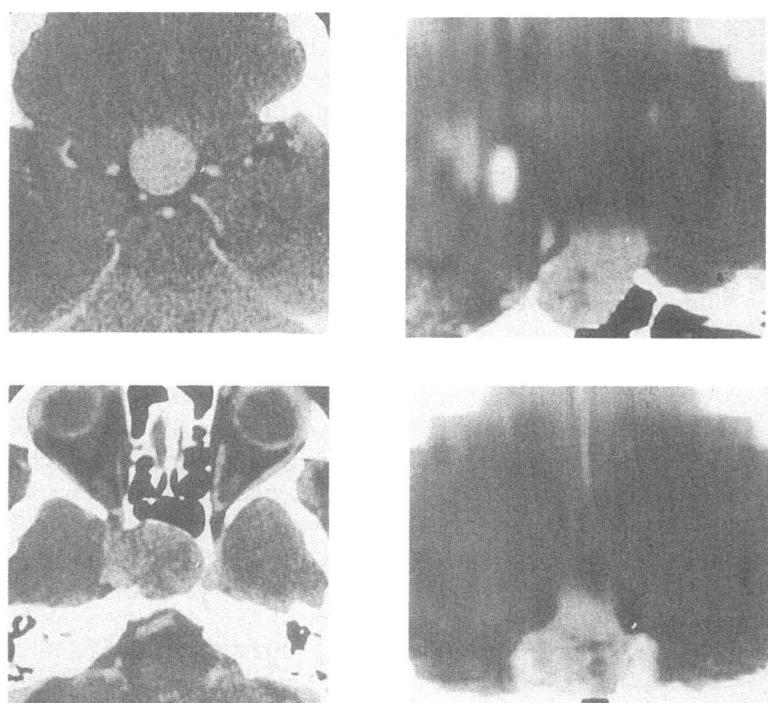

Fig. 7.3 CT scan after enhancement. Sagittal and coronal reconstructions showing almost homogeneous enhancement in a pituitary adenoma with supra-sellar extension

carotid or anterior communicating artery can extend into the sella turcica. The majority show a calcified rim sometimes enhancing after contrast injection. More diffuse enhancement may occur[46]. Though angiography is usually diagnostic, some aneurysms fail to fill[46]. Metastatic lesions involving the pituitary or the adjacent areas are not uncommon. CT reveals a uniformly enhancing mass in most patients[47]. Chaismatic gliomas are usually fairly well defined, iso- or hyperdense, contain no calcification and enhance to a degree dependent on their size.

MRI is clearly of value in the demonstration of para-sellar masses, and appears to be of at least equal diagnostic capacity to CT scanning[48].

Visual field analysis forms part of the investigation of lesions arising in the region of the sella. Indeed, visual failure is often the

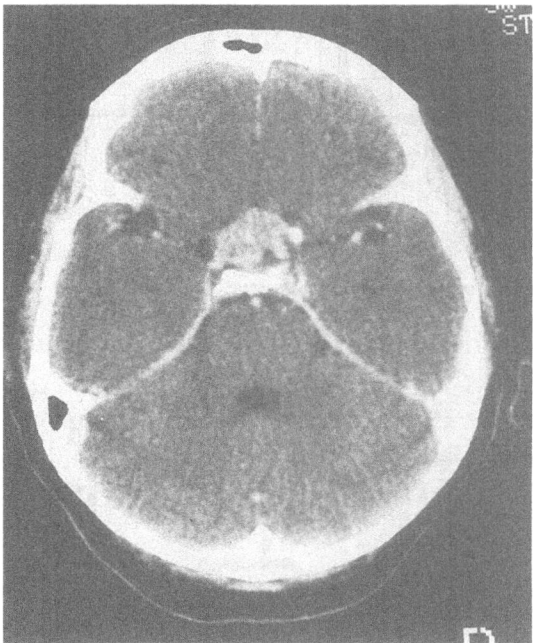

Fig. 7.4 CT scan after enhancement. Supra-sellar meningioma

presenting feature. Many patterns emerge, dependent on the relationship of the chiasm to the supra-sellar cistern, and the position of
the mass. More anteriorly placed lesions compromise the optic
nerve, more posteriorly the optic tract. Involvement of the chiasm
frequently results in asymmetry between the field defect of the two
eyes. Following decompression there may be a rapid improvement in
the visual field defect, its speed determined by the duration of
symptoms and the extent of optic and retinal nerve fibre atrophy.
Serial visual fields are indicated after surgery, since alterations in
visual function may be the first sign of tumour recurrence. When
prolactinomas are managed, at least initially, by the use of bromo-
criptine alone, serial fields serve as an accurate index to the response.

7.3.1 Recommendation (see flow chart A)

Plain skull X-rays, together with tomographic sections of the
pituitary fossa, are appropriate in all patients presenting with
evidence of a para-sellar or sellar syndrome. CT scanning should

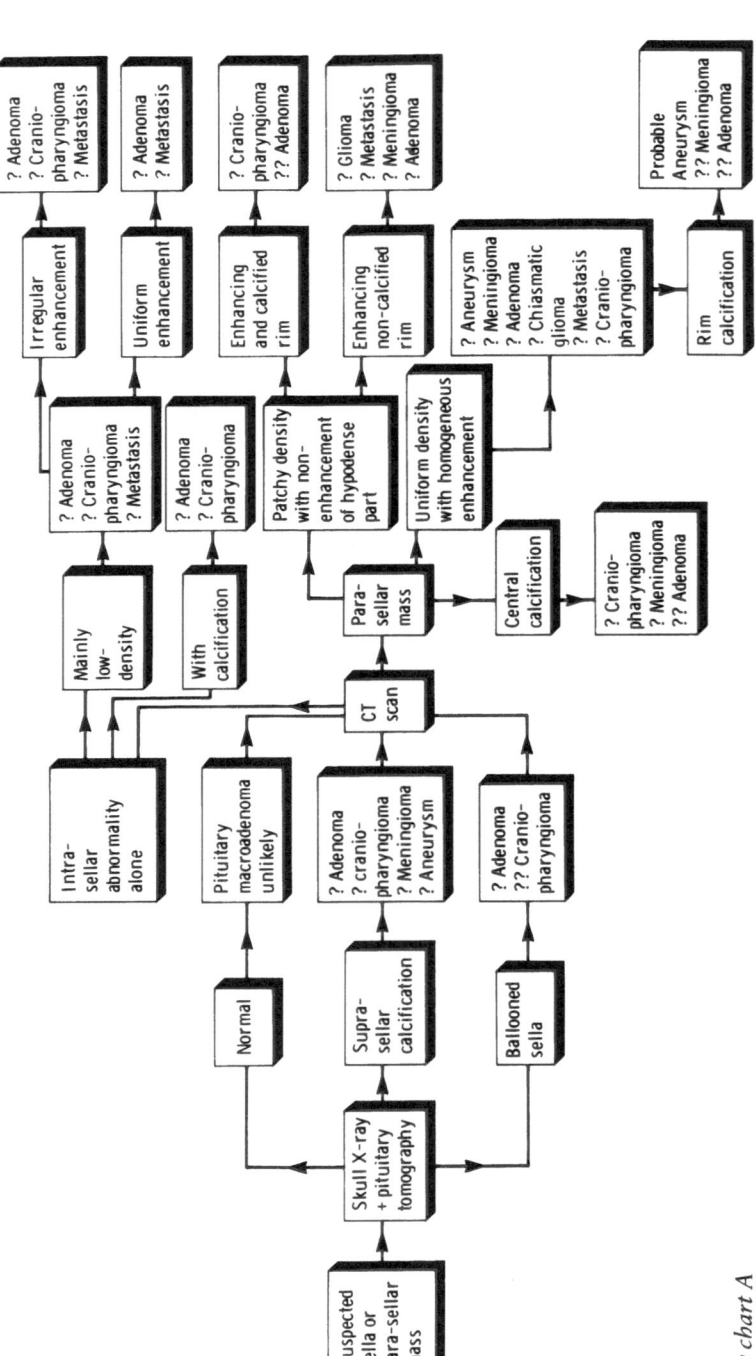

Flow chart A

then be pursued along with appropriate endocrinological investigation where there is evidence of pituitary expansion. CT or MR scanning will probably produce a definitive diagnosis in the majority of cases. If aneurysm is considered possible, angiography is mandatory, though in a small proportion of cases, the aneurysm will fail to fill due to thrombus occluding its neck.

Microadenomas are difficult to demonstrate. They are best assessed by coronal CT incorporating the use of contrast. They may then be demonstrated as iso- or hyperdense areas relative to the rest of the gland with varying patterns of enhancement [49].

7.4 CEREBELLO-PONTINE ANGLE LESIONS

Acoustic neuroma is, by far, the commonest tumour presenting in the cerebello-pontine angle, and accounts for up to 10% of all intracranial neoplasms. The commonest presenting symptom is progressive unilateral deafness associated with tinnitus. True vertigo is infrequent though dizziness is quite prominent by the time of diagnosis. Headache figures as the initial symptom in less than 10%, but is present in around a third by the time of diagnosis [50]. It may be generalized, suboccipital or retromastoid in distribution. At the time of diagnosis, clinical features are determined by the size of the tumour. Thus, in one review, ataxia was present in 42% of all cases at diagnosis, but in none of the cases with tumours less than 2 cm in diameter [50].

7.4.1 Investigation

With large tumours, plain X-rays demonstrate abnormalities in up to 90% of cases. Typically there is widening of the canal with asymmetry between the two sides. The yield falls sharply for smaller tumours. Though myodil cisternography is capable of detecting quite small protrusions into the cerebello-pontine angle, it is incapable of detecting intracanalicular neuromas, and its use has been superseded by other techniques. Vertebral angiography is sometimes employed to assess the vascularity of tumours, or to exclude aneurysm, but not as a first-line investigation.

The yield from CT scanning has increased dramatically with the improvement in scanning technique. In a large study published in 1981, of 237 acoustic neuromas, 71% were detected. For tumours exceeding 2.5 cm, the yield lay between 87 and 100%. When tumour size fell below 1.5 cm, the yield was only 5% [51]. Within a year, reports of the use of fourth generation scanners indicated that tumours protruding more than 1 cm beyond the meatus could be visualized [52]. Contrast studies in axial or coronal planes using thin overlapping sections through the internal auditory canal and cerebello-pontine angle were recommended. For the detection of smaller tumours, and those still confined to the canal, high-resolution gas or air cisternography has been advocated. In one report, 21 tumours, four of which were intracanalicular, were detected when routine scanning had been negative [53].

A review of this procedure and comparison with angiography, pantopaque cisternography and metrizamide cisternography has been performed [54]. It was concluded that metrizamide studies were unsatisfactory in demonstrating the presence or absence of canicular filling, only succeeding in outlining exclusively intracanalicular tumour when the acoustic canal was grossly enlarged. The value of angiography is restricted to tumours exceeding 1.5 cm in diameter. For tumours of less than 1 cm in diameter, enhancement is detected by conventional scanning in some 53% of cases. The authors concluded that for tumours with a diameter of less than 1.5 cm diameter air CT cisternography should be performed.

MR imaging appears to rival the resolution capacity of air CT cisternography (Fig. 7.5). Two recent reports have compared MRI with conventional CT. Where the tumour exceeds 1 cm in diameter, the two techniques produce comparable images though the extent of the tumour is better represented by MRI [55]. With smaller tumours, the appearances on MRI are similar to those obtained by air CT cisternography. MRI can separately visualize the seventh and eighth cranial nerves across the cerebello-pontine angle and within the internal auditory canal [56]. The imagery of meningiomas at the cerebello-pontine angle produces similar signal characteristics, differentiation from acoustic neuroma being achieved by the relationship of the mass to the facial/acoustic complex [56].

Tests designed to assess the function of the auditory and vestibular components of the eighth nerve are of value in the diagnosis of acoustic neuroma. Audiometry shows an abnormal pure tone deafness in 95%, typically high frequency. Speech discrimination is impaired in excess of the pure tone loss. In an analysis of the literature, the stapedial reflex was abnormal in 84% of cases, but in 77% where the tumour was less than 2 cm in diameter [50]. Similarly caloric responses were depressed overall in 87% of cases, but in only

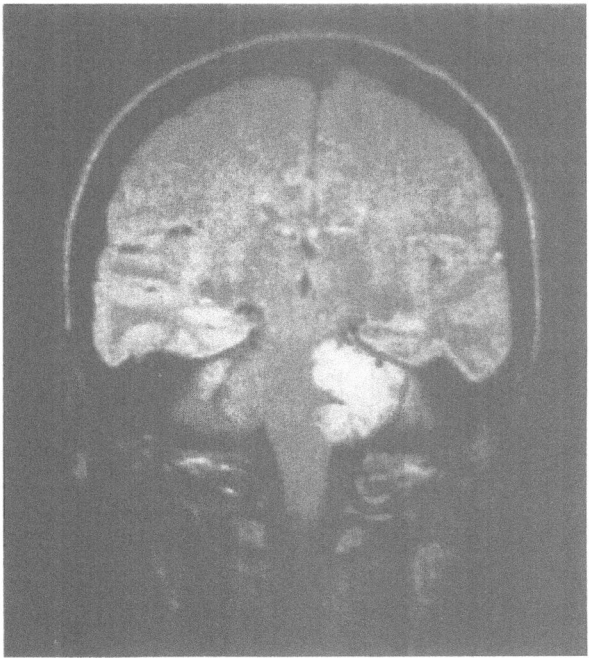

Fig. 7.5 MRI. Large left-sided acoustic neuroma

57% of the smaller tumour cases. Brain-stem evoked responses have proved of considerable value in diagnosis. In one analysis of 37 cases, evoked responses were abnormal in all of them. A variable pattern was described which differentiated between a cochlear and a retro-cochlear lesion in 24[57]. A delay between wave I and the following components (especially II) was considered particularly suggestive of an acoustic nerve lesion. In 10 patients, responses from the unaffected ear were abnormal, with a delay in the latency of wave V in seven. Bilateral abnormalities of the evoked response seem particularly associated with acoustic neuroma, since the finding is rare in other unilateral extrinsic space-occupying lesions[58]. Delayed latencies of the middle components of the BAER occur in about half the cases of cerebello-pontine angle tumour, are common in MS but rare in vascular lesions which mimic the clinical picture of a small acoustic neuroma[58].

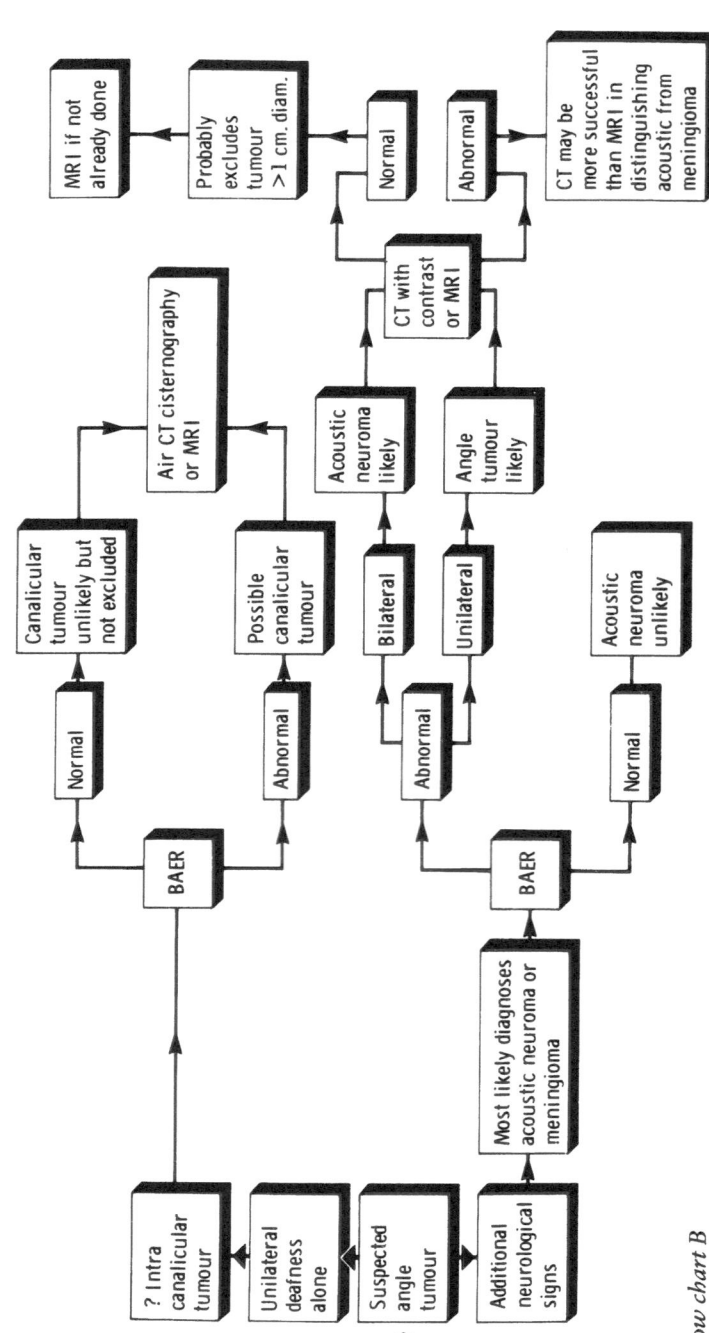

Flow chart B

7.4.2 Recommendation (see flow chart B)

Where there is a suspicion of an acoustic neuroma on the basis of the clinical syndrome of the cerebello-pontine angle, BAER represents a valuable screening procedure. A normal finding virtually excludes the diagnosis of acoustic neuroma. Alternatively high resolution scanning with enhancement should be performed, detection reaching 100% for tumours greater than about 1 cm in diameter. MR imaging will detect all such tumours. More vexing is the determination of the cause of isolated nerve deafness, and the best way to demonstrate a tumour confined to the canal, or barely protruding beyond it. Occasionally, BAER may be normal in such circumstances. If so, the alternative radiological procedures are either air cisternal CT, or MR imaging. Both are capable of detecting small intracanalicular tumours.

7.5 OTHER INTRACRANIAL TUMOURS

Many of the other, rarer, tumours of the CNS are partly suggested by the site of the abnormality on CT or MR imaging. Colloid cysts of the third ventricle generally appear as hyperdense masses with some degree of enhancement[59]. Calcification, though sometimes present on histological examination, is rarely evident radiologically. Epidermoid cysts tend to be located in the cerebello-pontine angle but can arise at other sites, for example the supra-sellar cisterns. They are of low density often with calcification in their wall[60]. They, and several other tumours can arise in the region of the pineal gland. The majority of tumours at this site are germinomas. They tend to be hyperdense and show prominent enhancement[61].

7.6 BENIGN INTRACRANIAL HYPERTENSION

The aetiology of this condition remains unsettled, though some cases are related to venous sinus thrombosis and others are drug induced (for example by the oral contraceptive, vitamin A, nalidixic acid and corticosteroids). The condition predominates in women. Neurological signs are limited to papilloedema, sixth nerve palsy and certain visual field defects related to papilloedema.

7.6.1 Investigation

Prior to CT scanning, patients were usually evaluated by cerebral angiography (to exclude hydrocephalus) followed, in some instances, by air encephalography. Despite popular belief that the ventricular system is more normally of reduced volume in this condition, ventricular volume in one series, based on encephalography, was rather above normal[62]. In a series of 17 patients, mean ventricular size was, in fact, similar to a control group[63], whereas in another report, of 28 patients, 18 had normal-sized ventricles and sub-arachnoid spaces[64]. A minimal increase in the latencies of visual evoked responses has been reported, with, in one instance, a futher increase antedating changes in visual acuity or the appearance of visual field defects[65]. The CSF is normally examined in benign intracranial hypertension, partly to confirm that the constituents are normal and partly in the hope that the procedure may have a therapeutic effect.

7.6.2 Recommendation

In the patient with suspected BIH, CT scanning is performed. The diagnosis is suggested by the absence of a mass lesion. The ventricular volume may be small, normal or slightly increased. CSF is then examined, any abnormal constituents refuting the diagnosis. Conceivably performance of serial visual evoked responses may early identify those patients at risk from visual failure.

7.7 NEOPLASTIC MENINGITIS

In general, the clinical picture produced by neoplastic infiltration of the meninges differs little according to whether the responsible process is lymphomatous, leukaemic or carcinomatous[66]. Typically there is a constellation of symptoms and signs, reflecting involvement of the neuraxis at cerebral, cranial nerve and spinal root levels. Headache is prominent, often with some change in the mental state. Visual failure and ophthalmoplegia are particularly frequent signs of cranial nerve infiltration. Spinal root involvement results in pain with segmental motor and sensory findings.

7.7.1 Investigation

Examination of the cerebrospinal fluid is likely to reveal abnormalities in all patients, although, in some, this will necessitate multiple assessment[66]. Protein concentration is elevated in the majority. There is frequently a pleocytosis, either lymphocytic or polymorphonuclear. A depressed glucose concentration is found in perhaps three-quarters of the patients. Examination of the fluid for malignant cells was successful, in one series, in 37 out of 47 patients, though if only a single lumbar puncture had been performed, positive findings would have been restricted to 21 patients[66]. Other CSF markers may point to the diagnosis. Elevated levels of β-glucuronidase in the CSF are highly suggestive of leptomeningeal carcinomatosis if acute bacterial meningitis has been excluded[67]. Levels are less commonly elevated with lymphomatous infiltration but may be abnormal in tuberculous and viral meningitis[68]. They are not consistently elevated in the presence of primary or secondary parenchymal tumours. Concentrations of carcino-embryonic antigen (CEA) are elevated in meningeal carcinomatosis, particularly that due to lung cancer. It has been suggested that if a CSF/serum concentration ratio of β_2-microglobulin exceeds 1 then CNS involvement by leukaemia or lymphoma is likely[69]. Furthermore, CSF levels decline with clinical remission with a fresh elevation sometimes antedating relapse.

Radiological investigation can add further support to the diagnosis. Multiple nodular defects were encountered in 7 of 18 patients studied by myelography[66]. A particular CT pattern has been described in patients with meningeal and ependymal infiltration. The basal cisterns and sulci are obliterated with enhancement of the ependyma, cisterns and sulci[70]. This relatively specific pattern has been confirmed, together with ventricular distention and periventricular oedema[71]. Serial scanning may be necessary to elicit an abnormality. In one series, multiple superficial enhancing cortical nodules represented an early radiological feature of leptomeningeal metastasis[71].

Not surprisingly, diffuse infiltration of spinal roots can lead to abnormalities of peripheral nerve conduction. In an analysis of 25 patients, 15 of whom had evidence of peripheral nerve or root involvement, lower limb conduction studies were abnormal in 20. The findings included slowed motor conduction velocities, prolongation of F wave latencies, but an absence of denervation[72].

Indeed, the authors suggested that, in symptomatic cancer patients, a delayed lower limb F wave latency, or an absent F wave, were suspicious of leptomeningeal metastases if root compression from other causes could be excluded [72].

7.7.2 Recommendation

CT scanning should be performed in patients suspected of having leptomeningeal carcinomatosis. Repeat scanning despite an initial negative study, is appropriate if the clinical picture is suggestive. Routine CSF studies, together with a search for neoplastic cells may suffice to confirm the diagnosis. If not, elevated β-glucuronidase levels strongly support the diagnosis of leptomeningeal carcinomatosis whereas an abnormal CSF/serum concentration ratio of β_2-microglobulin is suggestive of CNS infiltration by leukaemia or lymphoma. Abnormal F wave latencies in the lower limbs, assuming root compression has been excluded, indicate the likelihood of spinal root infiltration.

7.8 SYRINGOMYELIA

Though differing opinions are expressed regarding the aetiology of syringomyelia, there is uniform agreement that anomalies at the level of the foramen magnum are closely associated with cavity formation within the spinal cord. Other pathogenetic mechanisms include spinal cord trauma and intrinsic tumours. In one series of 209 autopsy proven cases of intramedullary tumour, 31% had syringomyelia. Radiological procedures in syringomyelia have concentrated on determining the presence of cord swelling and assessing the anatomical relationships at the level of the foramen magnum.

7.8.1 Investigation

The CSF is normal in the majority of cases, and is of no value in determining the correct diagnosis. Plain X-rays of the cervical spine and skull base may demonstrate a widened cervical canal, various fusion abnormalities of the spine or basilar impression. The value of oil-contrast myelography has been summarized for 92 patients. The results were normal in 13, showed a widened cervical cord in 34 and ectopic or abnormal cerebellar tonsils in 62 [73]. Neither this procedure nor vertebral angiography, designed to demonstrate

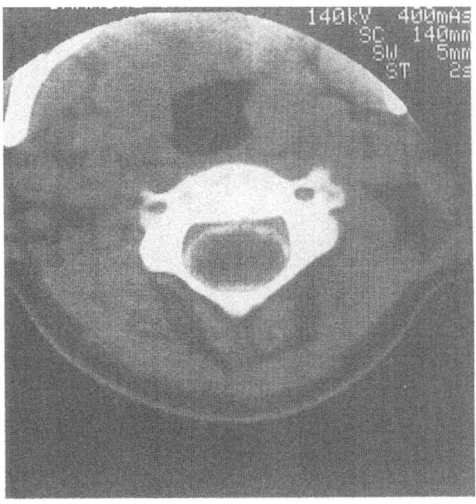

Fig. 7.6 CT scan with metrizamide. Expanded cervical cord in patient with syringomyelia associated with cord tumour

tonsillar herniation by showing displacement of the caudal loop of the posterior inferior cerebellar artery[74], are now performed. Using air, myelography can demonstrate, in some patients, an alteration of cord size according to position, a sign thought to be pathognomonic of syringomyelia[75]. Early experience with CT scanning established that it was as capable as myelography of demonstrating tonsillar herniation[76] (Fig. 7.6). In a study of 75 cases, 67 patients had cavities demonstrated within the cord[76]. A proportion of patients showed opacification of the cavity following intrathecal administration of metrizamide, and a similar result can occur in the syringomyelia secondary to cord tumour[77]. In a small-scale study of CT versus MRI the former was thought capable, using high resolution with metrizamide, of demonstrating 80–90% of syrinx cavities[78]. MRI identified cavities in all five patients, spin–echo sequences being more successful than inversion–recovery[78]. A more extensive study has been recently published[79]. It concluded that sagittal and parasagittal MRI was superior to CT in visualizing the rostrocaudal extent of tonsillar herniation and in distinguishing ectopic cerebellar tissue from brain stem and cervical spinal cord masses. Either technique sometimes proved superior to the other in demonstrating the syringomyelic

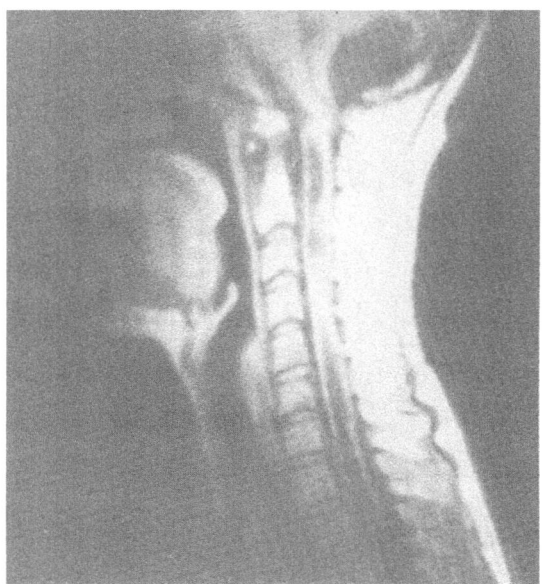

Fig. 7.7 MRI. Sagittal reconstruction illustrating cavitation within cervical spinal cord

cavity (Fig. 7.7). Electrophysiological investigation has a fairly limited role in the diagnosis of syringomyelia. Conduction studies in the upper limb are normal. Sampling of upper limb muscles demonstrates denervation with increased fibre density characteristic of reinnervation maximal in the small hand muscles [80].

7.8.2 Recommendation

Plain X-rays of the spine are of very limited value in diagnosis. Vertebral angiography and metrizamide myelography have been superseded by other techniques. The patient suspected of having a lesion at the cervico-medullary junction should have either metrizamide CT or MRI in sagittal and transverse planes. If syringomyelia is suspected, the CT should be repeated six hours after installation of metrizamide in an attempt to detect filling of the cavity. If the MRI is normal, or demonstrates either a syrinx or cerebellar ectopia, then CT is not required. Similarly, if CT demonstrates ectopia or a syrinx, then MRI is unnecessary. If MRI detects a mass, CT scanning with intravenous contrast can be helpful in determining the presence of calcification or enhancement. If metrizamide CT demonstrates a mass, or equivocal abnormalities, then MRI is indicated. There are fairly characteristic electrophysiological changes in syringomyelia which add support to the diagnosis.

REFERENCES

1. Baker, H.L. Jr, Houser, O.W. and Campbell, J.K. (1980) National Cancer Institute Study: Evaluation of computed tomography in the diagnosis of intracranial neoplasms. I. Overall results. *Radiology*, 136, 91–6.
2. Kalan, C. and Burrows, E.H. (1962) Calcification in intracranial gliomata. *Br. J. Radiol.*, 35, 589–602.
3. Moreno, J.B. and Deland, F.H. (1971) Brain scanning in the diagnosis of astrocytomas of the brain. *J. Nuclear Med.*, 12, 107–11.
4. Di Chiro, G. (1968) Relative value of air studies, angiography and radioisotope scanning in the diagnosis of glial intracranial tumours. *Progr. Neurol. Res.*, 2, 292–317.
5. Boller, F., Patten, D.H. and Howes, D. (1973) Correlation of brain-scan results with neuropathological findings. *Lancet*, i, 1143–6.
6. Bickford, R.G. (1957) Electroencephalographic diagnosis of brain tumors. *Am. J. Surg.*, 93, 946–51.
7. Bagchi, B.K., Kooi, K.A., Selving, B.T. and Calhoun, H.D. (1961) Subtentorial tumours and other lesions: an electroencephalographic study of 121 cases. *Electroencephalogr. Clin. Neurophysiol.*, 13, 180–92.
8. Small, J.G., Bagchi, B.K. and Kooi, K.A. (1961) Electro-clinical profile of 117 deep cerebral tumors. *Electroencephalogr. Clin. Neurophysiol.*, 13, 193–207.
9. Zachrisson, L. (1963) Angiography of cerebral metastases. *Acta Radiol. (Diagnosis)*, 1, 521–7.
10. Thomson, J.L.G. (1976) Computed axial tomography and the diagnosis of glioma: A study of 100 consecutive histologically proven cases. *Clin. Radiol.*, 27, 431–41.
11. Steinhoff, H., Lanksch, W., Kazner, E. *et al.* (1977) Computed tomography in the diagnosis and differential diagnosis of glioblastomas. A qualitative study of 295 cases. *Neuroradiology*, 14, 193–200.
12. Weisberg, L.A. (1984) Intracranial neoplasms. *Neurol. Clin.*, 2, 695–718.
13. Shalen, P.R., Hayman, L.A., Wallace, S. and Handel, S.F. (1981) Protocol for delayed contrast enhancement in computed tomography of cerebral neoplasia. *Radiology*, 139, 397–402.
14. Wulff, J.D., Proffitt, P.Q., Panszi, J.G. and Ziegler, D.K. (1982) False-negative CTs in astrocytomas: the value of repeat scanning. *Neurology*, 32, 766–9.
15. Bolender, N.F., Cromwell, L.D., Graves, U. *et al.* (1983) Interval

appearance of glioblastomas not evident in previous CT examinations. *J. Comput. Assist. Tomogr.*, 7, 599–603.

16. Potts, D.G., Abbott, G.F. and Von Sneidern, J.V. (1980) National Cancer Institute Study: Evaluation of computed tomography in the diagnosis of intracranial neoplasms. III. Metastatic tumours. *Radiology*, 136, 657–64.

17. Spillane, J.A., Kendall, B.E. and Moseley, I.F. (1982) Cerebral lymphoma: Clinical radiological correlation. *J. Neurol. Neurosurg. Psychiatry*, 45, 199–208.

18. Mendenhall, N.M., Thar, T.L., Agee, O.F. *et al.* (1983) Primary lymphoma of the central nervous system. Computerized tomography scan characteristics and treatment results for 12 cases. *Cancer*, 52, 1993–2000.

19. Masdeu, J.C. (1983) Infarct versus neoplasm on CT: Four helpful signs. *Am. J. Neuroradiol.*, 4, 522–4.

20. Monajati, A. and Heggeness, L. (1982) Patterns of edema in tumors vs infarcts: Visualization of white matter pathways. *Am. J. Neuroradiol.*, 3, 251–5.

21. Tanaka, R., Takeda, N., Okada, K. and Ueki, K. (1979) Computerized tomography of coagulation necrosis of the brain and brain tumours. *Surg. Neurol.*, 11, 9–12.

22. Burger, P.C., Dubois, P.J., Clifford Schold, S. Jr. *et al.* (1983) Computerized tomographic and pathologic studies of the untreated, quiescent, and recurrent glioblastoma multiforme. *J. Neurosurg.*, 58, 159–69.

23. Laster, D.W., Ball, M.R., Moody, D.M. *et al.* (1984) Results of nuclear magnetic resonance with cerebral glioma. Comparison with computed tomography. *Surg. Neurol.*, 22, 113–22.

24. Bradley, W.G. Jr, Waluch, V., Yadley, R.A. and Wycoff, R.R. (1984) Comparison of CT and MR in 400 patients with suspected disease of the brain and cervical spinal cord. *Radiology*, 152, 695–702.

25. Randell, C.P., Collins, A.G., Young, I.R. *et al.* (1983) Nuclear magnetic resonance imaging of posterior fossa tumors. *Am. J. Neuroradiol.*, 4, 1027–34.

26. McGinnis, B.D., Brady, T.J., New, P.F.J. *et al.* (1983) Nuclear magnetic resonance (NMR) imaging of tumors in the posterior fossa. *J. Comput. Assist. Tomogr.*, 7, 575–84.

27. Hueftle, M.G., Han, J.S., Kaufman, B. and Benson, J.E. (1985) MR imaging of brain stem gliomas. *J. Comput. Assist. Tomogr.*, 9, 263–7.

28. New, P.F.J., Aronon, S. and Hesselink, J.R. (1980) National Cancer Institute Study: Evaluation of computed tomography in the diagnosis of intracranial neoplasms. IV. Meningiomas. *Radiology*, 136, 665–75.

29. Gold, L.H.A., Kieffer, S.A. and Peterson, H.O. (1969) Intracranial meningiomas. A retrospective analysis of the diagnostic value of plain skull films. *Neurology*, 19, 873–8.

30. Sheldon, J.J., Smoak, W.M., Gargano, F.P. and Watson, D.D. (1973) Dynamic scintigraphy in intracranial meningiomas. *Radiology*, 109, 109–15.

31. Banna, M. and Appleby, A. (1969) Some observations on the angiography of supratentorial meningiomas. *Clin. Radiol.*, **20**, 375–86.
32. Sauer, J., Fiebach, O., Otto, H. *et al.* (1971) Comparative studies of cerebral scintigraphy, angiography and encephalography for detection of meningiomas. *Neuroradiology*, **2**, 102–6.
33. Pullicino, P., Kendall, B.E. and Jakubowski, J. (1980) Difficulties in diagnosis of intracranial meningiomas by computed tomography. *J. Neurol. Neurosurg. Psychiatry*, **43**, 1022–9.
34. New, P.F.J., Hesselink, J.R., O'Carroll, C.P. and Kleinman, G.M. (1982) Malignant meningiomas: CT and histologic criteria, including a new CT sign. *Am. J. Neuroradiol.*, **3**, 267–76.
35. Strother, C.M., Hoyt, W.F., Appen, R.E. and Newton, T.H. (1980) Meningiomatous changes in the optic canal. A polytomographic study. *Radiology*, **135**, 109–14.
36. Swenson, S.A., Forbes, G.S., Younge, B.R. and Campbell, R.J. (1982) Radiologic evaluation of tumors of the optic nerve. *Am. J. Neuroradiol.*, **3**, 319–26.
37. Daniels, D.L., Williams, A.L., Syvertsen, A. *et al.* (1982) CT recognition of optic nerve sheath meningioma: Abnormal sheath visualization. *Am. J. Neuroradiol.*, **3**, 181–3.
38. Bydder, G.M., Kingsley, D.P.E., Brown, J. *et al.* (1985) MR imaging of meningiomas including studies with and without gadolinium-DTPA. *J. Comput. Assist. Tomogr.*, **9**, 690–7.
39. Du Boulay, G. and Trickey, S. (1967) The choice of radiological investigations in the management of tumours around the sella. *Clin. Radiol.*, **18**, 349–65.
40. Evens, R.G., James, A.E. and Adatepe, M.H. (1971) Brain scans in pituitary tumours. *Neurology*, **21**, 806–9.
41. McLachlan, M.S.F., Lavender, J.P. and Edwards, C.R.W. (1971) Polytome-encephalography in the investigation of pituitary tumours. *Clin. Radiol.*, **22**, 361–9.
42. Powell, D.F., Baker, H.L. Jr and Laws, E.R. Jr. (1974) The primary angiographic findings in pituitary adenomas. *Radiology*, **110**, 589–95.
43. Kuuliala, I. (1981) Computed axial tomogrpahy of pituitary adenomas. *Clin. Radiol.*, **32**, 259–64.
44. Davis, P.C., Hoffman, J.C. Jr, Tindall, G.T. and Braun, I.F. (1985) CT-surgical correlation in pituitary adenomas: Evaluation in 113 patients. *Am. J. Neuroradiol.*, **6**, 711–16.
45. Fitz, C.R., Wortzman, G., Harwood-Nash, D.C. *et al.* (1978) Computed tomography in craniopharyngiomas. *Radiology*, **127**, 687–91.
46. O'Neill, M., Hope, T. and Thomson, G. (1980) Giant intracranial aneurysms: Diagnosis with special reference to compūterised tomography. *Clin. Radiol.*, **31**, 27–39.
47. Kattah, J.C., Silgals, R.M., Manz, H. *et al.* (1985) Presentation and management of parasellar and suprasellar metastatic mass lesions. *J. Neurol. Neurosurg. Psychiatry*, **48**, 44–9.
48. Hawkes, R.C., Holland, G.N., Moore, W.S. *et al.* (1983) The

application of NMR imaging to the evaluation of pituitary and juxtasellar tumors. *Am. J. Neuroradiol.*, 4, 221–2.

49. Gardeur, D., Naidich, T.P. and Metzger, J. (1981) CT analysis of intrasellar pituitary adenomas with emphasis on patterns of contrast enhancement. *Neuroradiology*, 20, 241–7.

50. Hart, R.G., Gardner, D.P. and Howieson, J. (1983) Acoustic tumors: Atypical features and recent diagnostic tests. *Neurology*, 33, 211–21.

51. Wong, M.L. and Brackmann, D.E. (1981) Computer cranial tomography in acoustic tumor diagnosis. *J. Am. Med. Assoc.*, 245, 2497–500.

52. Valavanis, A., Dabir, K., Hamdi, R. *et al.* (1982) The current state of the radiological diagnosis of acoustic neuroma. *Neuroradiology*, 23, 7–13.

53. Pinto, R.S., Kricheff, I.I., Bergeron, R.T. and Cohen, N. (1982) Small acoustic neuromas: Detection by high resolution gas CT cisternography. *Am. J. Neuroradiol.*, 3, 283–6.

54. Meijenohorst, G.C.H., van der Lande, B.A.E., Baretta-Kooi, H.H.J. *et al.* (1984) High-resolution CT and air CT cisternography in the diagnosis of acoustic neuromas. *Diagnostic imaging in Clin. Med.*, 53, 120–7.

55. Kingsley, D.P.E., Brooks, G.B., Leung, A.W-L. and Johnson, M.A. (1985) Acoustic neuromas: Evaluation by magnetic resonance imaging. *Am. J. Neuroradiol.*, 6, 1–5.

56. Mikhael, M.A., Ciric, I.S. and Wolff, A.P. (1985) Differentiation of cerebellopontine angle neuromas and meningiomas with MR imaging. *J. Comput. Assist. Tomogr.*, 9, 852–6.

57. Maurer, K., Strumpel, D. and Wende, S. (1982) Acoustic tumour detection with early auditory evoked potentials and neuroradiological methods. *J. Neurol.*, 227, 177–85.

58. Robinson, K. and Rudge, P. (1983) The differential diagnosis of cerebello-pontine angle lesions. A multidisciplinary approach with special emphasis on the brainstem auditory evoked potential. *J. Neurol. Sci.*, 60, 1–21.

59. Michels, L.G. and Rutz, D. (1982) Colloid cysts of the third ventricle. A radiologic-pathologic correlation. *Arch. Neurol.*, 39, 640–3.

60. Zimmerman, R.A., Bilaniuk, L.T. and Dolinhas, C. (1979) Cranial computed tomography of epidermoid and congenital fatty tumors of maldevelopmental origin. *J. Comput. Assist. Tomogr.*, 3, 40–50.

61. Futrell, N.N., Osborn, A.G. and Cheson, B.D. (1981) Pineal region tumors: Computed tomographic-pathologic spectrum. *Am. J. Neuroradiol.*, 2, 415–20.

62. Boddie, H.G., Banna, M. and Bradley, W.G. (1974) 'Benign' intracranial hypertension – A survey of the clinical and radiological features, and long-term prognosis. *Brain*, 97, 313–26.

63. Huckman, M.S., Fox, J.S., Ramsey, R.G. and Penn, R.D. (1976) Computed tomography in the diagnosis of pseudotumor cerebri. *Radiology*, 119, 593–7.

64. Weisberg, L.A. (1985) Computed tomography in benign intracranial hypertension. *Neurology*, 35, 1075–8.

References 179

65. Soelberg Sørensen, P., Trojaborg, W., Gjerris, F. and Krogsaa, B. (1985) Visual evoked potentials in pseudotumor cerebri. *Arch. Neurol.*, 42, 150–3.
66. Olson, M.E., Chernik, N.L. and Posner, J.B. (1974) Infiltration of the leptomeninges by systemic cancer. A clinical and pathologic study. *Arch. Neurol.*, 30, 122–37.
67. Schold, S.C., Wasserstrom, W.R., Fleisher, M. *et al.* (1980) Cerebrospinal fluid biochemical markers of central nervous system metastases. *Ann. Neurol.*, 8, 597–604.
68. Shuttleworth, E. and Allen, N. (1980) CSF β-glucuronidase assay in the diagnosis of neoplastic meningitis. *Arch. Neurol.*, 37, 684–7.
69. Mavligit, G.M., Stuckey, S.E., Cabanillas, F.F. *et al.* (1980) Diagnosis of leukaemia or lymphoma in the central nervous system by β_2-microglobulin determination. *N. Engl. J. Med.*, 303, 718–22.
70. Ascherl, G.F. Jr, Hilal, S.K. and Brisman, R. (1981) Computed tomography of disseminated meningeal and ependymal malignant neoplasms. *Neurology*, 31, 567–74.
71. Jaeckle, K.A., Krol, G. and Posner, J.B. (1985) Evolution of computed tomographic abnormalities in leptomeningeal metastases. *Ann. Neurol.*, 17, 85–9.
72. Argov, Z. and Siegal, T. (1985) Leptomeningeal metastases: Peripheral nerve and root involvement – clinical and electrophysiological study. *Ann. Neurol.*, 17, 593–6.
73. Barnett, H.J.M., Foster, J.B. and Hudgson, P. (eds) (1973) *Syringomyelia*. Saunders, London, Philadelphia, Toronto, pp. 55–63.
74. Occleshaw, J.V. (1970) The posterior inferior cerebellar arteries. Some quantitative observations in posterior cranial fossa tumours and the Arnold–Chiari malformation. *Clin. Radiol.*, 21, 1–9.
75. Bradac, G.B. (1972) The value of gas myelography in the diagnosis of syringomyelia. *Neuroradiology*, 4, 41–5.
76. Aubin, M.L., Vignaud, J., Jardin, C. and Bar, D. (1981) Computed tomography in 75 clinical cases of syringomyelia. *Am. J. Neuroradiol.*, 2, 199–204.
77. Kan, S., Fox, A.J., Vinvela, F. *et al.* (1983) Delayed CT metrizamide enhancement of syringomyelia secondary to tumor. *Am. J. Neuroradiol.*, 4, 73–8.
78. Yeates, A., Brant-Zawadzki, M., Norman, D. *et al.* (1983) Nuclear magnetic resonance imaging of syringomyelia. *Am. J. Neuroradiol.*, 4, 234–7.
79. Bosley, T.M., Cohen, D.A., Schatz, N.J. *et al.* (1985) Comparison of metrizamide computed tomography and magnetic resonance imaging in the evaluation of lesions at the cervicomedullary junction. *Neurology*, 35, 485–92.
80. Schwartz, M.S., Stålberg, E. and Swash, M. (1980) Pattern of segmental motor involvement in syringomyelia: A single fibre EMG study. *J. Neurol. Neurosurg. Psychiatry*, 43, 150–5.

8

Peripheral nerve disease

8.1 PERIPHERAL NEUROPATHY

Since there is a vast array of agents and conditions which can be associated with a peripheral neuropathy, extensive investigation is often advised in patients with this condition in an attempt to elicit the underlying cause. Such a wholesale approach to investigation can be partly avoided by better classification, on electrophysiological grounds, of the neuropathic process, and indeed the logic of comprehensive investigation can be questioned on the grounds of its likely success and consequent benefit to the patient.

Peripheral neuropathies can be classified according to whether the primary pathological event is in the axon (axonal neuropathy) or in the myelin sheath (demyelinating neuropathy). In the latter, differing pathological patterns of myelin loss are encountered, but all share certain electrodiagnostic features (including a marked slowing of conduction velocity), which separate them from the axonal neuropathies. The two pathological processes are not distinct, since some axonal neuropathies may be associated with secondary demyelination.

Typically, peripheral neuropathy manifests as a symmetrical distal sensory disturbance, usually predominantly affecting the lower limbs, associated with distal weakness and depression or loss of the tendon reflexes. The clinical pattern varies, sometimes showing a monophasic course with recovery, sometimes fluctuant, or, often, slowly progressive. Variations in the distribution of the pathological process result in sensory changes appearing alone, proximal involvement as a prominent feature or predominant involvement of the upper limbs.

Many processes disturb the function of the peripheral nerve. Most toxic neuropathies result in axonal degeneration. The genetically determined neuropathies, however, are less uniform in terms of their pathological effect. Indeed very similar clinical patterns in

Charcot–Marie–Tooth disease (hereditary motor and sensory neuropathy) can occur with demyelination (Type 1) or axonal involvement (Type 2). The type of familial disorder causing neuropathy is sometimes suggested by the presence of other neurological deficits. Adult onset metachromatic leucodystrophy, for example, is likely to produce both a peripheral neuropathy and dementia. A combination of ataxia and neuropathy, presenting in adult life, raises the possibility of Refsum's disease or the Roussy–Levy variant of Type 1 hereditary motor and sensory neuropathy. Suspicion that a neuropathy is genetically determined may be raised by a particular clinical picture, but is finally confirmed by demonstration of involvement in other family members.

At times certain clinical features suggest the pathogenesis of an acquired neuropathy. For example, porphyria can present as a rapidly evolving, predominantly motor neuropathy. In the neuropathy associated with amyloidosis, pain and prominent sensory involvement occur, along with autonomic disturbances. In general, however, clues to the possible pathogenesis are lacking, and it is then that debate is most encountered regarding the logic of extensive investigation.

8.1.1 Investigation

Electrophysiological evaluation is essential in the diagnosis and investigation of a peripheral neuropathy, allowing the first step in its classification. Though in theory an objective procedure, in reality numerous factors can influence the results of nerve conduction measurement and muscle sampling, quite apart from the capacity of the electrophysiologist. Variables to be taken into account include the influence of skin temperature (distal slowing in cold peripheries), age (decline in conduction velocity over the age of 40) and anatomical variants in nerve distribution (for example the Martin–Gruber anastomosis in the forearm between the median and ulnar nerves) [1]. The examination is designed to determine the presence or absence of denervation, the degree of slowing in conduction velocity and its uniformity, the presence or absence of conduction block, and the evidence for temporal dispersion of evoked potentials as the stimulus moves along the course of the nerve trunk [2]. Abnormalities may be detected in asymptomatic individuals, or may be more extensive than the clinical disability suggests. In diabetes, for example, changes in sensory action potentials (SAP) can be detected in the absence of sensory symptoms or signs [3].

When a comparison is made of the yield from testing individual peripheral nerves, most studies have concluded that analysis of conduction in the sural nerve is the most sensitive guide to the presence of a peripheral neuropathy. In one report of 300 patients with peripheral neuropathy, 107 had a normal median but an abnormal sural velocity but only 9 the reverse [4]. Depression of the sural sensory action potential amplitude is a poor discriminant between those with normal and those with abnormal nerve function, whereas, in the same study, 86.6% of patients with a polyneuropathy had a depressed sural conduction velocity [5]. Analysis of orthodromic is preferable to antidromic conduction and study of the proximal segment of the nerve (from lateral malleolus to mid-calf) more valuable than assessment of its distal segment [6]. In a small group of patients with peripheral neuropathy, the sensitivity of measurement of the sural was less than that of the medial plantar SAP [7]. Surprisingly, the same authors found a reduction of the sural SAP to be of no greater value in the diagnosis of peripheral neuropathy than changes in the median SAP.

Analysis of F and H waves allows measurement of conduction velocity in more proximal nerve segments. In one study of 50 neuropathic patients, nine had normal peripheral nerve conduction studies but abnormal F or H responses, whilst only two had the reverse pattern. Measurement of sural nerve conduction was not included [8]. Studies of nerve conduction not only serve to establish the presence of abnormal function but can indicate the type of pathological process producing it. Segmental demyelination results in slowing by 40% or more of normal values, compared to only slight reduction of velocities in axonal neuropathies. Despite this, axonal neuropathies are as readily detected by measurement of sural conduction velocities [5]. In familial demyelinating neuropathies, the degree of slowing tends to be uniform in all segments studied. In chronic inflammatory neuropathies, the degree of slowing is variable, the compound action potential is depressed with proximal stimulation, and conduction block (not found in familial cases) is sometimes apparent [9].

An initial classification of neuropathy can, therefore, be attempted on the basis of nerve conduction findings, and provides a rationale for further investigation. An acutely evolving demyelinating neuropathy of variable degree suggests the Guillain–Barré syndrome. A more chronically evolving demyelinating neuropathy can be subdivided into a group showing uniform slowing, and a group showing more patchy change, accompanied by evidence of conduction block. Finally, there are the axonal neuropathies, and neuropathies of mixed type.

8.2 GUILLAIN-BARRÉ SYNDROME

In this syndrome a rapidly evolving predominantly motor neuropathy develops, usually stabilizing within four weeks of the onset. Electrodiagnostic studies are helpful, but are normal in up to 20% of cases[10]. Estimation of F wave conduction velocity can reveal abnormalities not apparent from assessment of conduction in peripheral segments[11]. Typically the CSF shows an elevated protein concentration with a normal cell count. Exceptions occur, however. The rise in protein concentration may be delayed for two to three weeks, or may never occur, and an increased cell count, though seldom exceeding 50 cells/mm^3, can occur in otherwise typical cases. Variation in the clinical and laboratory findings is considerable, frustrating attempts to provide guidelines for the diagnosis[10,12].

In one study of 162 patients, 17.9% had serological evidence of recent infection with cytomegalovirus, Ebstein–Barr virus or mycoplasma[13]. Elevated serum IgM levels are a common finding. Evidence of preceding infection by *Campylobacter jejuni* was found in 38% of a group of 56 patients[14].

A condition closely resembling Guillain–Barré syndrome can occur in systemic lupus erythematosus, sarcoidosis and tick paralysis. Acute intermittent porphyria can present in a similar fashion, though with normal CSF protein levels.

No uniform opinion exists regarding a correlation between abnormalities of nerve conduction at onset and eventual outcome. The presence of fibrillation potentials, indicating denervation, carries a worse prognosis in terms of clinical recovery.

8.2.1 Recommendation

In many patients with Guillain–Barré syndrome the diagnosis is self-evident. If support for the diagnosis is pursued by CSF assessment and electrophysiological tests, it should be recalled that otherwise typical cases can have normal findings. Normal distal conduction studies should prompt study of proximal nerve segments, for example by measuring F-wave latency.

Serological tests are appropriate, though identification of a specific agent is unlikely to alter management. Appropriate investigations are those designed to exclude recent infection by cytomegalovirus, Ebstein–Barr virus, mycoplasma and *Campylobacter jejuni*. Sytemic lupus erythematosus and acute intermittent porphyria should be excluded.

8.3 CHRONIC DEMYELINATING NEUROPATHY

Electrical appraisal should identify whether there is uniform slowing of conduction, without block, or more patchy change with evidence of block. The former favours a familial disorder, particularly Type 1 hereditary motor and sensory neuropathy. Confirmation of a familial basis requires not simply a meticulous family history but, for many cases, clinical and electrophysiological appraisal of relatives[15]. Where the demyelinating neuropathy is associated with deafness, icthiosis and retinitis pigmentosa, Refsum's disease requires exclusion by the estimation of urinary phytanic acid. A demyelinating neuropathy of varying degree, with conduction block, is sometimes seen as the chronic counterpart of the Guillain–Barré syndrome (Fig. 8.1). HLA testing in these patients suggests an increased incidence of certain antigens, notably B8 and DRW3. It is also seen in association with monoclonal gammopathy, particularly of IgM type[16,17], and with Waldenstrom's macroglobulinaemia[18]. Osteosclerotic myeloma is a rarity but at least 50% of cases display a neuropathy of a similar type. Most of these myeloma cases have a serum or urine monoclonal protein, but, in some 25%, the diagnosis can be established only by radiological survey[19].

8.3.1 Recommendation

If a chronic variant of Guillain-Barré syndrome is suspected, CSF examination is worthwhile, since the protein concentration is likely to be elevated. Before proceeding to nerve biopsy, protein studies and skeletal survey are required to exclude a dysproteinaemia. Nerve biopsy reveals segmental demyelination with perivascular mononuclear cells. Where a familial basis for a chronic demyelinating neuropathy is suspected, meticulous examination and electrophysiological investigation of family members is indicated.

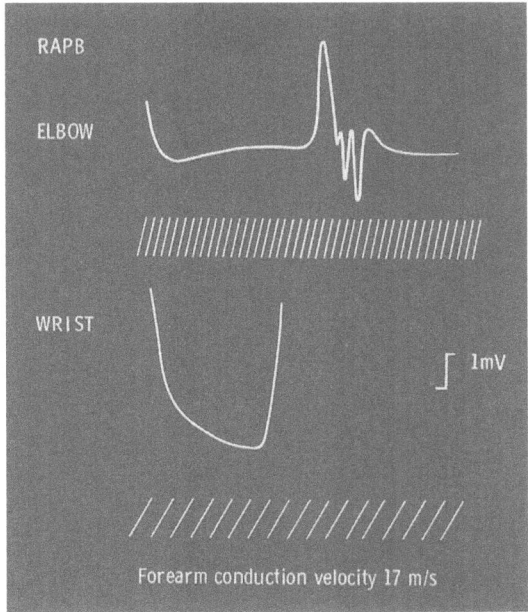

Fig. 8.1 Motor conduction studies in the right median nerve in a patient with Guillain–Barré syndrome

8.4 AXONAL AND MIXED NEUROPATHIES

It has to be recognized that in most patients presenting with a gradually evolving neuropathy the aetiological agent is not immediately apparent. Despite a considerable literature on the subject, the extent to which such patients should be investigated remains controversial. An extensive study by Prineas tends to defy analysis[20]. Of 278 cases of polyneuropathy, 107 were labelled as idiopathic, though of these, 69 appear to have had acute or chronic forms of Guillain–Barré syndrome, suggesting that 38 or 13.7% remained undiagnosed. However, within the 278 cases were 16 patients with 'atypical or doubtful forms' and 15 with 'neurological disorders simulating polyneuropathy'! The confusion is increased by the inclusion of a further 91 cases who were admitted for investigation. Of these, 32% were considered to be idiopathic. Familial disorders (including porphyria) accounted for 4.3% of the 278 cases. A recent, influential, paper considered that intensive evaluation of

Table 8.1 Diagnostic yield of various investigations
performed in a group of patients with polyneuropathy [22]

Investigation	Normal	Abnormal
Haemoglobin	89	2
Differential blood count	91	0
ESR	90	1
Platelet count	80	0
Creatinine	89	2
Bilirubin	87	0
Alkaline phosphatase	87	0
AST	91	0
ALT	88	3
Calcium	82	1
Albumin	79	4
B_{12}	89	2
Folate	83	1
ANF	78	1
Rheumatoid factor	76	4
TSH	52	0
Protein electrophoresis	65	14
Urine – albumin	89	2
– glucose	91	0
GTT	76	15
Chest X-ray	74	1

cases of peripheral neuropathy could discover the aetiology in
76% [15]. It was suggested that complaints of paraesthesiae or limb
discomfort were less frequent in the inherited neuropathies, which
accounted for 42% of the total. Great weight was attached to the
necessity for examination and investigation of relatives if the
diagnosis of a familial neuropathy was to be established. Sadly, the
authors failed to indicate the age distribution, what was the yield of
individual investigations, what proportion had nerve biopsy, and
how many had mononeuritis multiplex. Remarkably, nearly two-
thirds of the cases had either an inherited or inflammatory demyelinating neuropathy.

A study of 519 patients, all of whom had sural nerve biopsy, has
been reported [21]. Here, as in the other papers [15,20] no attempt
was made initially to classify the cases on electrophysiological
criteria. Though 67 patients remained undiagnosed, this number fell
to 50 (10% of the total) during a period of follow-up. Familial

Table 8.2 Initial investigation of a patient
with polyneuropathy

Haemoglobin
Full blood count
ESR
Calcium
Creatinine
Fasting glucose or GTT
Protein electrophoresis
Urinalysis
B_{12}
Chest X-ray

---

and inflammatory neuropathies accounted for 226 cases (43.5%).
The mean age at onset of symptoms was 50.6 years. No indication
was provided of the diagnostic yield from each of the investigations
performed, including the mandatory sural nerve biopsy. A more
valuable report in some ways, since it analyses the results of each of
the investigations performed, is that by Fagius [22]. The conclusions
could hardly be more different. Of 91 cases, all of whom had
developed symptoms in adult life, 74% were left without a diagnosis.
Cases of inflammatory polyneuropathy were exluded. Electrophysiological tests were performed in all the cases, but none had
sural nerve biopsy. Two cases were thought to have a familial
neuropathy though the author fails to indicate how rigorously the
search for a genetic basis was pursued. There is some value in
detailing the yield of the investigations performed (Table 8.1). How
valuable sural nerve biopsy would have been in this analysis can only
be conjectured. Biopsy can establish that a neuropathy is due to
amyloid, vasculitis or leprosy. It is clear, however, that the diagnostic
yield of performing nerve biopsy in a distal symmetrical polyneuropathy, whether subacute or chronic, axonal or demyelinating, once
appropriate screening tests have been performed, is unacceptably
low [23].

8.4.1 Recommendation

The symptomatology of peripheral neuropathy is of limited value in
assessing pathogenesis, though certain sensory symptoms are uncommon in the familial neuropathies. Exclusion of toxic factors
requires a meticulous history related to possible exposure. The

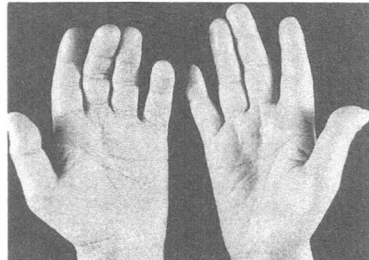 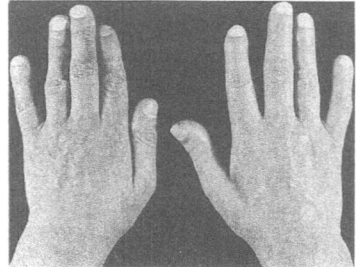

Fig. 8.2 Appearance of the hands in a patient with a mononeuritis multiplex principally affecting, in the upper limbs, the muscles supplied by the median nerves

establishment of a genetic basis for a neuropathy will require, in many instances, examination and investigation of family members. The vexed question of how far investigations should proceed is not readily answered from inspection of the literature. A limited group of tests can be recommended, with initial electrophysiological appraisal essential as a guide to mechanisms and distribution (Table 8.2). Sural nerve biopsy is only seldom justified.

8.5 MONONEURITIS MULTIPLEX

In mononeuritis multiplex, multiple individual peripheral nerves are affected. Leprosy is perhaps the commonest world-wide cause of this syndrome, though the disease is seldom encountered in the United Kingdom. Other causes include sarcoidosis, the dysproteinaemias, collagen vascular disease, and vasculitis, though all these conditions, including vasculitis[24] can produce a generalized neuropathy (Fig. 8.2). Screening tests for these conditions should be performed. Sural nerve biopsy may be necessary.

8.6 AUTONOMIC NEUROPATHY

Autonomic failure may occur in isolation, in association with other neurological disorders (either a pure Parkinsonian syndrome or multi-system atrophy) or as a complication of a systemic disorder, in particular diabetes. Failure of blood pressure control leads to increasingly severe postural hypotension. A vast array of tests has been devised to assess autonomic function[25] though, for most patients, the information obtained is of academic rather than therapeutic importance. Non-invasive tests of autonomic function have been developed, particularly for the study of diabetic patients. In general, disturbances of parasympathetic function are encountered more often than disturbances of sympathetic function. Continuous ECG recording during the Valsalva manoeuvre enables comparison of the R-R interval after the manoeuvre (as a measure of maximum bradycardia) with that during the procedure (as a measure of maximum tachycardia). In normal individuals, the ratio exceeds 1.20. Variation in heart-rate during deep breathing is controlled by vagal activity. In normal individuals, during slow deep inspiration and expiration, at a rate of six breaths per minute, the heart rate varies by at least 15 beats/minute, whereas, in the presence of autonomic neuropathy, the variation is less than 10 beats/minute. Measurements are taken from the ECG [26]. The increased heart rate that occurs after standing reaches a maximum about 15 beats later, followed by a slowing which peaks at about 30 beats. Again, the ratio is measurable from the ECG (30 : 15 ratio) by measuring R-R intervals. The normal exceeds 1.04 [27]. Sustained hand grip results in increased blood pressure in normal individuals. An increase in diastolic pressure of at least 15 mmHg occurs during hand grip over a maximum period of 5 minutes. In autonomic failure, the increase is lacking.

8.6.1 Recommendation

The above four screening tests, combined with measurement of postural hypotension, have proved of value in the assessment of early autonomic failure in diabetic patients. They are probably equally valid for the investigation of other causes of autonomic failure. More sophisticated tests of autonomic function are described, including measurement of sweating and pupillary responses, and the use of intra-arterial recording devices, but none can be recommended for screening purposes.

8.7 ENTRAPMENT NEUROPATHY

Entrapment neuropathy can result from compression of a nerve within a rigid canal (carpal tunnel syndrome), excessive angulation and stretch (a contributory factor to ulnar nerve lesions at the elbow), external pressure (for example with a radial nerve palsy at the level of the spiral groove) or from a combination of factors.

Short-lived compression of nerve causes damage predominantly from mechanical effects associated with local demyelination and conduction block. More chronic compression, though also leading to demyelination, is likely to result in Wallerian degeneration, with a corresponding influence on outcome.

Carpal tunnel syndrome is the commonest entrapment neuropathy, followed by ulnar nerve lesions at the level of the elbow. Though many entrapment neuropathies are readily diagnosed by clinical criteria, confirmation of the diagnosis, and localization of the site of compression, require electrophysiological investigation. The development of certain entrapment syndromes is accelerated by the presence of particular systemic disorders which may require exclusion.

8.7.1 The carpal tunnel syndrome

(a) Investigations

Electrophysiological investigation is vital in the diagnosis of carpal tunnel syndrome. Pathognomonic features include distal slowing of sensory conduction and distal slowing of motor conduction to APB. Varying recording techniques have led to some confusion in the literature regarding the most sensitive method. Generally abnormalities of sensory conduction are more common than those of motor conduction[28]. Sometimes a delay in sensory conduction is confined to a single digit. Repeating the tests after prolonged wrist flexion can increase the diagnostic yield[29]. In some studies, an alteration in the median/ulnar SAP amplitude ratio (normally greater than 1.1) has provided evidence for the presence of a carpal tunnel syndrome when other parameters were normal or minimally altered[30]. Since the major site of slowing in this condition is in the wrist segment, conduction studies have been performed by stimulating the nerve in the palm and recording at the wrist[31,32]. In one analysis of 72 cases, a prolonged distal latency to APB was found in 33%, a prolonged sensory action potential latency in 24%, but significant slowing of conduction in the palm to wrist fibres in 67% [32]. It is suggested that the procedure is no more painful than standard sensory techniques. Any evidence of denervation, a relatively uncommon finding, should be restricted to the muscles of the thenar eminence.

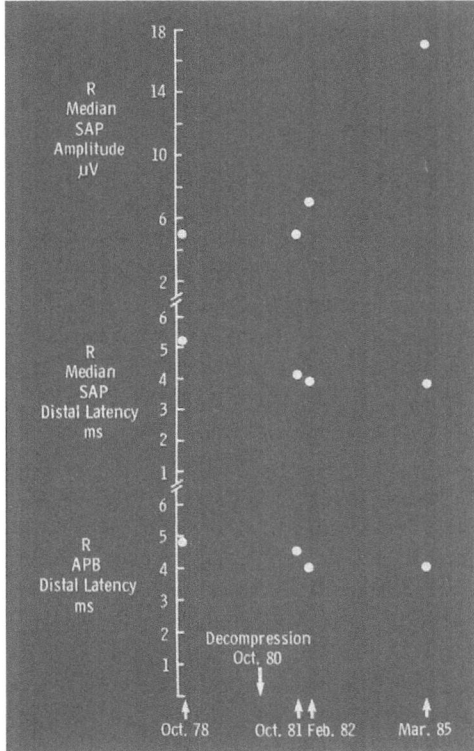

Fig. 8.3 Sequential EMG studies following carpal tunnel decompression

(b) Recommendation

Routine EMG findings are quite often normal in cases diagnosed clinically as carpal tunnel syndrome, even if sensory studies have included stimulation of all relevant digits. The diagnostic yield is improved if measurement of sensory conduction over the palm–wrist segment of the nerve is performed. Following decompression, recovery of nerve conduction to normal can be delayed over several months (Fig. 8.3). Acromegaly, myxoedema and rheumatoid arthritis may require exclusion.

8.7.2 Median nerve lesions at the elbow

Median nerve lesions at the elbow more often lead to evidence of denervation in muscles innervated by the nerve than changes in conduction studies in the forearm[28]. In the anterior interosseous syndrome, however, distal latency to pronator quadratus is prolonged with a normal latency to APB[33].

8.7.3 Ulnar nerve lesions at the elbow

Measurement techniques have been particularly critical in appraising abnormalities of conduction in the ulnar nerve. In normal subjects, with the elbow extended , conduction velocity across the elbow segment is slower than for the segment above or below. The slowing diminishes or disappears with the elbow flexed[34]. In a group of normal subjects, measuring motor conduction with the elbow flexed to 135°, velocity across the elbow exceeded 49 m/s, and did not fall short of the velocity in the forearm by more than 11.4 m/s. Similar findings were obtained for sensory conduction. The effects of elbow posture have been attributed to errors in measurement of nerve length with the elbow extended. Velocity measurement based on nerve segments of less than 10 cm, or with conduction times less than 2.5 ms, are susceptible to a high degree of error[34,35]. Absence of the ulnar sensory action potential at the wrist is a poor guide to the presence of an ulnar nerve lesion at the elbow[36]. Combining sensory and motor studies, slowing across the elbow was found in 95% of 63 cases with a mixed motor and sensory ulnar neuropathy[36]. On occasions motor slowing is confined to fibres supplying either the dorsal interossei or the hypothenar eminence. Clinical involvement of the forearm flexors is uncommon with ulnar nerve lesions at the elbow. One series, of 68 cases, reported weakness of flexor carpi ulnaris in five, and electrical evidence of denervation in eight. Despite this, measurement of latency to the muscle following stimulation 2 cm above the medial epicondyle showed abnormalities in 82.4% of cases[37]. Almost all patients with normal latencies had sensory deficits alone of short duration. These findings have been confirmed subsequently[36]. Measurement of change in the amplitude of the compound muscle action potential from the hypothenar eminence with stimulation of the ulnar nerve below and above the elbow has proved of disappointing value in localizing the site of entrapment[36].

(a) Recommendation

Measurement of sensory and motor conduction velocities across the elbow is well established as a sensitive guide to the presence of an ulnar nerve lesion at that level. The only additional electrophysiological test of value is the estimation of latency to flexor carpi ulnaris following stimulation of the ulnar nerve above the sulcus.

8.7.4 Distal ulnar nerve lesions

Ulnar nerve lesions in the hand are rare compared to those at a more proximal level. According to the site of involvement, there may be involvement of all the small hand muscles supplied by the nerve, with or without sensory loss, or weakness of the small hand muscles save those of the hypothenar eminence, and no sensory loss. Electrophysiological tests indicate marked distal slowing to the relevant hand muscles, with little or no alteration of conduction velocity in more proximal segments [38].

8.7.5 Radial nerve palsy

The majority of radial nerve palsies are the result of external pressure on the nerve at the level of the spiral groove. Most of these result in local conduction block alone, but more profound trauma results in Wallerian degeneration. In the former case, distal motor latency and sensory conduction velocity between wrist and elbow is likely to be normal, with slowing of conduction between the axilla and elbow [39]. In the latter, the sensory action potential is absent and no motor response is obtained from brachioradialis and the forearm extensors, both of which display denervation on sampling.

8.7.6 Brachial plexus neuropathy

The electrophysiological changes in brachial plexus neuropathy depend to some extent on its pathogenesis. In neuralgic amyotrophy distal conduction studies tend to be normal. Assessment of sensory conduction by recording from Erb's point is more likely to demonstrate abnormalities, as is measurement of the compound action potential from biceps following stimulation of musculocutaneous nerve fibres at Erb's point [40]. Where the brachial plexopathy results from trauma, irradiation or neoplastic infiltration, there is a high incidence of abnormal findings from assessment of musculocutaneous nerve function and loss of distal sensory action potentials is more common than in cases of neuralgic amyotrophy [40]. In both groups, denervation of affected muscle is common, but is lacking in cervical paraspinal muscles. CT scanning of the brachial plexus can

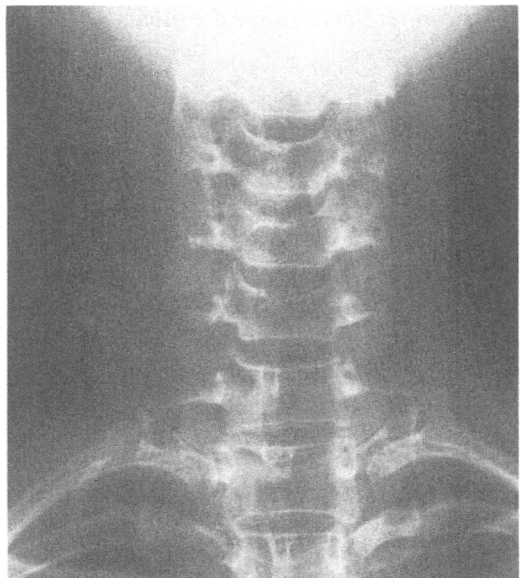

Fig. 8.4 Cervical spine X-ray demonstrating a right cervical rib and an elongated left C7 transverse process

aid differentiation of plexopathies secondary to irradiation from those due to neoplastic infiltration. The former produce a diffuse loss of soft tissue planes, the latter are identified by the presence of a circumscribed mass[41].

8.7.7 Thoracic outlet syndrome

The thoracic outlet syndrome results from stretching of the lower trunk of the brachial plexus (or its constituent roots) by a cervical rib or fibrous band passing from the C7 transverse process to the first rib (Fig. 8.4). Curiously the small hand muscle weakness and wasting which eventually develop predominantly affect the thenar eminence. Standard peripheral nerve conduction studies reveal an absent or depressed ulnar sensory action potential at the wrist, a delayed F wave recorded from abductor digiti minimi and evidence of denervation in the small hand muscles[42]. It is clear that the classical syndrome, described by Gilliatt and others[43], is rare, and that most patients with a cervical band have pain or paraesthesiae in the hand but little or no abnormality on physical examination. Normality of ulnar sensory action potentials and F waves is likely and has led to assessment of somatosensory evoked potentials as an alternative means to diagnosis. One study included 11 patients, all of whom had cervical ribs proven radiologically. In seven patients, there was pain and paraesthesiae alone, accompanied in the remainder by physical signs. Somatosensory responses following median and ulnar stimulation at the wrist were recorded from Erb's point (N9) and over the spinous process of C2 (N13). In seven patients, the responses were normal. In the remainder, some showed a normal N9 response but an abnormal or absent N13, the rest showed attenuation and prolongation of both N9 and N13 [44]. A further report of 18 patients, all of whom had normal radiological studies, indicated that 14 had symptoms alone, and, of the remainder, only one had motor deficit. Of 15 patients who had abnormal somatosensory responses, 12 had a depressed amplitude of N9 [45].

Recommendation

Radiological studies of the cervical spine are valuable in the diagnosis of the thoracic outlet syndrome associated with a cervical band. If there are classic features of the condition, studies of the ulnar SAP and F wave often suffice to confirm the diagnosis. Where there are prominent symptoms but a paucity of physical findings, these electrophysiological tests are usually normal. In such cases evaluation of somatosensory responses is likely to be of value, though a characteristic pattern of abnormality, and its relationship to clinical patterns of presentation, has yet to be established.

8.7.8 Sciatic nerve lesions

The sciatic nerve is susceptible to injury from trauma to the buttock or hip, intramuscular injections into the buttock and prolonged external pressure on the thigh, for example during drug-induced coma (Fig. 8.5). Normal conduction studies for the sciatic nerve have been published, employing stimulation at the gluteal fold (better with needle electrodes) with recording electrodes over the medial head of gastrocnemius [46].

8.7.9 Femoral nerve lesions

Proximal femoral nerve lesions, at the level of the psoas sheath, are often the result of haematoma, the consequence, for example, of

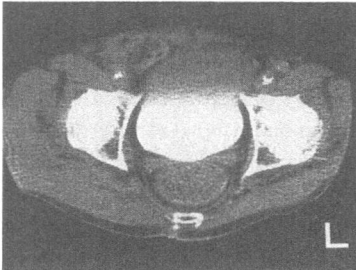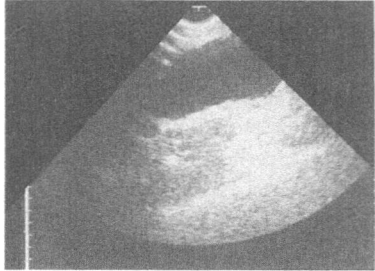

Fig. 8.5 CT scan (left) and ultrasound (right) of the buttock in a patient with a sciatic palsy secondary to a haematoma

anticoagulant therapy. More distal femoral nerve lesions can result from operative trauma. The femoral neuropathy of diabetics is more often a lumbar radiculopathy secondary to vasculitis. Normal values for conduction velocities have been calculated from a stimulation point just below the inguinal ligament to several levels in the quadriceps femoris[47].

Since both femoral and sciatic nerve palsies can result from haemorrhage within the pelvis, or in the thigh, CT scanning or ultrasound examination can be helpful in their evaluation.

8.7.10 Common peroneal lesions

The common peroneal nerve is particularly susceptible to external pressure as it winds round the neck of the fibula. Along with the lateral cutaneous nerve of thigh, it is the commonest nerve in the lower limb to be affected by a mononeuropathy. In a recent study, localization of a peroneal nerve lesion to the level of the knee was best achieved by measuring the fall in amplitude of the common muscle action potential recorded from extensor digitorum brevis following stimulation at the ankle, neck of fibula and popliteal fossa. In 61% of cases, the fall in amplitude exceeded 20%. An additional criterion, a fall in motor conduction velocity across the knee of more than 6 m/s, did not increase the diagnostic yield[48].

8.7.11 The tarsal tunnel syndrome

Compression of the posterior tibial nerve, or its branches, the medial and lateral plantar nerves, at the level of the flexor retinaculum in the foot results in paraesthesiae and burning discomfort in the distribution of the nerve, often associated with a positive Tinel's sign at the ankle. Techniques designed to assist diagnosis include measurement of distal motor latency to abductor hallucis (for the medial plantar nerve) and to abductor digiti minimi (for the lateral plantar nerve) together with measurement of sensory action potentials at the ankle following stimulation of the first and fifth toes. The discovery of denervation in the small foot muscles supplied by the nerve has to be interpreted with caution, since this can sometimes be detected in normal individuals. In a comparison of the diagnostic yield of motor and sensory studies, abnormal distal motor latencies were found in 52.4% of 17 subjects, but abnormal sensory nerve conduction (either absent or delayed potentials) in 90.5%. In some cases, abnormalities were confined to one of the constituent branches of the posterior tibial nerve[49]. If, in addition to measurement of sensory action potentials from the first and fifth toes, corresponding potentials from the interdigital nerves are assessed., the percentage of patients with abnormal findings rises to 96[50].

Recommendation

Electrophysiological investigation is essential for the diagnosis of the tarsal tunnel syndrome. Sensory studies are more productive than motor and should include, as a minimum, measurement of the medial and lateral plantar sensory action potentials following stimulation of the first and fifth toes.

8.7.12 Interdigital neuropathy (Morton's metatarsalgia)

The common plantar digital nerves are liable to entrapment by the deep transverse ligaments between the heads of the metatarsals. The nerve most commonly affected is that between the third and fourth metatarsals. The patient, usually female, experiences pain in the foot, exacerbated by walking or standing. The digital neuroma, described by Morton, is a pseudoneuroma proximal to the site of entrapment. Sensory loss is sometimes detectable in the toe clefts. The interdigital nerves can be stimulated, either with surface electrodes designed simultaneously to activate adjacent branches[51] or with needle electrodes[52]. The potentials are recorded with needle electrodes close to the posterior tibial nerve above the flexor retinaculum. Abnormalities, confined to the relevant digital nerve, include slowing of conduction, an abnormal wave form, and an absent or reduced amplitude of the action potential. There is a good correlation between the electrophysiological findings and evidence of entrapment at the time of surgery[52].

REFERENCES

1. Kimura, J. (1984) Principles and pitfalls of nerve conduction studies. *Ann. Neurol.*, **16**, 415–29.
2. Gilliatt, R.W. (1982) Electrophysiology of peripheral neuropathies – an overview. *Muscle Nerve*, **5**, S108–16.
3. Lamontagne, A. and Buchthal, F. (1970) Electrophysiological studies in diabetic neuropathy. *J. Neurol. Neurosurg. Psychiatry*, **33**, 442–52.
4. Burke, D., Skuse, N.F. and Lethlean, A.K. (1974) Sensory conduction of the sural nerve in polyneuropathy. *J. Neurol. Neurosurg. Psychiatry*, **37**, 647–52.
5. Kayser-Gatchalian, M.C. and Neundörfer, B. (1984) Sural nerve conduction in mild polyneuropathy. *J. Neurol.*, **231**, 122–5.
6. Kayed, K. and Røsjø, Ø. (1983) Two-segment sural nerve conduction measurement in polyneuropathy. *J. Neurol. Neurosurg. Psychiatry*, **46**, 867–70.
7. Guiloff, R.J. and Sherratt, R.M. (1977) Sensory conduction in medial plantar nerve. *J. Neurol. Neurosurg. Psychiatry*, **40**, 1168–81.
8. Lachman, T., Shahani, B.T. and Young, R.R. (1980) Late responses as aids to diagnosis in peripheral neuropathy. *J. Neurol. Neurosurg. Psychiatry*, **43**, 156–62.
9. Lewis, R.A. and Sumner, A.J. (1982) The electrodiagnostic distinctions between chronic familial and acquired demyelinating neuropathies. *Neurology*, **32**, 592–6.
10. Asbury, A.K. (1981) Diagnostic considerations in Guillain–Barré syndrome. *Ann. Neurol.*, **9** (Suppl), 1–5.
11. Kimura, J. and Butzer, J.F. (1975) F-wave conduction velocity in Guillain–Barré syndrome. Assessment of nerve segment between axilla and spinal cord. *Arch. Neurol.*, **32**, 524–9.
12. Posner, C.M. (1981) Criteria for the diagnosis of the Guillain–Barré syndrome. A critique of the NINCDS guidelines. *J. Neurol. Sci.*, **52**, 191–9.
13. Dowling, P.C., Bosch, V.V., Cook, S.D. and Chmel, H. (1982) Serum immunoglobulins in Guillain–Barré syndrome. *J. Neurol. Sci.*, **57**, 435–40.
14. Kaldor, J. and Speed, B.R. (1984) Guillain–Barré syndrome and *campylobacter jejuni*: A serological study. *Br. Med. J.*, **288**, 1867–70.
15. Dyck, P.J., Oviatt, K.F. and Lambert, E.H. (1981) Intensive evaluation of referred unclassified neuropathies yields improved diagnosis. *Ann. Neurol.*, **10**, 222–6.

16. Kelly, J.J. Jr (1983) The electrodiagnostic findings in peripheral neuropathy associated with monoclonal gammopathy. *Muscle Nerve*, 6, 504–9.
17. Smith, I.S., Kahn, S.N., Lacey, B.W. *et al.* (1983) Chronic demyelinating neuropathy associated with benign IgM paraproteinaemia. *Brain*, 106, 169–95.
18. Kelly, J.J. Jr, Kyle, R.A., O'Brien, P.C. and Dyck, P.J. (1981) Prevalence of monoclonal protein in peripheral neuropathy. *Neurology*, 31, 1480–3.
19. Kelly, J.J. Jr, Kyle, R.A., Miles, J.M. and Dyck, P.J. (1983) Osteosclerotic myeloma and peripheral neuropathy. *Neurology*, 33, 202–10.
20. Prineas, J. (1970) Polyneuropathies of undetermined cause. *Acta Neurol. Scand.*, Suppl. 44, 1–72.
21. McLeod, J.G., Tuck, R.R., Pollard, J.D. *et al.* (1984) Chronic polyneuropathy of undetermined cause. *J. Neurol. Neurosurg. Psychiatry*, 47, 530–5.
22. Fagius, J. (1983) Chronic cryptogenic polyneuropathy. *Acta Neurol. Scand.*, 67, 173–80.
23. Asbury, A.K. and Gilliatt, R.W. (1984) The clinical approach to neuropathy. in *Peripheral Nerve Disorders. A Practical Approach*, (ed. A.K. Asbury and R.W. Gilliatt), Butterworths, London, pp. 1–20.
24. Kissel, J.T., Slivka, A.P., Warmolts, J.R. and Mendell, J.R. (1985) The clinical spectrum of necrotizing angiopathy of the peripheral nervous system. *Ann. Neurol.*, 18, 251–7.
25. Testing autonomic reflexes. In *Autonomic Failure*. (ed. R. Bannister), Oxford University Press, 1983, pp. 52–63.
26. Hilsted, J. and Jensen, S.B. (1979) A simple test for autonomic neuropathy in juvenile diabetics. *Acta Med. Scand.*, 205, 385–7.
27. Ewing, D.J., Campbell, I.W., Murray, A. *et al.* (1978) Immediate heart-rate response to standing: simple test for autonomic neuropathy in diabetes. *Br. Med. J.*, 1, 145–7.
28. Buchthal, F., Rosenfalck, A. and Trojaborg, W. (1974) Electrophysiological findings in entrapment of the median nerve at wrist and elbow. *J. Neurol. Neurosurg. Psychiatry*, 37, 340–60.
29. Schwartz, M.S., Gordon, J.A. and Swash, M. (1980) Slowed nerve conduction with wrist flexion in carpal tunnel syndrome. *Ann. Neurol.*, 8, 69–71.
30. Loong, S.C. (1977) The carpal tunnel syndrome: A clinical and electrophysiological study in 250 patients. *Proc. Aust. Assoc. Neurol.*, 14, 51–65.
31. Tackmann, W., Kaeser, H.E. and Magun, H.G. (1981) Comparison of orthodromic and antidromic sensory nerve conduction velocity measurements in the carpal tunnel syndrome. *J. Neurol.*, 224, 257–66.
32. Mills, K.R. (1985) Orthodromic sensory action potentials from palmar stimulation in the diagnosis of carpal tunnel syndrome. *J. Neurol. Neurosurg. Psychiatry*, 48, 250–5.
33. Meya, U. and Hacke, W. (1983) Anterior interosseous nerve syndrome

following supracondylar lesions of the median nerve: clinical findings and electrophysiological investigations. *J. Neurol.*, **229**, 91–6.

34. Kincaid, J.C., Phillips, L.H. II and Daube, J.R. (1986) The evaluation of suspected ulnar neuropathy at the elbow. *Arch. Neurol.*, **43**, 44–7.
35. Eisen, A. (1974) Early diagnosis of ulnar nerve palsy. An electrophysiologic study. *Neurology*, **24**, 256–62.
36. Tackmann, W., Vogel, P., Kaeser, H.E. and Ettlin, Th. (1984) Sensitivity and localizing significance of motor and sensory electroneurographic parameters in the diagnosis of ulnar nerve lesions at the elbow. A reappraisal. *J. Neurol.*, **231**, 204–11.
37. Benecke, R. and Conrad, B. (1980) The value of electrophysiological examination of the flexor carpi ulnaris muscle in the diagnosis of ulnar nerve lesions at the elbow. *J. Neurol.*, **223**, 207–17.
38. Ebeling, P., Gilliatt, R.W. and Thomas, P.K. (1960) A clinical and electrical study of ulnar nerve lesions in the hand. *J. Neurol. Neurosurg. Psychiatry*, **23**, 1–9.
39. Trojaborg, W. (1970) Rate of recovery in motor and sensory fibres of the radial nerve: clinical and electrophysiological aspects. *J. Neurol. Neurosurg. Psychiatry*, **33**, 625–38.
40. Flaggman, P.D. and Kelly, J.J. Jr (1980) Brachial plexus neuropathy. An electrophysiologic evaluation. *Arch. Neurol.*, **37**, 160–4.
41. Cascino, T.L., Kori, S., Krol, G. and Foley, K.M. (1983) CT of the brachial plexus in patients with cancer. *Neurology*, **33**, 1553–7.
42. Yiannikas, C. and Walsh, J.C. (1983) Somatosensory evoked responses in the diagnosis of thoracic outlet syndrome. *J. Neurol. Neurosurg. Psychiatry*, **46**, 234–40.
43. Gilliatt, R.W., Le Quesne, P.M., Logue, V. and Sumner, A.J. (1970) Wasting of the hand associated with a cervical rib or band. *J. Neurol. Neurosurg. Psychiatry*, **33**, 615–24.
44. Yiannikas, C. and Walsh, J.C. (1983) Somatosensory evoked responses in the diagnosis of thoracic outlet syndrome. *J. Neurol. Neurosurg. Psychiatry*, **46**, 234–40.
45. Jerrett, S.A., Cuzzone, L.J. and Pasternak, B.M.(1984) Thoracic outlet syndrome. Electrophysiologic reappraisal. *Arch. Neurol.*, **41**, 960–3.
46. Yap, C.-B. and Hirota, T. (1967) Sciatic nerve motor conduction velocity study. *J. Neurol. Neurosurg. Psychiatry*, **30**, 233–9.
47. Gassel, M.M. (1963) A study of femoral nerve conduction time. *Arch. Neurol.*, **9**, 607–14.
48. Pickett, J.B. (1984) Localizing peroneal nerve lesions to the knee by motor conduction studies. *Arch. Neurol.*, **41**, 192–5.
49. Oh, S.J., Sarala, P.K., Kuba, T. and Elmore, R.S. (1979) Tarsal tunnel syndrome: electrophysiological study. *Ann. Neurol.*, **5**, 327–30.
50. Oh, S.J., Kim, H.S. and Ahmad, B.K. (1985) The near-near sensory nerve conduction in tarsal tunnel syndrome. *J. Neurol. Neurosurg. Psychiatry*, **48**, 999–1003.
51. Oh, S.J., Kim, H.S. and Ahmad, B.K. (1984) Electrophysiological diagnosis of interdigital neuropathy of the foot. *Muscle Nerve*, **7**, 218–25.

52. Falck, B., Hurme, M., Hakkarainen, S. and Aarnio, P. (1984) Sensory conduction velocity of plantar digital nerves in Morton's metatarsalgia. *Neurology*, **34**, 698–701.

9

Nerve root and muscle disease

9.1 RADICULOPATHY; PLEXOPATHY

In patients with limb pain associated with segmental sensory or motor abnormalities on examination, the diagnosis of radiculopathy is inescapable. Indeed, early discussion of the diagnosis of cervical and lumbar radiculopathy suggested that an accurate diagnosis was readily achieved by clinical examination supported by plain X-ray changes without recourse to contrast radiology. In one study, published in 1961, of patients with lumbar disc protrusions confirmed surgically, clinical diagnosis was correct in 77%. The lateral recess syndrome can prove a more troublesome diagnosis. Typically it causes severe leg pain characteristically triggered by standing or walking. Motor deficit on examination is common, but objective sensory change is unusual. The facet joint at L4/5 is the one most commonly affected. Lumbar canal stenosis is usually more readily diagnosed, almost all patients complaining of paroxysmal sensory symptoms, together with pain, during walking or standing. Neurological findings are often not prominent.

A variety of disorders can cause a brachial or lumbosacral plexopathy. The most troublesome dilemma in diagnosis occurs in patients with cancer who have had previous radiotherapy. Certain clinical characteristics help distinguish radiation from neoplastic plexopathy. The latter is more painful, more likely to be unilateral and to progress more rapidly. At times epidural metastases can closely simulate the effects of malignant plexopathy. A proximal, asymmetrical, lower limb weakness in diabetic patients has long been recognized. Though originally considered to be the consequence of femoral neuropathy, the almost inevitable finding of weakness of the thigh adductors indicates that the lesion is at plexus level. The finding of paraspinal fibrillations in some of these patients, and its association with elevated CSF protein levels, indicates that radicular involvement also occurs. Vasculitic and inflammatory disorders have been described as the cause of a lumbosacral plexopathy, both often accompanied by an elevated ESR. A lumbosacral plexus neuropathy, analogous to neuralgic amyotrophy, is characterized by pain followed by a predominant motor plexopathy. At times, the presence of paraspinal muscle denervation suggests an additional radicular component. Recently, a triad of polyradiculitis, cranial neuritis and meningitis has been described under various titles, including Lyme disease and Bannwarth's syndrome. Both conditions, which may, in fact, be identical, are caused by a Borrelia spirochaete transmitted by a tick bite. Additional clinical features include skin lesions, cardiac disturbances, and arthritis.

9.1.1 Investigations

(a) Plain X-rays

Interpretation of plain X-rays of the cervical and lumbar spine in patients with presumed radiculopathy must take account of the changes found in an age-matched control population. In a group of inpatients, over the age of 50, admitted for other neurological reasons, severe cervical canal narrowing was detected in 30%, and severe cervical foraminal narrowing in 12% [1]. Changes were as likely in those under as in those over the age of 65. The incidence of foraminal narrowing in patients with root signs was 82%. In an extensive population study of the frequency of cervical spondylosis, radiological evidence of a disc lesion (the criteria were not stated) was found in 83.5% of men, and 80.7% of women aged 55 or over [2]. In patients with suspected lumbar radiculopathy, less emphasis has been placed on the frequency of abnormal findings in asymptomatic individuals. In an early study, some abnormality on plain X-ray was detected in 66.9% of individuals who were subsequently shown to have a disc lesion at surgery [3]. Disc space narrowing, found in 31.2%, was found to correlate very closely with disc abnormalities at that level at the time of operation. Faith in the role of clinical evaluation, combined with plain X-rays, is typified by a review of 500 cases of lumbar disc protrusion treated surgically [4]. Plain X-rays indicated the presence and level of the protrusion in 57% and myelography was confined to 40 patients. Plain X-rays are less successful in confirming a diagnosis of the lateral recess

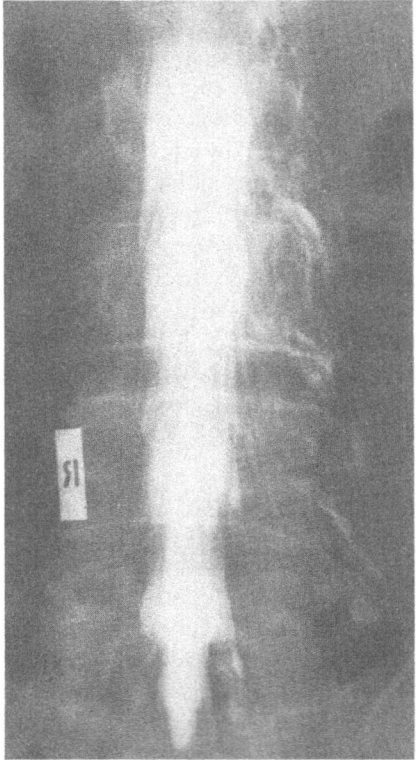

Fig. 9.1 Myelogram demonstrating L5 root compression (left sided)

syndrome but better results are achieved with lateral or transaxial polytomography of the lumbar spine[5]. Similarly, for patients with lumbar spinal stenosis, standard X-rays have proved of limited value[6] though, in an analysis of 68 patients, 70% had degenerative disc disease and 62% osteoarthritis of the facet joints[7]. Plain X-rays are helpful when attempting to distinguish radiation from tumour plexopathy of the pelvis. Changes are lacking in the former, but present in some 50% of the latter[8].

(b) Myelography

Until recently, the most definitive radiological procedure for the diagnosis of cervical or lumbar radiculopathy was myodil, and subsequently metrizamide, myelography. Whilst one analysis of lumbar disc prolapse identified myelographic abnormalities in 96%

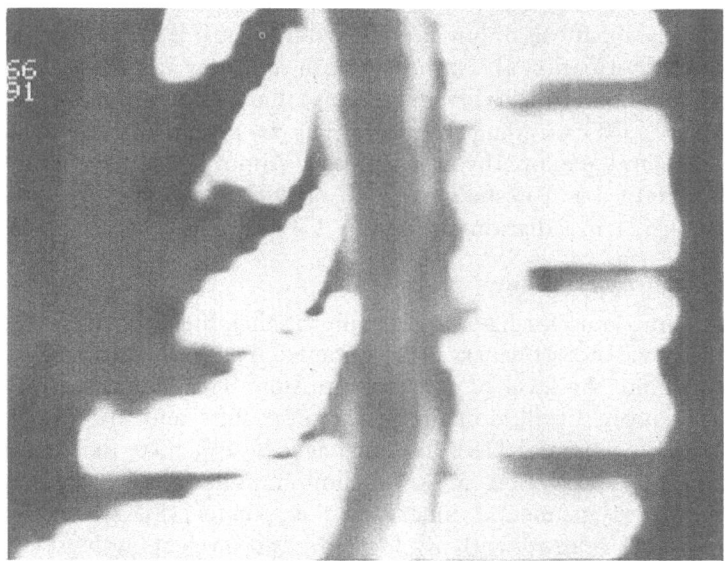

Fig. 9.2 CT with metrizamide demonstrating central disc protrusion at C5/6

of cases [9], another established abnormalities for L5/S1 disc herniations in 61.7%, but for L4/L5 herniations in 93.2% [10] (Fig. 9.1). In one prospective study, the sensitivity of myelography in the diagnosis of lumbar disc herniation was 75%, with a specificity of 90% [11]. When negative myelography coincides with the absence of neurological signs, the chance of finding a significant lumbar disc prolapse at surgery recedes further [12]. Myelography generally provides definitive evidence of lumbar canal stenosis [7]. Epidural metastases affecting the spinal cord or roots may mimic the features of malignant lumbosacral plexopathy. Myelography successfully demonstrates such lesions [13].

(c) CT scanning

It has been suggested that high-resolution CT scanning without contrast, is the investigation of choice for the evaluation of lumbar disc disease, lumbar canal stenosis and the lateral recess syndrome [14]. In one, prospective, comparison of CT with myelography the two methods achieved almost exactly the same level of diagnostic accuracy [15]. CT is probably superior to myelography in the diagnosis of lateral lumbar disc herniation [16]. CT scanning with metrizamide has not, as yet, replaced conventional myelography in the diagnosis of lumbar disc syndromes. It is likely to provide greater information about the extent of radicular and cord involvement secondary to cervical disc disease than can myelography (Fig. 9.2)[17]. CT scanning of the pelvis is essential if malignant lumbosacral plexopathy is suspected. Abnormalities include the presence of a soft-tissue mass with or without lymph node enlargement[13]. In radiation plexopathy, CT scanning is negative[8,13].

(d) Electrophysiology

Since limb muscles have a generally predictable segmental innervation, evidence of denervation, obtained by sampling, can be used to calculate the level of root compression. The evidence includes fasciculation, fibrillation, loss of motor units and an excess of polyphasic potentials[18]. Caution has to be applied to the interpretation of denervation in lower limb muscles, however, where variation in segmental innervation is greater[18]. In an early comparison of EMG with myelography and surgical findings, EMG correctly localized the relevant segment in 90.7% of cases, and myelography in 85.3%. Both cervical and lumbosacral disc protrusions were studied[19]. Among 48 patients with an L5/S1 disc protrusion, 80% had segmental denervation at the S1 level, whereas for 56 cases with an L4/L5 disc protrusion, 75.7% had segmental denervation of L5 muscles[10]. The same study concluded that segmental denervation might occur in the absence of clinical or myelographic evidence of root compression, and might suggest involvement at a single level alone when clinical examination had suggested more than one. When the localizing value of EMG has been compared with myelography, in patients with lumbar disc disease, the former has generally proved superior[20]. The yield of electromyography may be enhanced if paraspinal muscles are sampled. In one study, for patients with L5 root involvement, EMG abnormalities were confined to paraspinal muscles in a third[21]. Doubt has been expressed about the accuracy of a segmental prediction of denervation based on findings in muscles at a particular vertebral level. Furthermore, mono- and diphasic fibrillation recorded in spinal muscle may reflect normal spontaneous activity of the motor end-plate region[18]. Despite this, it has been suggested that sampling of muscle 2–3 cm from the midline and at a depth exceeding 3 cm allows prediction of segmental changes based on the adjacent vertebral level[21]. Sampling of paraspinal muscles carries an additional advantage. In disease processes affecting the lumbo-sacral plexus, abnormalities in the paraspinal muscles will be lacking[22,23]. Furthermore, sampling of limb muscles in such cases reveals denervation in muscles innervated by at least two lumbo-sacral segments and supplied by at least two peripheral nerves[22]. In irradiation plexopathy, on the other hand, more widespread damage may be reflected by evidence of paraspinal denervation. Furthermore, myokymia is encountered on sampling of lower limb muscles in the majority[8].

Evaluation of peripheral conduction can also be of value in the differential diagnosis of radiculopathy and plexopathy. Cervical root compression is almost always preganglionic, resulting in preservation of median and ulnar sensory action potentials[24]. Comparison of F and M wave latencies provides a reliable guide to the presence of proximal nerve or root entrapment in the upper limb. Thus, an absent F wave, recorded from APB or ADM, or one with slowed conduction between spinal cord and elbow, in the presence of normal conduction between elbow and wrist is indicative of a proximal lesion[25]. Besides root compression due to disc disease, the technique can detect evidence of metastatic root involve-ment[26]. H-reflex latency obtained by stimulating the median nerve at the elbow and recording from flexor carpi radialis with needle electrodes was abnormal in 17 of 24 C6 or C7 root lesions (confirmed myelographically) but normal in root lesions affecting C5 or C8[27]. In a comparable lower limb study, of 20 patients with a surgically confirmed S1 root lesion, 18 had an abnormal H index, calculated as (height of subject in cm ÷ time interval H-M in ms)^2 × 2. The other two had an abnormal index compared to the normal side[28]. When conduction studies are performed in the peroneal nerve, the nerve action potential is likely to be absent in lumbosacral plexopathy but present in the case of an L5 radiculo-pathy[29]. Evidence of abnormal conduction in the cauda equina can be obtained by the use of transcutaneous spinal stimulation at the L1 and L4 vertebral levels, with recording from puborectalis via an electrode inserted in the rectum[30].

Measurement of somatosensory responses has proved disappoint-ing in the evaluation of radiculopathy. In 12 patients with clinical evidence of cervical radiculopathy, confirmed by myelography in ten, the N14 amplitude was depressed with prolongation of N9/N14 conduction time[31]. In a more recent study, however, somato-sensory responses recorded from the supraclavicula fossa (N9), over the seventh cervical vertebra (N13) and over the cortex (N20) following stimulation of the median and ulnar nerves, failed to correlate with radiological changes or clinical features of radiculopathy [32].

Dermatomal somatosensory responses have been analysed in patients with unilateral lumbosacral radiculopathy. The lesion was correctly identified by the technique in a quarter of the patients. Peroneal somatosensory responses were normal in all of them [33]. A comparison of EMG, late responses and somatosensory potentials has been performed in patients with lumbosacral radiculopathy [34]. Peroneal somatosensory responses were normal in all patients, and, whilst dermatomal somatosensory responses were abnormal in 25%, all these patients had clearly defined sensory changes in the distribution of the affected or adjacent nerve root. Other authors have claimed a higher yield from dermatomal responses, but only by using less rigid criteria for abnormality. Abnormal F wave responses were found in five of 28 patients, and an abnormal H reflex in approximately 50%. Segmental denervation, however, found in 75% was often the only abnormal electrophysiological finding and was sometimes abnormal in the absence of any clinical signs.

(e) Other investigations

CSF examination is of limited value in the investigation of radiculopathy. It was normal in 216 of 296 patients in one series [9]. Generally the only abnormality discovered is a modest increase in protein concentration. Similarly a mild increase in protein concentration may occur in both irradiation and tumour plexopathy [8]. In patients with diabetic proximal neuropathy, an elevated protein concentration correlates with the presence of paraspinal fibrillation [35]. The neuropathic complications of diabetes are mixed, some patients presenting with the acute onset of a picture resembling lumbar plexopathy. Evidence of a more generalized neuropathy may be lacking. Besides, therefore, performing glucose tolerance in patients with acute onset lumbar plexopathy, other diagnostic possibilities have to be considered. A painful lumbosacral plexopathy associated with an elevated ESR has been described [23]. The findings on sural nerve biopsy suggested an inflammatory disorder. A vasculitic syndrome can produce a similar picture [23]. In Lyme disease, the CSF is inflammatory with a predominantly lymphocytic pleocytosis [36]. In addition the IgG and IgM indices are elevated with an oligoclonal IgG pattern [37]. IgM and IgG antibodies to

Borrelia burgdorferi are elevated in both serum and CSF in typical cases[38]. An association with HLA-DR2 is described[39].

9.1.2 Recommendations (see flow chart A)

9.2 RADICULOPATHY

In patients with a clinically typical radicular syndrome, plain X-rays of the spine are valuable for identification of cervical disc disease but less so for lumbar spondylosis. The radiological procedure of choice for cervical radiculopathy is probably CT scanning with metrizamide, with conventional myelography the alternative. For lumbar radiculopathy, plain CT is the investigation of choice, if availaible, followed by myelography if the findings are uncertain. If CT is unavailable, conventional myelography is required. For the lateral recess syndrome, and spinal stenosis, CT scanning is often diagnostic. The alternative procedure for the former is polytomography of the spine. For the latter, metrizamide CT or myelography are diagnostic. If the radicular signs are less clear cut, electrophysiological investigation is of value. Probably the most sensitive technique is EMG to elicit evidence of segmental denervation. Demonstration of abnormalities in paraspinal muscles favours a radicular rather than plexus lesion. Tests of peripheral conduction will be normal. Measurement of F and H wave latencies are worthwhile, though, in most hands, they provide less diagnostic information than EMG. Somatosensory evoked responses have generally proved disappointing in the diagnosis of cervical and lumbar radiculopathy.

9.3 LUMBOSACRAL PLEXOPATHY

Clinical appraisal may indicate the likelihood of a plexus rather than root syndrome. EMG is invaluable in such cases. Peripheral conduction studies are appropriate and are likely to be abnormal. EMG is required to indicate the extent of segmental denervation. For most conditions causing plexopathy (though not irradiation or diabetes) denervation of paraspinal muscles will be lacking. CT scanning of the plexus is required and will generally provide diagnostic information in cases of neoplastic plexopathy. Glucose tolerance should be tested to exclude diabetes. An elevated ESR suggests neoplastic plexopathy, vasculitis, or the syndrome of inflammatory plexopathy.

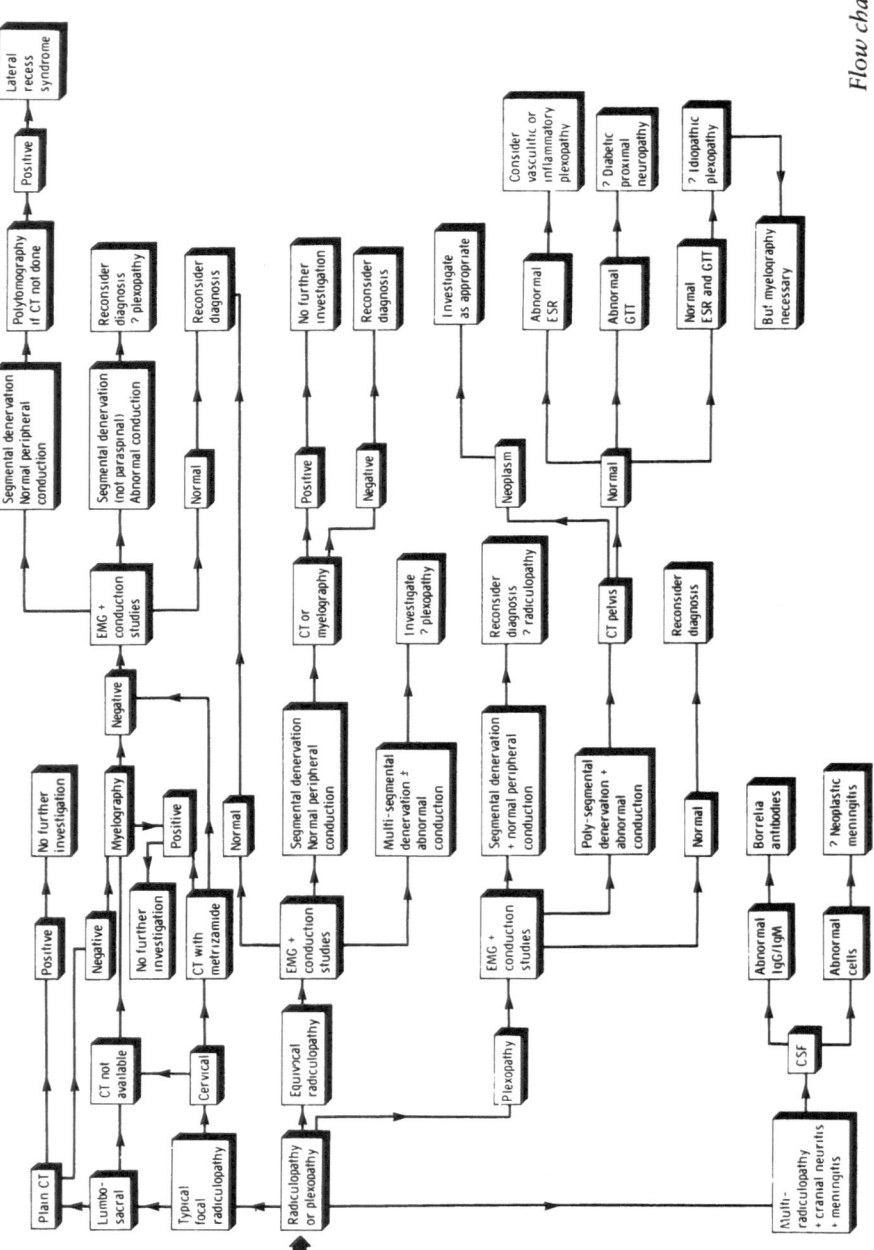

Flow chart A

Since a cauda equina syndrome can mimic the effects of plexo-pathy, myelography may be required if CT scanning of the pelvis is negative. The association of a polyradicular syndrome with cranial neuritis can occur in both neoplastic meningitis and Lyme disease. CSF examination is usually diagnostic in their differentiation.

9.4 MUSCLE DISEASE

Certain clinical characteristics have been used as a guide to determining whether a patient with muscle weakness has a myo-pathic or neurogenic disorder. Some features, for example distal sensory loss, would generally exclude a myopathic disorder, except that on occasions, particularly in patients with cancer, a neuromyo-pathic syndrome emerges which embraces manifestations of both primary muscle and nerve disease. Symmetry is held to be more characteristic of a myopathic than neurogenic disorder though certain muscle diseases, for example polymyositis, can be sur-prisingly focal. The simple concept of proximal weakness having a myopathic basis, and distal weakness being neurogenic does not withstand critical examination. Many patients previously diagnosed as cases of limb-girdle dystrophy, have, in fact, a form of chronic spinal muscular atrophy. Distal weakness with proximal sparing is certainly more often neurogenic than myopathic in origin but exceptions occur, for example with cases of adult onset debrancher deficiency. With the aid of increasingly sophisticated investigative techniques, it is recognized that a particular distribution of weakness can no longer be automatically categorized as either myopathic or neurogenic. For example, patients with a facio-scapulo-humoral distribution of weakness may have muscular dystrophy, polymyo-sitis or, exceptionally, spinal muscular atrophy. Pseudo-hypertrophy is automatically associated with certain myopathic disorders, par-ticularly Duchenne's and Becker's muscular dystrophies, but the same finding has been described in patients with spinal muscular atrophy[40]. Tendon reflexes are lost earlier in the course of neurogenic than myopathic disease.

The muscular dystrophies are genetically determined diseases of muscle. A group of relatively benign myopathies, presenting in childhood, has been classified according to the findings on muscle biopsy. These, and Duchenne's dystrophy, present early in life, and will not be considered in further detail. Forms of muscular dystrophy presenting in adult life include limb-girdle dystrophy, with both autosomal recessive [41] and dominant forms [42], scapulo-peroneal dystrophy [43] and a rare, distal myopathy, with both dominant and recessive forms [44]. Thyrotoxicosis is the most common endocrinological disorder associated with muscle disease. In one review of 50 patients, 40 had evidence of muscle weakness [46], which represented the principal complaint in three of them [45]. Muscle weakness, thought to be on a myopathic basis, is also encountered in myxoedema, though seldom to a severe degree [46]. In a review of 189 cases of Cushing's syndrome collected from the literature, 50% had muscle weakness as a symptom or sign [47]. A more common problem is muscle weakness occurring during the course of steroid therapy. Proximal lower limb involvement predominates, occasionally with pain [48]. The importance of the identification of an endocrine myopathy lies in its potential reversibility. Though many of the metabolic myopathies present in childhood, the expression of some forms is delayed until adult life. In general, metabolic myopathies present either as progressive muscle weakness or as episodic paralysis usually related to exercise [49]. Acid maltase deficiency can present as proximal muscle weakness in adult life and rarely as late as the fifth or sixth decade [50]. The clinical pattern can closely resemble limb-girdle dystrophy or polymositis, except that up to 50% of cases have prominent respiratory involvement, sometimes as a presenting feature [50,51]. In a recently described family with evidence of a lysosomal glycogen storage disease of muscle, acid maltase levels were normal. Inheritance was by a dominant trait with mild limb weakness but severe cardiac involvement [52]. Debrancher deficiency (Type III glycogenosis – Cori's disease) usually presents in childhood with evidence of liver dysfunction. Rarely, adult onset of a progressive distal weakness and wasting occurs, often mistakenly diagnosed as neuropathic in origin [53]. Systemic carnitine deficiency appears in childhood, but the syndrome of muscle carnitine deficiency is dominated by a slowly progressive myopathy which, though usually appearing in childhood, is occasionally delayed until adult life. Weakness of neck muscle is sometimes prominent [54]. Carnitine deficiency has also been described in association with glutaric aciduria type II. Again, onset is usually in childhood, but isolated cases with adult-onset have been described, usually with evidence of hepatic disease as well as proximal weakness. Biopsy shows accumulation of lipid in muscle with low carnitine levels. The importance of recognition relates to the fact that the muscle disturbance is reversed by riboflavin[55]. Defects affecting the mitochondrial respiratory chain principally affect the central nervous system but other tissues, including skeletal muscle can be involved. Again, most of these conditions present in childhood. Late-onset cases occur, however, typically with a multisystem disorder producing dementia, myoclonic seizures, involuntary movements, ataxia, disorders of higher cortical function and weakness[56]. At times the muscle involvement is inconspicuous or subclinical. Causes of exercise-induced muscle weakness include McArdle's disease, Tarui's disease and carnitine palmityltransferase deficiency. Except for rare cases of the first[57], these conditions do not present in adult life. The periodic paralysis syndromes result in paroxysmal muscle weakness which is typically triggered after, rather than during exercise. The diagnosis is usually suggested by evidence of familial involvement, since only some 5% of cases are sporadic[58]. Congenital myotonia, and paramyotonia congenita are almost always recognized in childhood, the latter sharing clinical features with hyperkalaemic periodic paralysis. Dystrophia myotonica, however, may not declare itself until middle life. In affected sibships, partial forms of the disease are encountered, recognized most often by the presence of facial weakness and upper limb reflex depression[59].

Inflammatory muscle disease is uncommon. Specific clinical and laboratory criteria have been devised for the diagnosis of polymyositis which typically presents with proximal limb weakness[60]. Muscle pain and tenderness are inconstant[61]. Cardiac abnormalities occur, including myocardial necrosis and various arrhythmias[62]. By definition, evidence of neurogenic involvement is lacking though rare cases combining polymyositis and peripheral nerve disease, unrelated to an underlying collagen vascular disease or carcinoma, are described[63]. A number of conditions can simulate polymyositis, provoking a syndrome of muscle pain and weakness, sometimes of rapid evolution. In developed countries, viral myositis requires consideration, whereas, in third world countries, bacterial fungal and parasitic involvement of muscle are still encountered[64]. D-Penicillamine can provoke an inflammatory myopathy. Inclusion body myositis shares many clinical and biochemical features with polymyositis, but appears resistant to corticosteroid therapy[65]. Though proximal muscle pain is prominent in polymyalgia rheumatica, sometimes with muscle tenderness, weakness is lacking[66].

A number of muscle disorders occur in alcoholics, including a rapidly evolving syndrome embracing pain, tenderness and weakness, associated with high serum levels of muscle-associated enzymes and myoglobinuria [67].

An almost endless list of other disorders may be associated with muscle disease. Proximal weakness is sometimes a prominent feature of primary hyperparathyroidism and osteomalacia. Bone pain suggests the diagnosis of metabolic bone disease [68]. Involvement of the musculoskeletal system in sarcoidosis is well recognized. At times, the muscle syndrome is the presenting feature and may remain so throughout life [69]. In patients receiving haemodialysis proximal limb weakness has been found to be associated with evidence of iron deposition on biopsy together with evidence of severe iron overload [70]. Carcinoma can disturb muscle function by its direct infiltration [71], or as a non-metastatic phenomenon. The latter can result in a neuromyopathic syndrome with proximal weakness of a myopathic nature combined with distal sensory abnormalities [72].

9.4.1 Investigation

(a) Muscle enzymes

Creatine kinase (CK) is the enzyme most commonly studied in patients with suspected muscle disease. Interpretation of the findings must take account of the ease with which a moderate increase in CK levels occurs in normal people after excercise and variability between laboratories in their reporting of the enzyme activity [73]. In muscle disease with an associated myocarditis or cardiomyopathy, measurement of the MB fraction of CK (derived from cardiac muscle) helps identify those patients with cardiac involvement [62]. Aspartate aminotransferase (GOT) can be separated into cytoplasmic (sGOT) and mitochondrial (mGOT) fractions. Both enzyme levels correlate well with muscle weakness in polymyositis and mGOT levels appear resistant to the effects of exercise [74]. CK levels are high in Duchenne's dystrophy, particularly in the early stages, but the elevations are less dramatic in the other muscular dystrophies, and are sometimes absent. Surprisingly high CK levels are encountered in some cases of chronic spinal muscular atrophy [75]. Muscle enzymes are usually normal in patients with endocrine myopathy though increased levels have been described in the muscle disorders complicating thyroid and pituitary disease. They are unchanged in polymyalgia rheumatica. Patients with metabolic myopathies presenting with persistent weakness almost inevitably have altered CK levels, whereas, in those with paroxysmal, exercise-related, weakness, elevations are less consistent. Increases occur during the paroxysms of weakness in the periodic paralysis syndromes.

Abnormal muscle enzyme activity is particularly prominent in polymyositis. Indeed the criteria for diagnosis include an elevated level of CK (MM isoenzyme), aldolase or myoglobin[60]. Normal enzyme values throughout the course of the illness are found in no more than 1% of cases[76]. With treatment, levels fall to 50% of initial values over the course of 4–5 weeks, and fresh elevation may antedate clinical relapse by several weeks[60]. Inclusion body myositis is similarly associated with abnormal CK levels, though to a lesser degree than occurs with polymyositis[65].

(b) EMG

Certain criteria have been described by which proximal weakness due to myopathic disorders can be distinguished from that associated with chronic spinal muscular atrophy. The finding of widespread fasciculation is strongly in favour of chronic spinal muscular atrophy but is absent in the majority of cases[77]. Though fibrillation potentials are characteristically associated with neurogenic disorders, they have been described as a fairly common feature in muscular dystrophy[78], and in polymyositis. High-frequency discharges (pseudo-myotonia) occur in the muscular dystrophies, polymyositis and chronic spinal muscular atrophy. The interference pattern in patients with primary muscle disease is characteristically composed of an increased proportion of polyphasic potentials, typically of shorter duration and reduced amplitude (Fig. 9.3). In spinal muscular atrophy, on the other hand, the potentials tend to be prolonged and polyphasic, with some of increased amplitude. Particular emphasis has been placed on the value of the EMG in diagnosing the cause of a slowly evolving proximal weakness beginning in adult life. Routine studies, however, are apt to be misleading. Amongst 17 cases of spinal muscular atrophy, three had myopathic features alone on sampling[75]. In other cases, although the EMG may show neuropathic abnormalities, the muscle biopsy suggests a myopathy[79]. Single fibre EMG has been used to aid the differentiation of myopathic proximal weakness from spinal muscular atrophy[77]. In the former, there is lower fibre density, less jitter, and a lower percentage of abnormal pairs (the percentage of

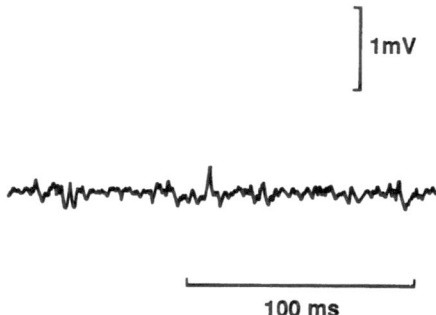

Fig. 9.3 EMG in Becker's muscular dystrophy. Low-voltage interference pattern with increased polyphasia

muscle fibre pairs with high jitter or blocking) than in the latter. The EMG findings in acid maltase deficiency are similar to those found in polymyositis. In debrancher deficiency a mixed neuropathic and myopathic picture is seen [54]. The EMG is generally normal in the metabolic myopathies producing exercise-induced weakness, unless persistent weakness has supervened. In attacks of periodic paralysis, muscle fibres are inexcitable, whereas in patients with hyperkalaemic periodic paralysis, both pseudomyotonic and myotonic discharges are seen. Certain EMG characteristics distinguish congenital myotonia from paramyotonia congenita [80]. In the former, the compound muscle action potential is unaffected by cooling, in the latter, the amplitude falls. Cooling provokes an exaggerated decremental response to 2 Hz stimulation in paramyotonia but not in congenital myotonia. In dystrophia myotonica, myopathic changes are accompanied by myotonic discharges which are sometimes elicited by cooling the muscle. In addition, minor changes in motor conduction have been reported. EMG changes are often not prominent in the endocrine myopathies but in thyrotoxic myopathy, the interference pattern usually shows low amplitude polyphasic potentials. Similar appearances occur in some of the muscle disorders accompanying hypothyroidism, disorders of calcium metabolism, and Cushing's disease. EMG criteria are important in the diagnosis of polymyositis. In a survey of 140 definite cases, small amplitude, short-duration polyphasic potentials were present in 90%, fibrillation potentials, sharp waves and increased insertional activity in 74%, and bizarre, high-frequency discharges in 38% [76]. A normal EMG was encountered in 10.7% of cases. Rarely, despite widespread weakness, EMG changes have been confined to paraspinal muscles. When the disease has been established for some time, the pattern alters, with the appearance of large, prolonged motorunit potentials, fall out of units, and increased territory of those surviving[81].

(c) Muscle biopsy

As with the EMG, certain histological features have been used to distinguish myopathic from neurogenic disorders of muscle. In the myopathies, necrotic fibres are common, there is an increased variability in fibre size, and an increased proportion of central nuclei. Infiltration by fat and fibrous tissue is prominent, particularly in Duchenne's dystrophy. Neurogenic disorders produce grouping of fibre types, constellations of small, angulated, fibres and fibre type atrophy. In certain chronic neurogenic disorders, however, myopathic changes appear on biopsy. In a review of 375 cases of chronic spinal muscular atrophy from the literature, myopathic biopsies were encountered in 19% [75]. Vital staining with methylene blue of a muscle bundle in the terminal innervation area allows calculation of the terminal innervation ratio, the number of muscle fibres innervated by a given number of subterminal axons. The ratio is normal in myopathy but high in neurogenic disorders[82]. Choice of site for biopsy is of some importance, since the changes in severely affected muscle may be so profound that diagnostic features are lost. In a study of biopsy site for patients with facioscapulohumeral dystrophy, the supraspinatus was considered the best candidate[83]. The findings in endocrine myopathy are generally non-specific and seldom add usefully to the diagnosis. In steroid myopathy, however, type II fibre atrophy predominates. In some of the metabolic myopathies, specific changes on biopsy are crucial in establishing the diagnosis. Vastus medialis was found to yield most abnormalities in a biopsy study of acid maltase deficiency[50]. Vacuolation, tending to predominate in type I fibres[84], stains positively for periodic-acid–Schiff and acid phosphatase (Fig. 9.4). Muscle acid maltase levels are depressed. Light microscopy of peripheral blood lymphocytes, revealing prominent discrete glycogen deposits, is reported to be a highly specific screening test for all forms of acid maltase deficiency[51]. In a dominantly inherited lysosomal glycogen storage disease, with cardiac involvement predominating over limb weakness, a similar vacuolar myopathy is found but with normal

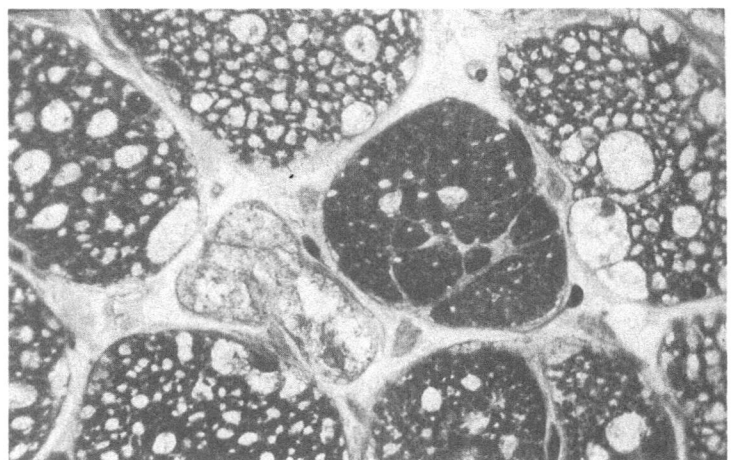

Fig. 9.4 Muscle biopsy demonstrating vacuolation in patient with acid maltase deficiency

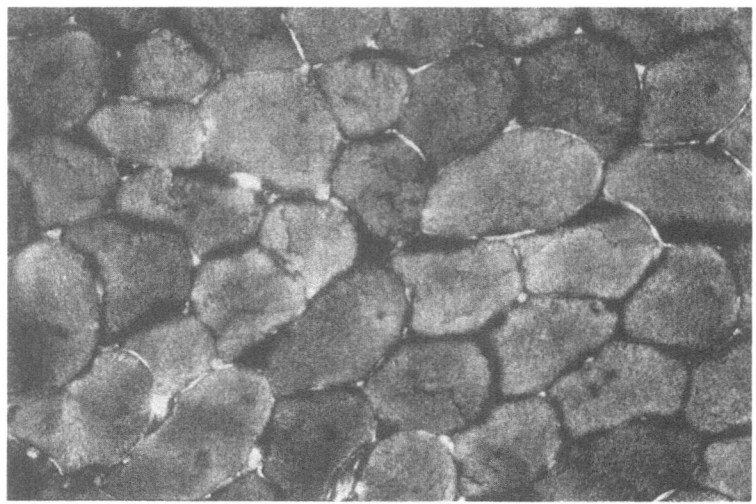

Fig. 9.5 McArdle's disease. Muscle biopsy (PAS-stain) demonstrating sarcolemmal glycogen (×64)

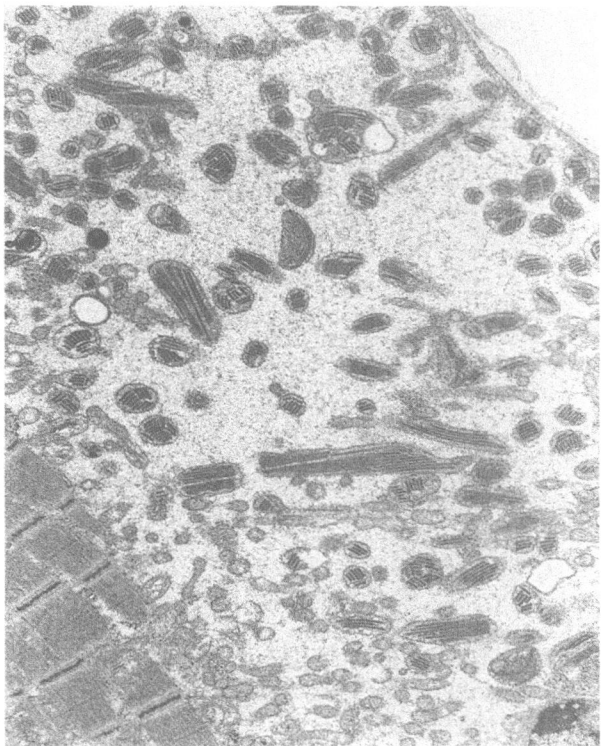

Fig. 9.6 Mitochondrial myopathy: Abnormal mitochondria beneath sarcolemma of a muscle fibre (EM × 7900)

assays for acid maltase [52]. Vacuolar myopathy is encountered in debrancher deficiency, with accumulation of abnormally short peripheral chains of polysaccharide [53]. Deficiency of debrancher enzyme can be demonstrated in muscle, liver, or peripheral leucocytes. The vacuoles found in adult onset muscle carnitine deficiency occur in both type I and type II fibres and stain intensely for neutral lipids [49]. Muscle carnitine levels are depressed as they are in the lipid-storage myopathy associated with glutaric aciduria [55]. The diagnoses of McArdle's disease and Tarui's disease are confirmed by the finding of depressed muscle levels of phosphorylase and phosphofructokinase respectively (Fig. 9.5). Deficiency of carnitine palmityl transferase can be established from muscle biopsy, or from assay of leucocytes, lymphocytes, platelets or cultured fibroblasts [49].

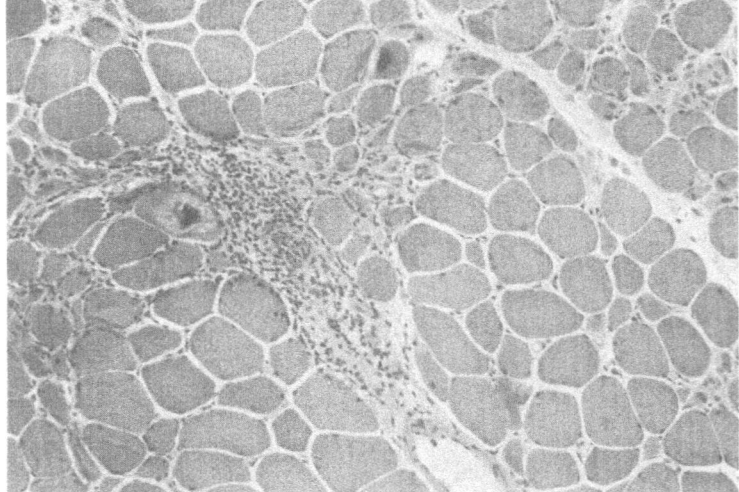

Fig. 9.7 Polymyositis. Muscle biopsy (HE stain) demonstrating foci of inflammatory cells (×10)

In the mitochondrial myopathies, dense subsarcolemmal deposits of red staining material positive for succinic dehydrogenase are found, predominantly in type I fibres[56]. On electron microscopy, these areas reveal enlarged, deformed mitochondria containing linear crystalline structures (Fig. 9.6). Muscle biopsy changes are usually lacking in cases of periodic paralysis unless specimens are obtained in attacks. Then, vacuolation is found which is likely to become permanent in cases who develop persistent weakness[58]. A relative reduction in the size of type I fibres is an early feature in dystrophia myotonica, accompanied by a striking increase in the number of central nuclei. Evidence of muscle fibre necrosis, together with cellular infiltration, is a vital element to the diagnosis of polymyositis. Some biopsy abnormality occurs in 90% of cases with polymyositis fulfilling the other diagnostic criteria, but with inflammatory change in perhaps 75% [60] (Fig. 9.7). The yield from a single site biopsy, however, is limited[61]. The correlation between clinical features and histological change has proved disappointing though one study suggested an inverse correlation between clinical response to steroids and the percentage of fibres with central nuclei on initial biopsy [85]. In inclusion body myositis, vacuoles lined with small basophilic granules are found within the muscle fibres. A mononuclear inflammatory cell infiltrate is inevitable[65]. For several other disorders affecting muscle, for example sarcoidosis or malignant invasion, diagnosis is finally established by biopsy.

(d) Other investigations

Electrocardiographic changes are common in Duchenne's dystrophy. Cardiac dysfunction was reported in 60% of one series of cases of polymyositis, almost all of whom had elevated levels of CK-MB (the cardiac specific enzyme of CK)[86]. It has been suggested that any patient with polymyositis and either elevated CK-MB levels, or an abnormal ECG, should have Holter monitoring to detect episodic cardiac arrhythmias[62]. Ironically, in a post-mortem study of one patient with confirmed spinal muscular atrophy, a severe cardiomyopathy was found of the type seen in Duchenne's dystrophy[87].

An elevated ESR has proved to be an inconstant feature of polymyositis, nor does its level correlate with disease activity[61,76]. In polymyalgia rheumatica, however, the ESR was above 42 in all 21 cases in one series[66]. Protein electrophoresis, reported to be abnormal in all six patients with polymyositis in one study[88], proved of limited diagnostic value in a larger cohort[61]. Evidence of collagen vascular disease is found in about 20% of cases of polymyositis[64,76]. About 10% have evidence of a malignancy, rising to 20% for patients presenting above the age of 50[64]. A recommended screen for malignancy in patients with polymyositis (and, more particularly, for dermatomyositis) includes haematological and biochemical investigation, chest X-ray and mammography[64]. Serum myoglobin levels are elevated in polymyositis, and increases in anticipation of clinical relapse, may antedate elevation of CK[89]. Abnormal muscle uptake of ^{99m}technetium has been found in polymyositis but similar changes occur in a proportion of patients with other muscle disease and in isolated cases of myasthenia and neurogenic disorder[90]. Myoglobinuria is typically associated with any situation where rapid muscle breakdown is occuring and tends to be associated with marked elevations of CK levels.

In McArdle's disease, muscle is unable to convert glycogen into lactate during ischaemic exercise. A standardized exercise test has been formulated in which normal individuals show a three- to five-fold increase in venous lactate levels over baseline values[91]. Lactate levels fail to rise in McArdle's disease, Tarui's disease and in most cases of debrancher deficiency, but show a normal response in carnitine palmityltransferase deficiency.

Many other systems are affected in myotonic dystrophy, reflected by a frequently abnormal ECG, evidence of abnormal gastrointestinal motility and a variety of endocrinological disorders, sometimes with overt diabetes.

CT scanning has been utilized for the study of a number of muscle disorders. Low density areas tend to appear in clinically affected muscle [92]. In neurogenic disorders, a reduction of muscle volume is seen earlier than is the case with primary muscle disease but the overlap is considerable [93].

The diagnosis of steroid myopathy is sometimes difficult, particularly if the drug is being used for the treatment of polymyositis. Creatine excretion is said to increase consistently whenever steroid myopathy develops [94].

9.4.2 Recommendation

For certain muscle diseases, the clinical pattern is sufficiently suggestive to establish the diagnosis. EMG analysis is appropriate in suspected myotonia but other investigations are not critical to the diagnosis. Investigative strategies are more relevant in patients presenting with acute, painful weakness, with periodic attacks of muscle weakness and particularly, with a sub-acute proximal weakness.

9.4.3 Acute painful weakness

Most patients with this complaint prove to have polymyositis. A history of alcoholism suggests the diagnosis of an acute alcoholic myopathy. Initial investigation should include ESR and CK levels. A normal CK level makes the diagnosis of polymyositis unlikely, but not impossible. Support for the diagnosis should be sought from EMG and biopsy studies though, in otherwise typical cases, either can be normal. Investigation for collagen vascular disease is appropriate. In patients over the age of 50, particularly if skin changes accompany the polymyositis, screening tests for cancer are indicated. At the least, these should include haematological and biochemical tests, chest X-ray and, possibly, mammography. In addition to CK, its cardiac isoenzyme CK-MB should be measured, together with ECG. If either is abnormal, Holter monitoring is probably indicated.

The finding of an eosinophilia will suggest the possibility of eosinophilic polymyositis or a parasite infestation of muscle. Vacuolation on muscle biopsy indicates the likely diagnosis of inclusion body myositis. Infiltration of muscle by carcinoma cells or granuloma indicates the need for investigation of an underlying cancer and sarcoidosis, respectively.

Myoglobinuria, although a non-specific consequence of acute muscle necrosis, is nevertheless of importance because of its association with the subsequent development of acute renal failure.

9.4.4 Periodic paralysis (flow chart B)

Where attacks of muscle weakness appear after physical activity, then one of the periodic syndromes should be suspected. Rarely, thyrotoxicosis can present in this way, and should be excluded. The designation of the syndrome is achieved by measuring serum $[K^+]$ during attacks. If necessary, known triggering factors can be tested. EMG and muscle biopsy are not essential for diagnosis.

Muscle weakness, often accompanied by cramps, which occurs during exercise suggests the diagnosis of metabolic myopathy. A lactate tolerance test is required. An abnormal result prompts measurement of muscle phosphorylase and phosphofructokinase. If both are normal, a diagnosis of debrancher deficiency should be considered, though the clinical appraisal should have already suggested this possibility. If the lactate tolerance test is normal, then carnitine palmityl transferase deficiency can be excluded by measurement of the enzyme in leucocytes or fibroblasts.

9.4.5 Sub-acute proximal weakness (flow chart C)

A sub-acute proximal weakness, arising in adult life, is the commonest of the diagnostic problems discussed in this section. Many of the endocrine myopathies are recognized early by the features of the primary disorder. Screening tests for these, and disorders of calcium metabolism should be performed first, however. A drug enquiry is necessary though other than for steroid myopathy (and the muscle syndromes associated with alcoholism) this seldom provides diagnostic information. Combined EMG and muscle biopsy studies are then performed, sometimes in themselves allowing a confident diagnosis of limb-girdle dystrophy, polymyositis or spinal muscular atrophy. Where the EMG is neuropathic, but the biopsy myopathic

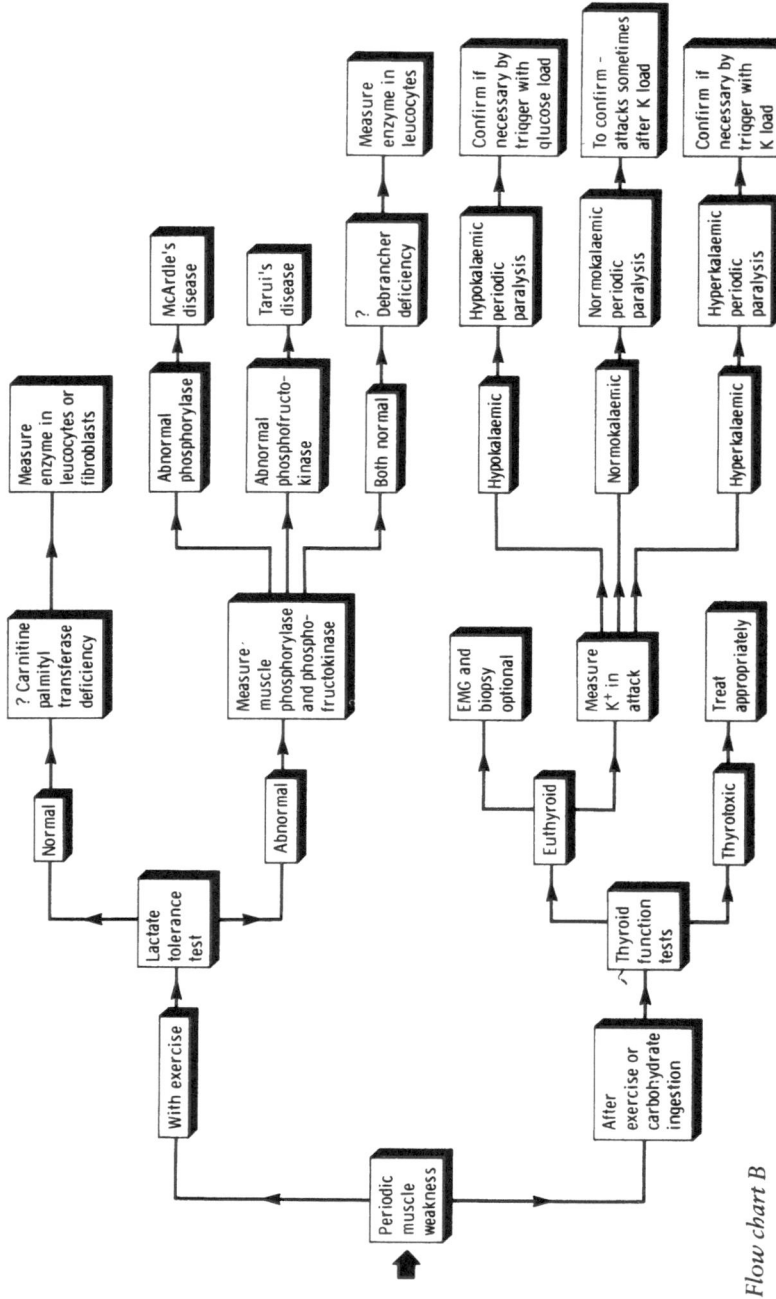

Flow chart B

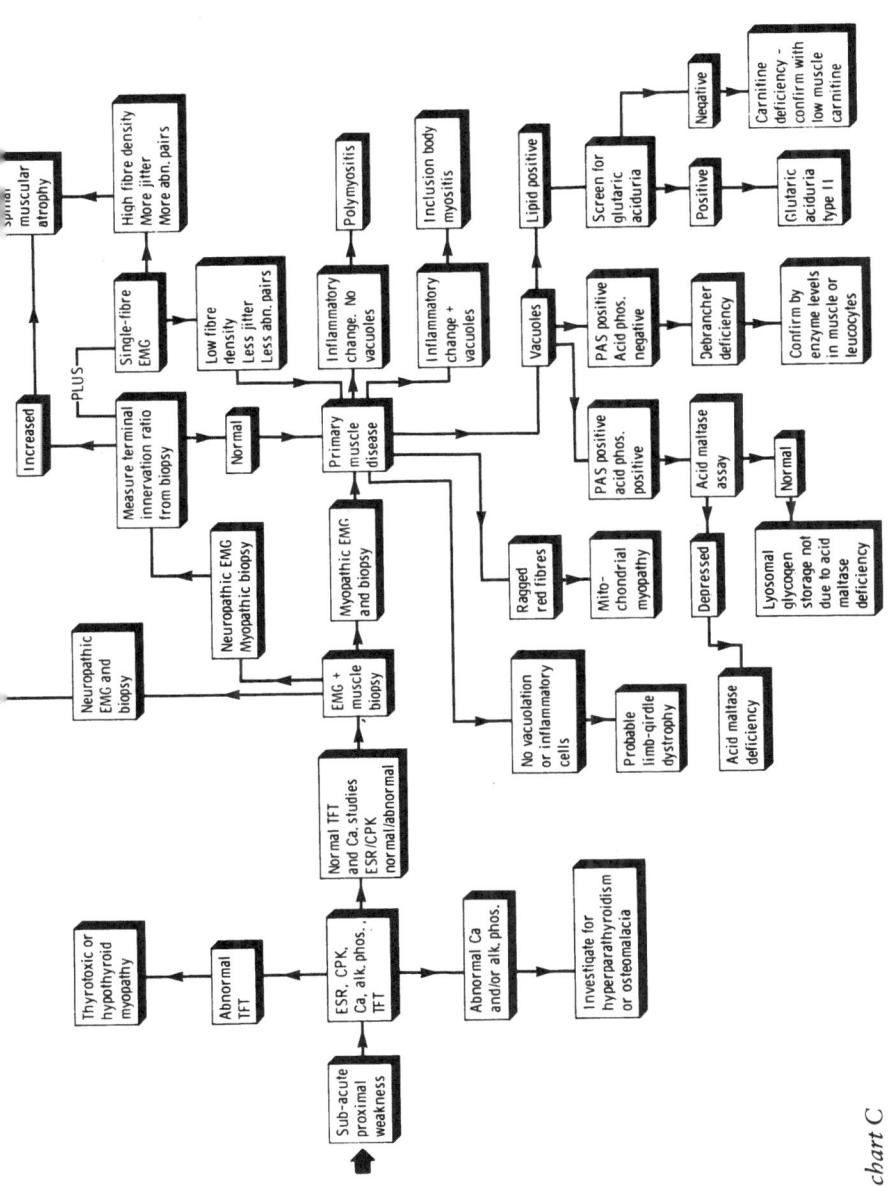

Flow chart C

specialized histological techniques, combined with single fibre EMG generally allows appropriate classification. If a vacuolar myopathy is discovered, special staining techniques, followed, where appropriate, by enzyme analysis aids the attainment of a specific diagnosis.

9.4.6 Carrier status

In the past, methods for detecting carriers, or for early detection of affected individuals with muscular dystrophy have proved disappointing. CK levels are elevated in about two-thirds of the gene carriers of Duchenne's dystrophy, and in about a half of the carriers of Becker's dystrophy [95]. Measurement of fetal serum CK has not proved reliable for the antenatal diagnosis of Duchenne's dystrophy [96]. Ultrasound and CT scanning of thigh muscle detects a proportion of carriers for Duchenne's dystrophy though with the latter technique, abnormalities are not usually detected before the age of 40 [97]. The use of DNA probes has now localized the gene for Duchenne's dystrophy to the short arm of the X-chromosome. It is probably allelic with the gene responsible for Becker's dystrophy. In the near future, more accurate localization will allow a confident prenatal diagnosis of either condition. Early diagnosis of myotonic dystrophy has proved difficult. Whilst the gene for this condition, and the secretor gene (which determines capacity to secrete ABH blood group substances in saliva and body fluids) are situated close to each other on the same chromosome, prenatal prediction using this knowledge is probably feasible in only 5–10% of families [99]. A recent report suggests a close linkage between the genes for myotonic dystrophy and apolipoprotein C11, both on chromosome 19. If the individual is heterozygous for the Apo C11 marker, amniocentesis with Apo C11 haplotype determination may show, with 96–98% accuracy that the foetus is not affected [100]. A combination of clinical and EMG appraisal has achieved a 50% diagnosis of at-risk offspring by the end of the second decade of life, allowing genetic counselling for affected individuals before they embark on a family [101]. Levels of acid maltase can be estimated in fetal amniotic cells allowing a reliable prenatal diagnosis of acid maltase deficiency [49].

REFERENCES

1. Pallis, C., Jones, A.M. and Spillane, J.D. (1954) Cervical spondylosis. Incidence and implications. *Brain*, 77, 274–89.

2. Lord Brain (1963) Some unsolved problems of cervical spondylosis. *Br. Med. J.*, **1**, 771–7.
3. Gillespie, H.W. (1946) Radiological diagnosis of lumbar intervertebral disc lesions. A report on 160 cases. *Br. J. Radiol.*, **19**, 420–8.
4. O'Connell, J.E.A. (1951) Protrusions of the lumbar intervertebral discs. A clinical review based on five hundred cases treated by excision of the protrusion. *J. Bone Jt Surg.*, **33B**, 8–30.
5. Ciric, I., Mikhael, M.A., Tarkington, J.A. and Vick, N.A. (1980) The lateral recess syndrome. A variant of spinal stenosis. *J. Neurosurg.*, **53**, 433–43.
6. Yates, D.A.H. (1981) Spinal stenosis. *J. R. Soc. Med.*, **74**, 334–42.
7. Hall, S., Bartleson, J.D., Onofrio, B.M. *et al.* (1985) Lumbar spinal stenosis. Clinical features, diagnostic procedures, and results of surgical treatment in 68 patients. *Ann. Intern. Med.*, **103**, 271–5.
8. Thomas, J.E., Cascino, T.L. and Earle, J.D. (1985) Differential diagnosis between radiation and tumor plexopathy of the pelvis. *Neurology*, **35**, 1–7.
9. Dinakar, I. and Balaparameswararao, S. (1972) Lumbar disk prolapse. Study of 300 surgical cases. *Int. Surg.*, **57**, 299–302.
10. Knutsson, B. (1961) Comparative value of electromyographic, myelographic and clinical neurological examinations in diagnosis of lumbar root compression syndrome. *Acta Orthopaed. Scand. Suppl.* **49**.
11. Hudgins, W.R. (1970) The predictive value of myelography in the diagnosis of ruptured lumbar discs. *J. Neurosurg.*, **32**, 152–62.
12. Hirsch, C. and Nachemson, A. (1963) The reliability of lumbar disk surgery. *Clin. Orth. Relat. Res.*, **29**, 189–95.
13. Pettigrew, L.C., Glass, J.P., Maor, M. and Zornoza, J. (1984) Diagnosis and treatment of lumbosacral plexopathies in patients with cancer. *Arch. Neurol.*, **41**, 1282–5.
14. Barrow, D.L., Wood, J.H. and Hoffman, J.C. Jr (1983) Clinical indications for computer-assisted myelography. *Neurosurgery*, **12**, 47–57.
15. Haughton, V.M., Eldevik, O.P., Magnaes, B. and Amundsen, P. (1982) A prospective comparison of computed tomography and myelography in the diagnosis of herniated lumbar disks. *Radiology*, **142**, 103–10.
16. Williams, A.L., Haughton, V.M., Daniels, D.L. and Thornton, R.S. (1982) CT recognition of lateral lumbar disk herniation. *Am. J. Neuroradiol.*, **3**, 211–13.
17. Yu, Y.L., du Boulay, G.H., Stevens, J.M. and Kendall, B.E. (1986) Computer-assisted myelography in cervical spondylotic myelopathy and radiculopathy. Clinical correlations and pathogenetic mechanisms. *Brain*, **109**, 259–78.
18. Trojaborg, W. (1981) Electrodiagnosis in the rheumatic diseases. *Clin. Rheum. Dis.*, **7**, 349–63.
19. Shea, P.A., Woods, W.W. and Werden, D.H. (1950) Electromyography

in diagnosis of nerve root compression syndrome. *Arch. Neurol. Psychiatry*, **64**, 93–104.

20. Mendelsohn, R.A. and Sola, A. (1958) Electromyography in herniated lumbar disks. *Arch. Neurol. Psychiatry*, **79**, 142–5.

21. Johnson, E.W. and Melvin, J.L. (1971) Value of electromyography in lumbar radiculopathy. *Arch. Phys. Med. Rehab.*, **52**, 239–43.

22. Evans, B.A., Stevens, J.C. and Dyck, P.J. (1981) Lumbosacral plexus neuropathy. *Neurology*, **31**, 1327–30.

23. Bradley, W.G., Chad, D., Verghese, J.P. *et al.* (1984) Painful lumbosacral plexopathy with elevated erythrocyte sedimentation rate: A treatable inflammatory syndrome. *Ann. Neurol.*, **15**, 457–64.

24. Benecke, R. and Conrad, B. (1980) The distal sensory nerve action potential as a diagnostic tool for the differentiation of lesions in dorsal roots and peripheral nerves. *J. Neurol.*, **223**, 231–9.

25. Eisen, A., Schomer, D. and Melmed, C. (1977) The application of F-wave measurements in the differentiation of proximal and distal upper limb entrapments. *Neurology*, **27**, 662–8.

26. Ongerboer de Visser, B.W., van der Sande, J.J. and Kemp, B. (1982) Ulnar F-wave conduction velocity in epidural metastatic root lesions. *Ann. Neurol.*, **11**, 142–6.

27. Schimsheimer, R.J., Ongerboer de Visser, B.W. and Kemp, B. (1985) The flexor carpi radialis H-reflex in lesions of the sixth and seventh cervical nerve roots. *J. Neurol. Neurosurg. Psychiatry*, **48**, 445–9.

28. Aiello, I., Rosati, G., Serra, G. and Manca, M. (1981) The diagnostic value of H-index in S1 root compression. *J. Neurol. Neurosurg. Psychiatry*, **44**, 171–2.

29. Levin, K.H., Stevens, J.C. and Daube, J.R. (1986) Superficial peroneal nerve conduction studies for electromyographic diagnosis. *Muscle Nerve*, **9**, 322–6.

30. Swash, M. and Snooks, S.J. (1986) Slowed motor conduction in lumbosacral nerve roots in cauda equina lesions: A new diagnostic technique. *J. Neurol. Neurosurg. Psychiatry*, **49**, 808–16.

31. Ganes, T. (1980) Somatosensory conduction times and peripheral, cervical and cortical evoked potentials in patients with cervical spondylosis. *J. Neurol. Neurosurg. Psychiatry*, **43**, 683–9.

32. Yu, Y.L. and Jones, S.J. (1985) Somatosensory evoked potentials in cervical spondylosis: correlation of median, ulnar and posterior tibial nerve responses with clinical and radiological findings. *Brain*, **108**, 273–300.

33. Aminoff, M.J., Goodin, D.S., Barbaro, N.M. *et al.* (1985) Dermatomal somatosensory evoked potentials in unilateral lumbosacral radiculopathy. *Ann. Neurol.*, **17**, 171–6.

34. Aminoff, M.J., Goodin, D.S., Parry, G.J. *et al.* (1985) Electrophysiologic evaluation of lumbosacral radiculopathies: electromyography, late responses, and somatosensory evoked potentials. *Neurology*, **35**, 1514–18.

35. Subramony, S.H. and Wilbourn, A.J. (1982) Diabetic proximal

neuropathy. Clinical and electromyographic studies. *J. Neurol. Sci.,* **53**, 293–304.

36. Pachner, A.R. and Steere, A.C. (1985) The triad of neurologic manifestations of Lyme disease, meningitis, cranial neuritis and radiculoneuritis. *Neurology*, **35**, 47–53.

37. Henriksson, A., Link, H., Cruz, M. and Stiernstedt, G. (1986) Immunoglobulin abnormalities in cerebrospinal fluid and blood over the course of lymphocytic meningoradiculitis (Bannwarth's syndrome). *Ann. Neurol.,* **20**, 337–45.

38. Muhlemann, M.F. and Wright, D.J.M. (1987) Emerging pattern of Lyme disease in the United Kingdom and Irish Republic. *Lancet,* i, 260–2.

39. Kristoferitsch, W. and Mayr, W.R. (1984) HLA-DR in meningo-polyneuritis of Garin–Bujadoux–Bannwarth: contrast to Lyme disease? *J. Neurol.,* **231**, 271–2.

40. Pearn, J. and Hudgson, P. (1978) Anterior-horn cell degeneration and gross calf hypertrophy with adolescent onset. A new spinal muscular atrophy syndrome. *Lancet,* i, 1059–61.

41. Walton, J.N. and Nattrass, F.J. (1954) On the classification, natural history and treatment of the myopathies. *Brain,* **77**, 169–231.

42. Chutkow, J.G., Heffner, R.R. Jr, Kramer, A.A. and Edwards, J.A. (1986) Adult-onset autosomal dominant limb-girdle muscular dystrophy. *Ann. Neurol.,* **20**, 240–8.

43. Thomas, P.K., Schott, G.D. and Morgan-Hughes, J.A. (1975) Adult onset scapuloperoneal myopathy. *J. Neurol. Neurosurg. Psychiatry,* **38**, 1008–15.

44. Miyoshi, K., Kawai, H., Iwasa, M. *et al.* (1986) Autosomal recessive distal muscular dystrophy as a new type of progressive muscular dystrophy. Seventeen cases in eight families including an autopsied case. *Brain,* **109**, 31–54.

45. Havard, C.W.H., Campbell, E.D.R., Ross, H.B. and Spence, A.W. (1963) Electromyographic and histological findings in the muscles of patients with thyrotoxicosis. *Q. J. Med.,* **32**, 145–63.

46. Astrom, K.-E., Kugelberg, E. and Muller, R. (1961) Hypothyroid myopathy. *Arch. Neurol.,* **5**, 472–82.

47. Plotz, C.M., Knowlton, A.I. and Ragan, C. (1952) The natural history of Cushing's syndrome. *Am. J. Med.,* **13**, 597–614.

48. Perkoff, G.T., Silber, R., Tyler, F.H. *et al.* (1959) Studies in disorders of muscle. XII. Myopathy due to the administration of therapeutic amounts of 17-hydroxycorticosteroids. *Am. J. Med.,* **26**, 891–8.

49. Cornelio, F. and Di Donato, S. (1985) Myopathies due to enzyme deficiencies. *J. Neurol.,* **232**, 329–40.

50. Swash, M., Schwartz, M.S. and Apps, M.C.P. (1985) Adult onset acid maltase deficiency. Distribution and progression of clinical and pathological abnormality in a family. *J. Neurol. Sci.,* **68**, 61–74.

51. Trend, P. St. J., Wiles, C.M., Spencer, G.T. *et al.* (1985) Acid

maltase deficiency in adults. Diagnosis and management in five cases. *Brain*, **108**, 845–60.

52. Byrne, E., Dennett, X., Crotty, B. *et al.* (1986) Dominantly inherited cardioskeletal myopathy with lysosomal glycogen storage and normal acid maltase levels. *Brain*, **109**, 523–36.

53. Cornelio, F., Bresolin, N., Singer, P.A. *et al.* (1984) Clinical varieties of neuromuscular disease in debrancher deficiency. *Arch. Neurol.*, **41**, 1027–32.

54. Bosch, E.P. and Munsat, T.L. (1979) Metabolic myopathies. *Med. Clin. N. Am.*, **63**, 759–82.

55. de Visser, M., Scholte, H.R., Schutgens, R.B.H. *et al.* (1986) Riboflavin-responsive lipid-storage myopathy and glutaric aciduria type II of early adult onset. *Neurology*, **36**, 367–72.

56. Morgan-Hughes, J.A., Hayes, D.J., Clark, J.B. *et al.* (1982) Mitochondrial encephalomyopathies. Biochemical studies in two cases revealing defects in the respiratory chain. *Brain*, **105**, 553–82.

57. Engel, W.K., Eyerman, E.L. and Williams, H.E. (1963) Late onset type of skeletal muscle phosphorylase deficiency. A new familial variety with completely and partially affected subjects. *N. Engl. J. Med.*, **268**, 135–7.

58. Pearson, C.M. (1964) The periodic paralyses: differential features and pathological observations in permanent myopathic weakness. *Brain*, **87**, 341–54.

59. Pryse-Phillips, W., Johnson, G.J. and Larsen, B. (1982) Incomplete manifestations of myotonic dystrophy in a large kinship in Labrador. *Ann. Neurol.*, **11**, 582–91.

60. Mastaglia, F.L. and Ojeda, V.J. (1985) Inflammatory myopathies: Part 2. *Ann. Neurol.*, **17**, 317–23.

61. Barwick, D.D. and Walton, J.N. (1963) Polymyositis. *Am. J. Med.*, **35**, 646–60.

62. Askari, A.D. (1984) Inflammatory disorders of muscle. Cardiac abnormalities. *Clinics in Rheumatic Diseases.*, **10.**, 131–149.

63. McEntee, W.J. and Mancall, E.L. (1965) Neuromyositis: a reappraisal. *Neurology*, **15**, 69–75.

64. Mastaglia, F.L. and Ojeda, V.J. (1985) Inflammatory myopathies: Part 1. *Ann. Neurol.*, **17**, 215–17.

65. Danon, M.J., Reyes, M.G., Perurena, O.H. *et al.* (1982) Inclusion body myositis. A corticosteroid-resistant idiopathic inflammatory myopathy. *Arch. Neurology*, **39**, 760–4.

66. Gordon, I. (1960) Polymyalgia rheumatica. A clinical study of 21 cases. *Q. J. Med.*, **29**, 473–88.

67. Hed, R., Lundmark, C., Fahlgren, H. and Orell, S. (1962) Acute muscular syndrome in chronic alcoholism. *Acta Med. Scand.*, **171**, 585–99.

68. Prineas, J.W., Mason, A.S. and Henson, R.A. (1965) Myopathy in metabolic bone disease. *Br. Med. J.*, **1**, 1034–6.

69. Crompton, M.R. and MacDermot, V. (1961) Sarcoidosis associated

with progressive muscular wasting and weakness. *Brain*, **84**, 62–74.
70. Bregman, H., Gelfand, M.C., Winchester, J.F. *et al.* (1980) Iron-overload-associated myopathy in patients on maintenance haemodialysis: A histocompatibility-linked disorder. *Lancet*, ii, 882–5.
71. Doshi, R. and Fowler, T. (1983) Proximal myopathy due to discrete carcinomatous metastases in muscle. *J. Neurol. Neurosurg. Psychiatry*, **46**, 358–60.
72. Shy, G.M. and Silverstein, I. (1965) A study of the effects upon the motor unit by remote malignancy. *Brain*, **88**, 515–28.
73. Bullock, D.G., McSweeney, F.M., Whitehead, T.P. and Edwards, J.H. (1979) Serum creatine kinase activity and carrier status for Duchenne muscular dystrophy. *Lancet*, ii, 1370.
74. Ogasahara, S., Takahashi, M., Kang, J. *et al.* (1983) Serum mitochondrial aspartate aminotransferase in patients with polymyositis. *Ann. Neurol.*, **13**, 100–3.
75. Mastaglia, F.L. and Walton, J.N. (1971) Histological and histochemical changes in skeletal muscle from cases of chronic juvenile and early adult spinal muscular atrophy (the Kugelberg–Welander syndrome). *J. Neurol. Sci.*, **12**, 15–44.
76. Bohan, A., Peter, J.B., Bowman, R.L. and Pearson, C.M. (1977) A computer-assisted analysis of 153 patients with polymyositis and dermatomyositis. *Medicine*, **56**, 255–86.
77. Shields, R.W. Jr (1984) Single fiber electromyography in the differential diagnosis of myopathic limb girdle syndromes and chronic spinal muscular atrophy. *Muscle Nerve*, **7**, 265–72.
78. Buchthal, F. and Rosenfalck, P. (1966) Spontaneous electrical activity of human muscle. *Electroencephalogr. Clin. Neurophysiol.*, **20**, 321–36.
79. Black, J.T., Bhatt, G.B., Dejesus, P.V. *et al.* (1974) Diagnostic accuracy of clinical data, quantitative electromyography and histochemistry in neuromuscular disease. *J. Neurol. Sci.*, **21**, 59–70.
80. Subramony, S.H., Malhotra, C.P. and Mishra, S.K. (1983) Distinguishing paramyotonia congenita and myotonia congenita by electromyography. *Muscle Nerve*, **6**, 374–9.
81. Payan, J. (1984) Electromyography in polymyositis and some related disorders. *Clin. Rheum. Dis.*, **10**, 75–83.
82. Coërs, C. and Telerman-Toppet, N. (1979) Differential diagnosis of limb-girdle muscular dystrophy and spinal muscular atrophy. *Neurology*, **29**, 957–72.
83. Bodensteiner, J.B. and Schochet, S.S. (1986) Facioscapulohumeral muscular dystrophy: the choice of a biopsy site. *Muscle Nerve*, **9**, 544–7.
84. Papapetropoulos, T., Paschalis, C. and Manda, P. (1984) Myopathy due to juvenile acid maltase deficiency affecting exclusively the type I fibres. *J. Neurol. Neurosurg. Psychiatry*, **47**, 213–15.
85. Schwarz, H.A., Slavin, G., Ward, P. and Ansell, B.M. (1980) Muscle biopsy in polymyositis and dermatomyositis: A clinico-

pathological study. *Ann. Rheum. Dis.*, **39**, 500–7.

86. Strongwater, S.L., Annesley, T. and Schnitzer, T.J. (1983) Myocardial involvement in polymyositis. *J. Rheumatol.*, **10**, 459–63.

87. Tomlinson, B.E., Walton, J.N. and Irving, D. (1974) Spinal cord limb motor neurones in muscular dystrophy. *J. Neurol. Sci.*, **22**, 305–27.

88. Gavrilescu, K. and Small, J.M. (1962) Serum electrophoretic changes in polymyositis. *Br. Med. J.*, **2**, 1720–3.

89. Nishikai, M. and Reichlin, M. (1977) Radioimmunoassay of serum myoglobin in polymyositis and other conditions. *Arth. Rheum.*, **20**, 1514–18.

90. Messina, C., Bonanno, N., Baldari, S. and Vita, G. (1982) Muscle uptake of ^{99m}technetium pyrophosphate in patients with neuromuscular disorders. A quantitative study. *J. Neurol. Sci.*, **53**, 1–7.

91. Munsat, T.L. (1970) A standardized forearm ischemic exercise test. *Neurology*, **20**, 1171–8.

92. de Visser, M. (1983) Computed tomographic findings of the skeletal musculature in sporadic distal myopathy with early adult onset. *J. Neurol. Sci.*, **59**, 331–9.

93. Serratrice, G., Salamon, G,. Jiddane, M. *et al.* (1985) Résultats du scanner X musculaire dans 145 cas de maladies neuro-musculaires. *Rev. Neurol.*, **141**, 404–12.

94. Askari, A., Vignos, P.J. Jr and Moskowitz, R.W. (1976) Steroid myopathy in connective tissue disease. *Am. J. Med.*,**61**, 485–92.

95. Emery, A.E.H., Clack, E.R., Simon, S. and Taylor, J.L. (1967) Detection of carriers of benign X-linked muscular dystrophy. *Br. Med. J.*, **4**, 522–3.

96. Emery, A.E.H., Burt, D., Dubowitz, V. *et al.* (1979) Antenatal diagnosis of Duchenne muscular dystrophy. *Lancet*, i, 847–9.

97. Rott, H.-D., Santellani, M., Rödl, W. and Nebel, G. (1983) Duchenne muscular dystrophy: carrier detection by ultrasound and computerised tomography. *Lancet*, ii, 1199–200.

98. Kingston, H.M., Harper, P.S., Pearson, P.L. *et al.* (1983) Localisation of gene for Becker muscular dystrophy. *Lancet*, ii, 1200.

99. Schrott, H.G. and Omenn, G.S. (1975) Myotonic dystrophy: opportunities for prenatal prediction. *Neurology*, **25**, 789–91.

100. Bird, T.D., Boehnke, M., Schellenberg, G.D. *et al.* (1987) The use of apolipoprotein C11 as a genetic marker for myotonic dystrophy. *Arch. Neurol.*, **44**, 273–5.

101. Schubert, T., Jerusalem, F., Martenet, A.-C., *et al.* (1980) Myotonic dystrophy – early detection and genetic counselling. *J. Neurol.*, **223**, 13–22.

10

Myasthenia gravis
Anterior horn cell disease

10.1 MYASTHENIA GRAVIS

Myasthenia gravis is a rare condition. Perhaps as a consequence, there is sometimes considerable delay before the diagnosis is established. In some patients, the disorder is confined, at least clinically, to the ocular muscles, resulting in ptosis and diplopia. If this localization persists for two years, the condition is unlikely then to become generalized. Myasthenia may also present with generalized muscle weakness and fatiguability, sometimes in a fulminating fashion. Reversal of weakness by intravenous injection of edrophonium (Tensilon) supports the diagnosis but a small proportion of myasthenic patients (perhaps 5–10%) fail to respond[1]. There is an association between myasthenia and various auto-immune disorders, including pernicious anaemia and thyroid disease. Myasthenic patients have an increased incidence of thymic hyperplasia and some 10% are found to have a thymoma. Younger myasthenic patients, without thymoma, have a higher incidence of HLA antigens A1, B8 and DRW3, whereas in older patients (over 40 years) without thymoma, the association is with A3, B7 and DRW2[2].

10.1.1 Investigations

Assessment of thyroid function in one series of myasthenic patients revealed thyrotoxicosis in 5.7% and hypothyroidism in 1.9%[3]. Thyroid antibodies were found in 32% and anti-DNA antibodies in 62% of patients in one study, a correlation existing between the presence of these antibodies, the possession of HLA antigen B8 and the female sex[4]. Antibody to striated muscle is found in the vast majority of patient with thymoma[2].

An analysis of the prevalence of acetylcholine receptor antibodies amongst 153 patients has indicated that 88% of those with generalized disease had the antibody, and 60% of those with ocular myasthenia [5]. The antibody is sometimes not found in the early stages of the disease. There is some correlation between antibody levels and severity of the disease, with a tendency for the levels to mirror clinical fluctuation [6].

Many electrophysiological techniques have been assessed for their ability to add weight to the clinical diagnosis. Conventional EMG techniques are of limited value. When repetitive stimulation is applied to a peripheral nerve at 2–3 Hz, the amplitude of the response evoked from the muscle it innervates shows an abnormal decrement. The yield of abnormal results is higher when proximal muscles are tested [7]. Some two-thirds of patients have abnormal findings, the figure rising in severe cases, but falling to as low as 17.2% in ocular myasthenia [8]. The findings tend to revert to normal when the patient enters a remission. Exercise, increasing muscle temperature and ischaemia have all been used as provocative factors designed to increase the diagnostic yield.

Single fibre techniques are used to record activity from two muscle fibres belonging to the same motor unit. A slight time gap normally exists between the two potentials depending on difference in propagation time between the branching of the nerve and the recording electrode. With consecutive discharges, some variability in this interpotential interval occurs, and is entitled jitter. Generally extensor digitorum communis (EDC) is used to record jitter [7]. Twenty separate recordings are used to determine a mean jitter interval. In one series of 164 myasthenic patients, 94% had abnormal jitter [7]. If the measurements from EDC are normal in patients with ocular myasthenia, then frontalis or orbicularis oculi should be tested.

The stapedius reflex is measured by assessment of the acoustic impedance of the tympanic membrane. In the normal individual, using either 200 or 500 ms sound pulses and assessing impedance during the first and last 10 s period of a 300 s train, there is a slight increment for 500 ms pulses and a slight decrement for 200 ms pulses. Decrement at one or both frequencies is found in up to 96% of myasthenic patients [7]. The reflex may be less positive in more advanced cases, but has been reported to be positive in up to 90% of ocular cases [9].

Comparison of the various diagnostic techniques has been made [9,10]. In one study the percentage of positive yield from the three

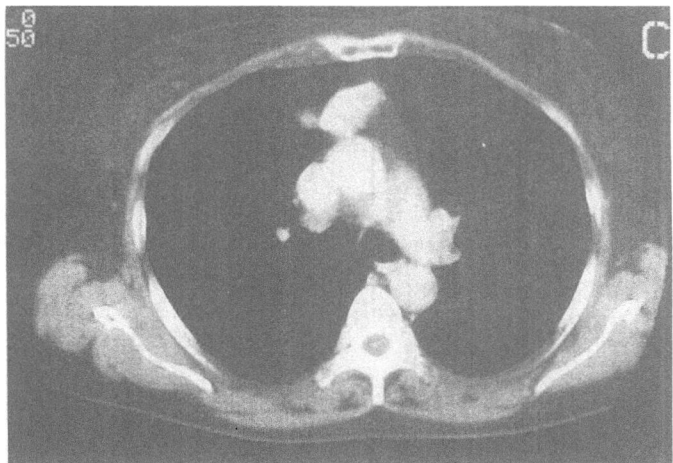

Fig. 10.1 CT demonstrating thymoma in a patient with myasthenia gravis

techniques, repetitive stimulation, stapedial reflex and single fibre study was 56, 84 and 91 respectively. Put another way, if patients with myasthenia and negative repetitive stimulation studies are subjected to either single fibre studies or stapedial reflex testing, some three-quarters will be found to be abnormal[10].

Electromyography of ocular muscle is uncomfortable and cannot be recommended for the investigation of ocular myasthenia. Following the administration of edrophonium, intra-ocular tension rises in patients with ocular myasthenia, but the same response may occur in normal subjects. Measurement of the amplitude or velocity of the saccadic phase of optokinetic nystagmus by infrared techniques, before and after edrophonium, appears to be a sensitive technique for detecting subclinical ocular muscle involvement[11].

Studies of methods for the detection of thymoma have compared routine chest radiography, mediastinal tomography and mediastinal CT scanning. Conflicting opinions have been expressed as to whether tomography provides a higher yield than chest radiography[12,13]. CT detects all thymomas, but may also demonstrate abnormalities due to thymic hyperplasia (Fig. 10.1). One study concluded that a mass detected by CT but not by tomography was almost certainly not a thymoma, unless the mass was calcified, or there was evidence of metastatic disease[13].

There appear to be two forms of ocular myasthenia. One group,

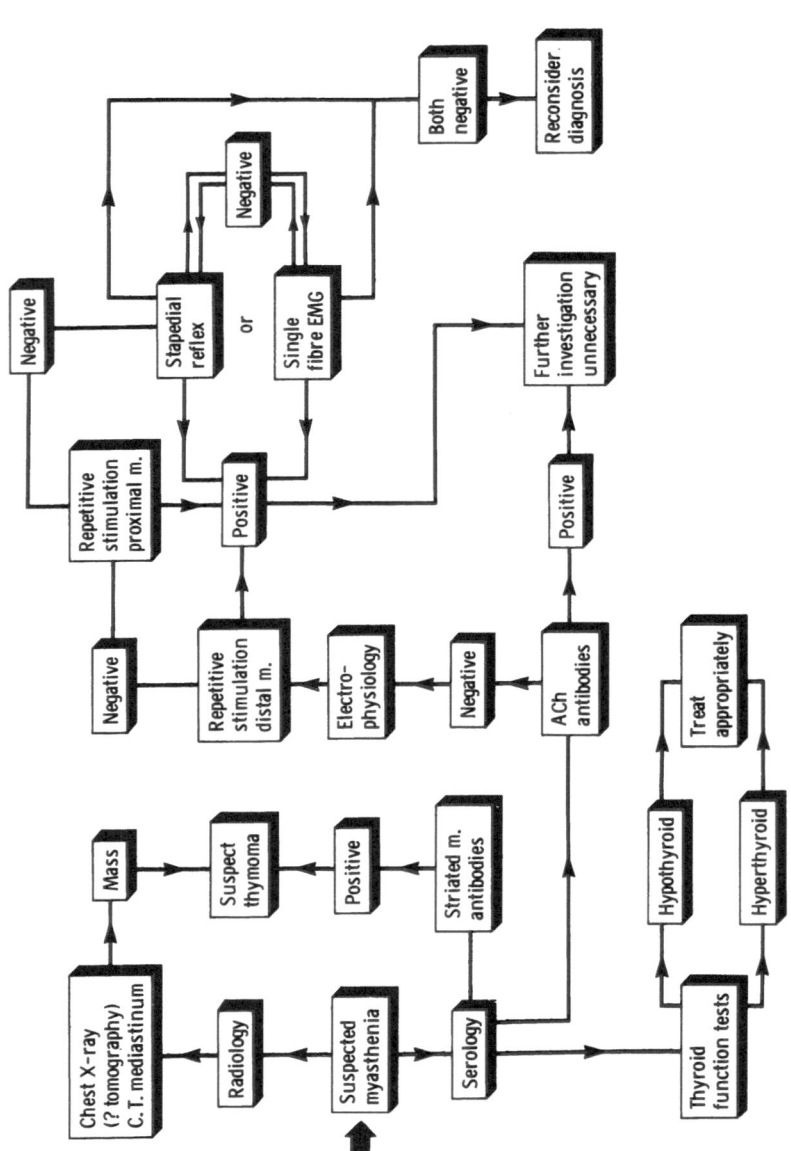

Flow chart

predominantly female, is likely to have AChR antibody, other auto-antibodies, abnormal EMG findings and evidence of thymic hyperplasia. The other group, mainly male, has negative antibody and EMG studies and a normal thymus.

10.1.2 Recommendation (see flow chart)

Where the diagnosis is likely on clinical grounds, and the signs respond to edrophonium, little further investigation is necessary. Thyroid function tests should be performed, and radiological investigation to exclude an associated thymoma. If there is some clinical doubt, then antibody to acetylcholine receptor should be estimated. If this is absent, electrophysiological assessment will be necessary.

10.2 LAMBERT–EATON SYNDROME

Patients with the Lambert–Eaton (myasthenic) syndrome may complain of muscle fatiguability but often their more prominent complaint is proximal muscle weakness and pain. Other symptoms include paraesthesiae and a dry mouth. Bulbar involvement is unusual and ocular muscle symptomatology fairly rare. Despite this, oculography may demonstrate subclinical involvement, with response to edrophonium [14]. In the myasthenic syndrome, however, the electrophysiological defect lies in impaired release of acetylcholine and is not associated with the presence of circulating acetylcholine receptor antibody. Many patients with the myasthenic syndrome have an underlying cancer, particularly oat cell carcinoma of the lung. Those without cancer show an increased incidence of the antigens HLA, B8 and DRW3 [2].

10.2.1 Investigations

In the myasthenic syndrome, the compound muscle action potential evoked in rested muscle by a single shock to the peripheral nerve supplying it has a depressed amplitude. At slow rates of stimulation (2–10 Hz) there is a further fall in the amplitude of successive responses, particularly if stimulation follows 2–3 min after sustained contraction for 60 s. At rapid stimulus rates (20–40 Hz) there is an increment of the amplitude of the initial response of two to twenty times, the maximum amplitude being reached within 7 s (Fig. 10.2). Finally, if the patient sustains a voluntary muscle contraction

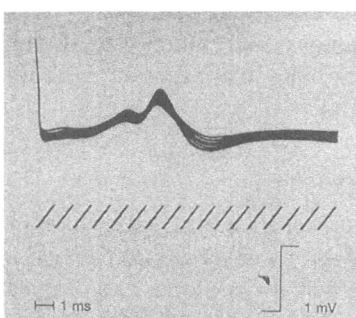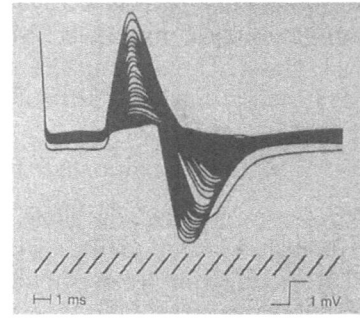

Fig. 10.2 Lambert–Eaton syndrome. EMG showing augmentation of muscle action potential amplitude during repetitive stimulation at 10 Hz and 50 Hz

for 10 s, the amplitude of the compound muscle action potential obtained from a single shock applied 3 s later is between 220 and 1100% greater than the pre-contraction amplitude[15]. Single fibre studies show similar jitter and blocking of impulse transmission to that found in myasthenia gravis, but with rapid stimulation rates, the jitter diminishes in the myasthenic syndrome, whereas it increases in myasthenia gravis[16].

10.2.2 Recommendation

Electrophysiological tests as detailed above should be performed in any patient suspected of having the myasthenic syndrome. If the diagnosis is confirmed, chest radiography is essential in order to exclude, as far as possible, an underlying lung cancer.

10.3 MOTOR NEURONE DISEASE

The prevalence of motor neurone disease has been estimated to lie between 2 and 7 cases per 100 000. The aetiology of the condition is unknown. Suggested, but unproven, factors have included previous polio, trauma, electric shocks and exposure to heavy metals. Although the clinical features reflect the pathological changes in the upper and lower motor neurone systems, post-mortem studies have revealed demyelination of certain ascending pathways sparing, except rarely, the posterior columns, Differing clinical subtypes of motor neurone disease are described, reflecting an initial pattern of involvement predominantly in the upper or lower motor neurone, and at bulbar or spinal level. Eventually all the subtypes merge into a common pattern. Dementia does not occur, nor is there involvement of sphincter function. Only rarely is there any evidence of ocular motor disturbance.

10.3.1 Investigations

Some patients show a moderate increase in the level of the enzyme CK[17]. In one study, 39% of patients had an elevated CSF protein concentration, but seldom did this exceed 1.0 g/l[18]. Slightly elevated lead concentrations in the CSF are of little diagnostic or pathogenic significance[19]. Though peripheral sensory conduction is almost inevitably normal, measurement of somatosensory evoked responses indicates a delay in central conduction, both in the cord and in the lemniscal pathway[20].

Electrophysiological assessment is of great value in supporting or even suggesting the diagnosis. Typically, widespread fibrillation and fasciculation potentials are found, with positive sharp waves and a reduction in the number, but an increase in size, of the motor unit action potential. Motor conduction velocity is either normal or marginally reduced.

Single fibre EMG demonstrates an increased fibre density, together with abnormal jitter, indicating an abnormality of conduction in the most peripheral part of the nerve or at the neuromuscular junction.

Muscle biopsy demonstrates neurogenic atrophy, with small, angular fibres and grouping of fibre-types. In up to two-thirds of patients, secondary myopathic change is found, including variation in fibre size and infiltration by fat and fibrous tissue[21].

10.3.2 Recommendation

EMG and nerve conduction studies are usually the only investigations required. Use of surface electrodes for detecting multiple sites of fasciculation in the upper and lower limbs is particularly useful[22].

10.4 SPINAL MUSCULAR ATROPHY

Though the predominant pathological change in spinal muscular atrophy is sited in the anterior horn cell, the resulting clinical picture shows substantial differences from motor neurone disease. Typically,

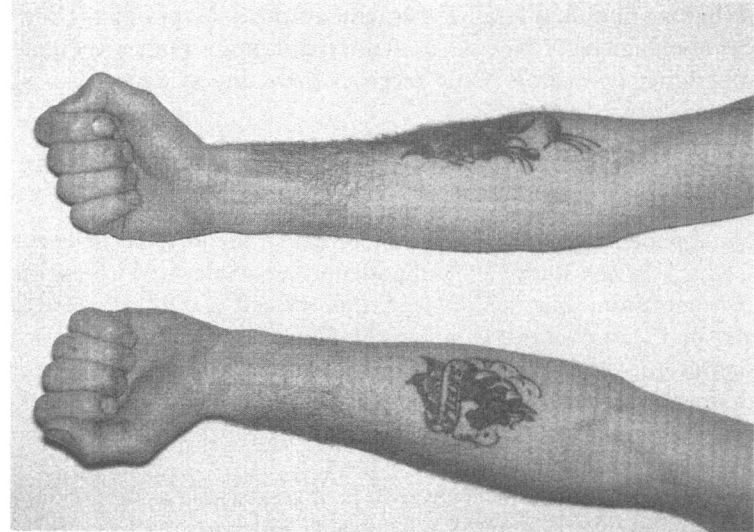

Fig. 10.3 Selective wasting of the right arm in a patient with asymmetric spinal muscular atrophy

bulbar and pyramidal signs are inconspicuous or absent[23]. Classification is based partly on age of onset, clinical distribution, and mode of inheritance[24]. In some patients, the signs remain remarkably asymmetrical[25] (Fig. 10.3). The findings on laboratory investigation are similar to those of motor neurone disease[26]. A slightly atypical form of spinal muscular atrophy with, in some cases, dementia, cerebellar signs or neuropathy can occur in individuals with hexosaminidase A deficiency. Onset is usually in adolescence[27].

10.4.1 Investigations

In essence, the findings on EMG and muscle biopsy are similar to those described for motor neurone disease, though fasciculation is less prominent, and, in more chronic cases, myopathic features on both EMG and muscle biopsy are likely. CK levels may be elevated, but seldom to the degree encountered in patients with muscular dystrophy.

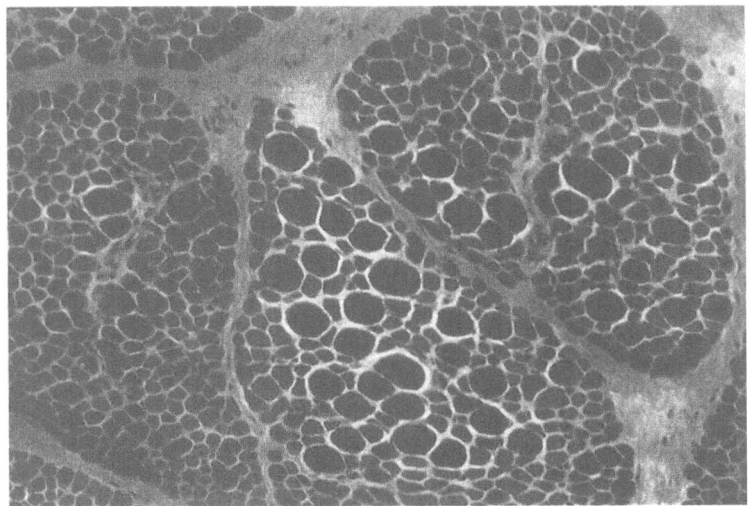

Fig. 10.4 Muscle biopsy demonstrating grouped fibre atophy in Werdnig–
Hoffman disease

10.4.2 Recommendation

Both EMG and muscle biopsy are necessary in patients suspected of
having spinal muscular atrophy (Fig. 10.4). Secondary myopathic
change is sometimes prominent[28], and since a similar clinical
syndrome, for example the scapulo-peroneal syndrome, can have
either a myopathic or neurogenic basis, differentiation can prove
difficult (see Chapter 9).

REFERENCES

1. Osserman, K.E. and Genkins, G. (1966) Critical reappraisal of the use
   of edrophonium (Tensilon) chloride tests in myasthenia gravis and
   significance of clinical observation. *Ann. N. Y. Acad. Sci.*, **135**, 312–26.
2. Engel, A.G. (1984) Myasthenia gravis and myasthenic syndromes. *Ann.
   Neurol.*, **16**, 519–34.
3. Kiessling, W.R., Pflughaupt, K.W., Ricker, K. *et al.* (1981) Thyroid
   function and circulating antithyroid antibodies in myasthenia gravis.
   Neurology, **31**, 771–4.
4. Sagar, H.J., Gelsthorpe, K., Milford-Ward, A. and Davies-Jones,
   G.A.B. (1980) Clinical and immunological associations in myasthenia
   gravis, 1: autoantibodies. *J. Neurol. Neurosurg. Psychiatry*, **43**,
   967–70.

5. Vincent, A. and Newsom-Davis, J. (1985) Acetylcholine receptor antibody as a diagnostic test for myasthenia gravis: results in 153 validated cases and 2967 diagnostic assays. *J. Neurol. Neurosurg. Psychiatry*, 48, 1246–52.

6. Oosterhuis, H.J.G.H., Limburg, P.C., Hummel-Tappel, E. and The, T.H. (1983) Anti-acetylcholine receptor antibodies in myasthenia gravis. II. Clinical and serological follow-up of individual patients. *J. Neurol. Sci.*, 58, 371–85.

7. Stalberg, E. (1980) Clinical electrophysiology in myasthenia gravis. *J. Neurol. Neurosurg. Psychiatry*, 43, 622–33.

8. Oh, S.J., Eslami, N., Nishihira, T. *et al.* (1982) Electrophysiological and clinical correlation in myasthenia gravis. *Ann. Neurol.*, 12, 348–54.

9. Kramer, L.D., Ruth, R.A., Johns, M.E. and Sanders, D.B. (1981) A comparison of stapedial reflex fatigue with repetitive stimulation and single-fiber EMG in myasthenia gravis. *Ann. Neurol.*, 9, 531–6.

10. Kelly, J.J. Jr, Daube, J.R., Lennon, V.A. *et al.* (1982) The laboratory diagnosis of mild myasthenia gravis. *Ann. Neurol.*, 12, 238–42.

11. Spector, R.H. and Daroff, R.B. (1976) Edrophonium infra-red opto-kinetic nystagmography in the diagnosis of myasthenia gravis. *Ann. N. Y. Acad. Sci.*, 274, 642–51.

12. Keesey, J., Bein, M., Mink, J. (1980) Detection of thymoma in myasthenia gravis. *Neurology*, 30, 233–9.

13. Janssen, R.S., Kaye, A.D., Lisak, R.P. *et al.* (1983) Radiologic evaluation of the mediastinum in myasthenia gravis. *Neurology*, 33, 534–9.

14. Dell'Osso, L.F., Ayyar, D.R., Daroff, R.B. and Abel, L.A. (1983) Edrophonium test in Eaton–Lambert syndrome: quantitative oculography. *Neurology*, 33, 1157–63.

15. Ablecki, C.J. (1984) Lambert–Eaton myasthenic syndrome. *Muscle Nerve*, 7, 250–7.

16. Stalberg, E. and Sanders, D.B. (1981) Electrophysiological tests of neuromuscular transmission, in *Clinical Neurophysiology* (eds E. Stalberg and R.R. Young) Butterworths, London, pp. 88–116.

17. Williams, E.R. and Bruford, A. (1970) Creatine phosphokinase in motor neurone disease. *Clin. Chim. Acta*, 27, 53–6.

18. Guiloff, R.J., McGregor, B., Thompson, E. *et al.* (1980) Motor neurone disease with elevated cerebrospinal fluid protein. *J. Neurol. Neurosurg. Psychiatry*, 43, 390–6.

19. Conradi, S., Ronnevi, L.-O., Nise, G. and Vesterberg, O. (1980) Abnormal distribution of lead in amyotrophic lateral sclerosis. Reestimation of lead in the cerebrospinal fluid. *J. Neurol. Sci.*, 48, 413–18.

20. Cosi, V., Poloni, M., Mazzini, L. and Callieco, R. (1984) Somato-sensory evoked potentials in amyotrophic lateral sclerosis. *J. Neurol. Neurosurg. Psychiatry*, 47, 857–61.

21. Achari, A.N. and Anderson, M.S. (1974) Myopathic changes in amyotrophic lateral sclerosis. Pathologic analysis of muscle biopsy changes in 111 cases. *Neurology*, 24, 477–81.

22. Hjorth, R.J., Walsh, J.C. and Willison, R.G. (1973) The distribution and frequency of spontaneous fasciculations in motor neurone disease. *J. Neurol. Sci.,* 18, 469–74.
23. Kugelberg, E. and Welander, L. (1956) Heredofamilial juvenile muscular atrophy simulating muscular dystrophy. *Arch. Neurol. Psychiatry,* 75, 500–9.
24. Pearn, J. (1980) Classification of spinal muscular atrophies. *Lancet,* i, 919–22.
25. Harding, A.E., Bradbury, P.G. and Murray, N.M.F. (1983) Chronic asymmetrical spinal muscular atrophy. *J. Neurol. Sci.,* 59, 69–83.
26. Pearn, J.H., Hudgson, P. and Walton, J.N. (1978) A clinical and genetic study of spinal muscular atrophy of adult onset. The autosomal recessive form as a discrete disease entity. *Brain,* 101, 591-606.
27. Mitsumoto, H., Sliman, R.J., Schafer, I.A. *et al.* (1985) Motor neuron disease and adult hexosaminidase A deficiency in two families: evidence for multisystem degeneration. *Ann. Neurol.,* 17, 378–85.
28. Schwartz, M.S., Sargeant, M. and Swash, M. (1976) Longitudinal fibre splitting in neurogenic muscular disorders – its relation to the pathogenesis of 'myopathic' change. *Brain,* 99, 617–36.

11

Neurological emergencies – 1

11.1 BACTERIAL MENINGITIS

In most surveys of bacterial meningitis, the meningococcus, pneumococcus and *Haemophilus influenzae* have been the predominant organisms [1–3]. *Haemophilus* infection mainly occurs in children under the age of six years. In a proportion of cases, especially those already receiving antibiotics, the organism is not isolated. The clinical features seldom allow a confident diagnosis of the causative agent, the majority of patients experiencing headache, fever, drowsiness, neck stiffness and vomiting. A petechial rash is, however, of diagnostic value, occuring in perhaps 50% of cases of meningococcal meningitis, but only rarely in other bacterial forms or with ECHO virus infection [2].

The vast majority of patients have signs of meningeal irritation, though these may be lacking in the elderly or very young. Mortality rates rise with a decreasing level of consciousness at the time of presentation. Many patients will exhibit signs of middle ear or respiratory tract infection.

11.1.1 Investigations at onset

Cultures from the upper respiratory tract are likely to be misleading. In one series, pneumococci were isolated from the throat as frequently in patients with meningococcal as in those with pneumococcal meningitis [3]. Overall, blood cultures are positive in perhaps 50% of cases of meningitis, a higher figure being obtained in some series for *Haemophilus* infection [3].

Analysis of the cerebrospinal fluid is mandatory in suspected meningitis, though the procedure is not without risk. The pressure is usually elevated. The cell count may rarely exceed 50 000/mm³, but most patients have a count between 1000 and 10 000 polymorphonuclear leucocytes/mm³. Normal cell counts have exceptionally been reported in cases of bacterial meningitis proven on culture. The cell count is not related to outcome, nor is the protein concentration which seldom exceeds 5 g/l. Levels tend to be higher in pneumococcal meningitis. In one series, 20% of cases of meningococcal meningitis had normal protein concentrations[4]. A depressed glucose concentration helps to distinguish bacterial from viral meningitis, though mildly depressed levels are sometimes encountered in the latter. A concentration below 2.2 mmol/l is found in at least half the cases of bacterial meningitis. Alternatively, the level can be considered significantly depressed if less than 40% of a simultaneously measured blood level. It must be recognized that a delay of at least 30 min exists before changes in blood glucose levels are mirrored in the CSF. Despite this, measurement of the ratio is relevant, since some cases of meningitis occur in diabetic patients.

The yield from examining a gram stain of the CSF has been variously reported. In one study, gram staining correctly identified the organism subsequently isolated on culture in 73%, and, in another, in over 75% of cases[3]. In the three series already referred to, the causative organism was not identified, even after culture, in 10.5, 9 and 23% respectively[1–3]. Prior antibiotic therapy is a common factor in such cases.

The delay in establishing the causative organism by culture has stimulated the search for bacterial antigen by counter immunoelectrophoresis[5] or latex agglutination[6]. In two studies[5,6], the techniques identified between 82 and 98% of the organisms responsible (as shown by subsequent culture) for bacterial meningitis. The results are available within an hour. Antibiotic sensitivities cannot be determined, and the techniques are not a substitute for culture. The two methods may be identifying slightly different antigens. A heavily blood-stained fluid sometimes gives a false positive reaction.

A number of other CSF changes have been described in meningitis. In one study of CSF lactate concentrations, all patients with untreated bacterial meningitis had a level over 2.98 mmol/l, whereas all the cases of viral meningitis had a level below 2.8 mmol/l. The test is simple and rapid to perform, and requires only 0.1 cm³ of CSF[7]. CSF lactate levels rise in the presence of other conditions, including cerebral abscess, traumatic haemorrhage and tuberculous meningitis.

Alterations in CSF amino acid concentrations occur in meningitis[8]. In bacterial meningitis, glutamic acid levels are normal, but glutamine levels rise, reaching a maximum in the first week of the illness, then rapidly declining. It has been suggested that a markedly elevated serum level of C-reactive protein is inevitable in bacterial meningitis but uncommon in viral meningitis[9], and that if levels fail to fall within 7–10 days, or rise again, a complication of the meningitis, for example subdural effusion, should be suspected.

In one series of 106 patients with bacterial meningitis who had lumbar puncture performed on the day of admission, the mean CSF pressure was 307 mm[10]. Despite this, papilloedema is rare in the early stages of meningitis, and demands radiological investigation. In a proportion of patients dying with meningitis, tonsillar or temporal lobe herniation is found and, in some of these, death may be precipitated by the performance of lumbar puncture.

CT scanning in acute bacterial meningitis is unlikely to show any parenchymal abnormalities in the initial stages, though there may be evidence of gyral enhancement.

11.1.2 Recommendation (see flow chart A)

If bacterial meningitis is suspected, immediate lumbar puncture is necessary, though the presence of papilloedema (suggesting focal intracranial sepsis) would favour prior CT scanning, providing that it can be performed without delay. A normal cell count makes the diagnosis highly unlikely, but not impossible, and should not deter the search for bacteria by gram stain. If the gram stain is negative, bacterial antigen should be sought by latex agglutination or counter immunoelectrophoresis. Problems arise if the cell count and glucose concentration are suggestive of bacterial meningitis but immediate attempts to identify the responsible organism fail. Where available, estimations of CSF lactate or glutamine levels or serum C-reactive protein are valuable, since if any or all of these are normal, the diagnosis of bacterial meningitis becomes correspondingly less likely. If these investigations are not available, blind antibiotic therapy is justified, at least while results of CSF culture materialize.

11.1.3 Subsequent investigations

Many physicians choose to re-examine the CSF during the course of treatment, assuming that normal, or near normal, findings correlate

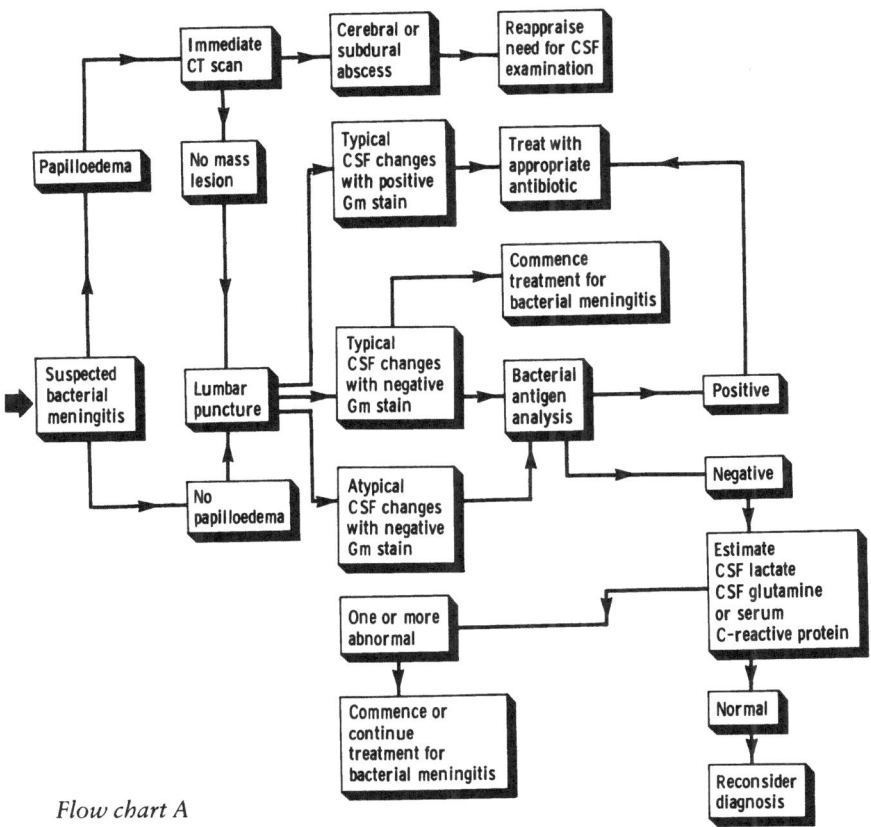

Flow chart A

with clinical recovery with persisting abnormalities reflecting the development of complications. A study based on CSF analysis after completion of therapy for bacterial meningitis was unable to confirm that glucose concentration below 2.2 mmol/l, a protein concentration above 1.0 g/l or an elevated white cell count were of any significance with respect to the development of complications[11]. Clearly, routine sequential CSF examination, when the clinical course is satisfactory, cannot be justified.

Certain developments during the course of treatment require further investigation. Seizures are relatively common in infants with meningitis but less common in the adult, in whom their appearance may reflect water intoxication due to inappropriate ADH production. In patients with seizures, focal neurological signs or late

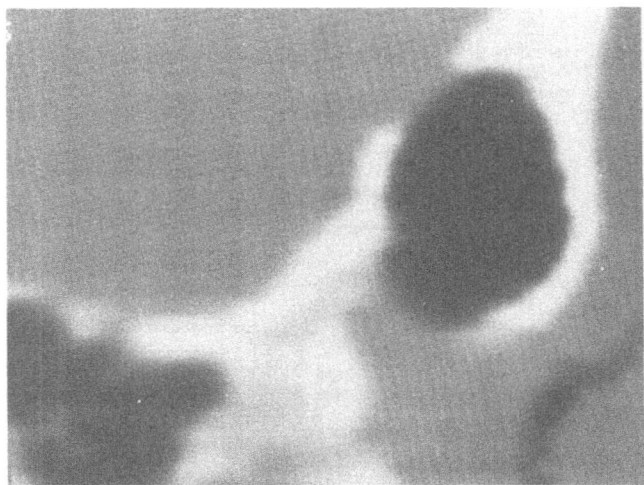

Fig. 11.1 CT scan showing a defect in the posterior wall of the frontal sinus, in a patient with recurrent pneumococcal meningitis

deterioration in the conscious level after initial response, CT scanning is necessary [12]. Subdural empyema is relatively common in infants, more so in those with *Haemophilus* meningitis, but is probably rare in the adult. Abnormalities in the adult accounting for these various complications include focal intracerebral sepsis and cortical venous thrombosis. The latter complication tends to appear during the second or third week of the illness after apparent clinical recovery [10].

11.1.4 The problem of recurrent meningitis

Recurrent bacterial meningitis is rare. Its development suggests either an anatomical defect allowing access of organisms to the central nervous system, a parameningeal focus of infection, or an immunological defect [13]. Most patients with recurrent meningitis have an anatomical defect, often post-traumatic in origin. Typical defects include fistulas into the frontal or ethmoid sinuses, or through the cribriform plate (Fig. 11.1). Specialized tomographic techniques are required to detect these abnormalities [14]. Congenital defects allowing ingress of organisms include myelomeningocoele and cranial or spinal dermoid sinuses. Patients with immunoparesis, for example due to AIDS, are liable to develop infection due to unusual organisms. In cases with recurrent meningitis careful clinical examination for cranial or spinal defects is required, along with immunological appraisal and radiological studies including skull X-ray and CT scan.

11.2 VIRAL MENINGITIS

The clinical presentation of viral meningitis is fairly uniform. Most patients experience headache, fever, neck rigidity and vomiting, with fever and signs of meningeal irritation the sole clinical findings [15]. The symptoms resolve rapidly, disappearing, in the vast majority, within two weeks. A small proportion of patients will have evidence of a concomitant encephalitis, with seizures, coma or involuntary movements. Follow-up studies reveal a surprisingly high incidence of protracted limb pains, irritability and fatigue. In one analysis of 430 cases of aseptic meningitis, a specific diagnosis was achieved in 71% of cases [16], but in another study of 111 patients the aetiology was identified in only 45% [17]. Enteroviruses or mumps account for at least half of these [15,16].

11.2.1 Investigations

Typically the CSF contains between 10 and 2000 white cells/mm^3. The earlier the CSF is examined, the more likely is the finding of a predominance of polymorphonuclear leucocytes [15,18]. Where this is the case, the transformation to a predominance of mononuclear cells occurs within 8 hours in the vast majority [18]. Protein concentrations are normal in a third, and, if elevated, usually do not exceed 1 g/l. Typically glucose concentrations are normal but, in a small proportion of cases (6% in one series), levels are slightly depressed. Cytopathic effects on cell culture develop more rapidly than is often appreciated. In one study, the mean delay, for cases due to enterovirus, before CSF produced abnormalities in cell culture was 3.7 days [17]. If enterovirus is suspected as the cause of aseptic meningitis, cultures from the nasopharynx and rectum are of value.

11.2.2 Recommendation

In suspected viral meningitis, CSF examination is essential. If the findings are characteristic, culture, though often undertaken, is unlikely to alter management. If the clinical picture is typical, but the

CSF contains an excess of polymorphonuclear leucocytes, repeat CSF examination after 8–12 hours should be performed, providing the clinical status is stable. Culture from the throat and rectum should be undertaken if enterovirus infection is suspected.

11.3 TUBERCULOUS MENINGITIS

Typically tuberculous meningitis presents as a subacute illness with malaise, headache and fever, followed by a deterioration in the conscious level, signs of meningeal irritation and focal neurological signs[19]. Outcome is related to the speed with which the diagnosis is established, and therapy initiated. Difficulties in diagnosis arise when the condition presents atypically, for example acutely[20], and where the results of investigation are misleading.

11.3.1 Investigations

In four separate studies of tuberculous meningitis, an abnormal chest X-ray suggestive of tuberculous infection was found in 47, 44, 40 and 56% respectively[19,21–23]. Tuberculin skin tests are often negative (in 59% of one group of patients[23]).

CSF examination is again essential. The majority of cases have a cell count between 100 and 400/mm^3. A small proportion of patients will have a cell count less than 50/mm^3 and, rarely, particularly in patients with inhibited tuberculin sensitivity, the cell count is normal[20]. Conversely, in patients with acute onset, the cell count may exceed 1000/mm^3 and can then contain a high proportion of polymorphonuclear leucocytes[20]. Normally these are in the minority, with a predominance of lymphocytes. The protein concentration usually lies between 1.0 and 5.0 g/l but again can be normal. In one study, of 52 patients, 48% had a glucose concentration between 1.7 and 2.5 mmol/l[21]. A normal concentration is compatible with the diagnosis.

Ziehl–Nielsen staining of CSF identified acid-fast bacilli in between 12 and 37% of cases according to one review[23]. The frequency with which acid-fast bacilli are cultured depends on the criteria chosen for accepting the diagnosis of tuberculous meningitis. In one series, culture of the first CSF specimen obtained was positive in 52%[21]. Sequential CSF examination is of value where the diagnosis remains uncertain. After four sequential examinations, the percentages of positive identifications by microscopy or culture had

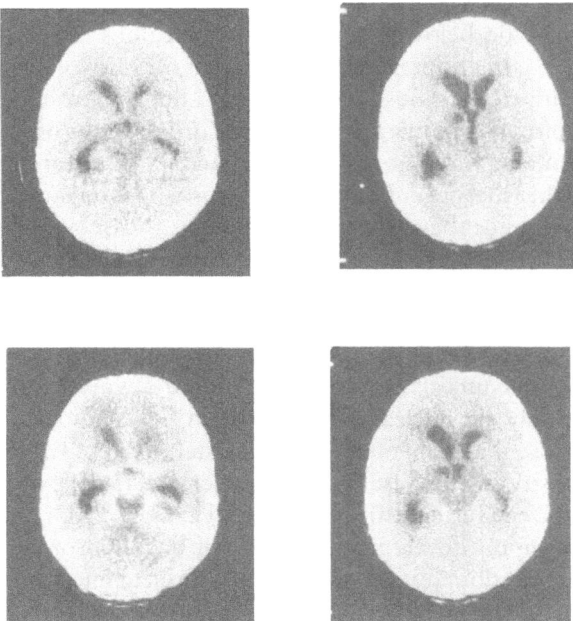

Fig. 11.2 CT scan demonstrating enhancement of the basal cisterns in a patient with tuberculous meningitis (lower pair are contrast views)

reached 87 and 83 in one study [21]. Positive identification was achieved in some 43% of cases after anti-tuberculous therapy had been initiated.

Remaining uncertainty in diagnosis has led to the search for mycobacterial antigen in the CSF using either an enzyme-linked immunosorbent assay [24] or latex particle agglutination [25]. Using the latter technique, antigen was detected in the initial CSF sample of 17 out of 18 patients with tuberculous meningitis, and in subsequent samples in the remainder. Amongst 134 'control' subjects only one, a child with *Haemophilus influenzae* meningitis, was positive. Tuberculostearic acid, a constituent of mycobacteria, has been demonstrated in the CSF in tuberculous meningitis [26].

An alteration of the blood–brain–CSF barrier in tuberculous meningitis is reflected by changes in the partition of orally administered bromide between serum and CSF. The chemical method of bromide estimation has proved unreliable with frequent false positive results [27]. Using radioactive bromide (^{82}Br) it was suggested that, in patients with a lymphocytic meningitis, a serum cerebrospinal fluid ratio below 1.6 indicated tuberculous rather than viral infection [28]. In another study, using a cut off ratio of 1.9, 40 of 42 patients with tuberculous meningitis had abnormal values, together with four out of 44 patients with other disorders, three of which were pyogenic meningitis. The test is performed 48 hours after administration of the isotope and does not appear to be influenced by recent initiation of anti-tuberculous therapy.

CSF lactate and amino acid levels have been studied in tuberculous meningitis. Both glutamine [8] and lactate [7] concentrations are increased.

Radiological investigation has proved valuable in patients with tuberculous meningitis. Chest X-ray should always be performed, though it may be misleadingly normal. CT scanning is likely to demonstrate enhancement of the basal cisterns (Fig. 11.2) with areas of low density in the basal regions. Later, areas of low density of lacunar type can be identified in the basal ganglia [29]. Hydrocephalus is a common development following bacterial or tuberculous meningitis, but does not usually warrant surgical intervention.

11.3.2 Subsequent investigations

Inappropriate ADH production is not uncommon during the course of tuberculous meningitis, contributing then to imperfect response to treatment or to unexpected deterioration after initial clinical response. The latter development should initiate repeat CT scanning since it may reflect the appearance of cerebral tuberculomas [30].

11.3.3 Recommendation (see flow chart B)

Skin testing is of limited value in the diagnosis of tuberculous meningitis. Results are apt to be misleading and are not available for 48 hours after testing. CSF examination should be performed immediately. The finding of a lymphocytic pleocytosis, elevated protein and depressed glucose concentration demands immediate anti-tuberculous therapy whether or not acid-fast bacilli are detected in the CSF smear. Sequential CSF examination increases the chance of isolating the responsible organism. CT scanning at this stage, with the finding of basal enhancement, would strongly favour the diagnosis even if the bacillus was absent on CSF staining. Continuing diagnostic uncertainty is likely if the CSF changes are atypical. Since

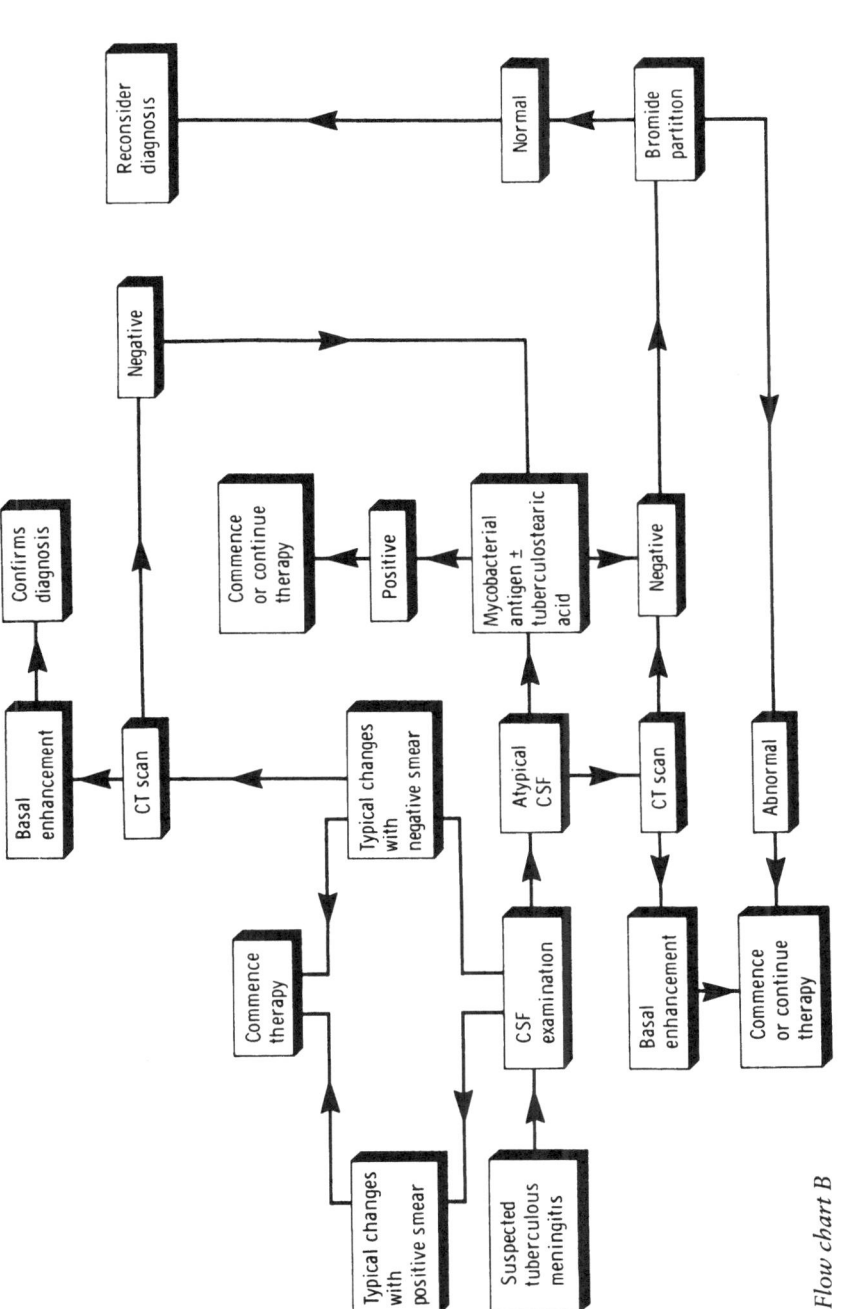

Flow chart B

'blind' therapy implies the use of potentially toxic drugs for at least a six-week period (until the results of culture are available) other diagnostic techniques merit consideration. If available, tests for plasma membrane antigen should be performed and are preferred to estimation of tuberculostearic acid, a more complex and less verified technique. The use of bromide partition is worth considering, particularly since the results are not influenced by the recent initiation of therapy. Only the radioactive technique can be recommended and results are delayed for 48 hours after the administration of the oral dose.

11.4 CRYPTOCOCCAL MENINGITIS

Cryptococcal meningitis shares many clinical features with tuberculous infection[23]. Headache, fever, nausea and vomiting are equally common in the two conditions, but changes in the mental state and nuchal rigidity are twice as common in tuberculous meningitis. Though some authors have stressed predisposing factors[23,31], another study, of 25 patients, found such factors in only one[32]. Headache is almost inevitable but fever is present in less than half at the time of presentation. Neurological signs, other than those reflecting meningeal irritation, are lacking initially, though papilloedema appeared in 45% of patients later in the course of the disease in one series.

11.4.1 Investigations

Chest X-ray opacities are detected in about a quarter of patients. Hyponatraemia due to inappropriate ADH production is considerably less common than in tuberculous meningitis[23]. The ESR is usually normal[32]. As with other forms of meningitis, CSF examination is mandatory. The pressure is usually elevated. In one study, the mean cell count was 130/mm³[23]. In rare instances, the count is normal, or exceeds 1000 cells/mm³. Lymphocytes predominate though, as in tuberculous meningitis, an excess of polymorphonuclear leucocytes can occur. The protein concentration is elevated in the majority but seldom above 2 g/l. A depression of glucose concentration is encountered of the order seen in tuberculous meningitis, but is absent in perhaps a third[32].

Indian ink staining is seldom positive in more than 50% of cases at initial CSF examination though the yield increases if serial specimens

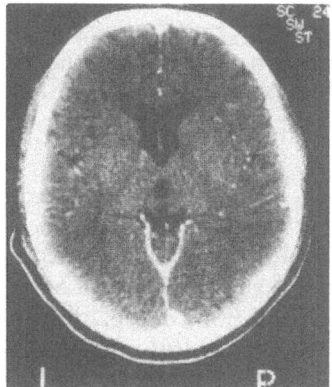 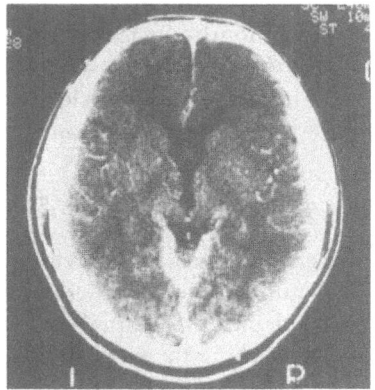

Fig. 11.3 CT scan demonstrating meningeal enhancement in a case of cryptococcal meningitis (left) subsequently resolving (right)

are examined. Indeed some authors have recommended at least three separate CSF examinations if the initial one is negative [32]. Cryptoccocal polysaccharide antigen is detectable by a latex agglutination test, and was found in 12 of 13 cases in one study [23]. Both false positive and false negative results are encountered.

CT scanning tends to show non-specific changes including cerebral oedema and hydrocephalus though in some cases meningeal enhancement is found [32] (Fig. 11.3).

11.4.2 Recommendation

In patients with suspected cryptococcal meningitis, the clinical features and CSF changes are such that concomitant investigation for tuberculous infection is appropriate. Repeat lumbar puncture is of value if Indian ink staining is initially negative. Though false positive antigen studies are recorded, the finding necessitates initiation of therapy.

11.5 ENCEPHALITIS

Herpes simplex virus is the commonest cause of sporadic encephalitis in the United Kingdom. In adults, type 1 virus is usually responsible. When encephalitis is diagnosed on clinical criteria alone, it is frequently incorrect [33]. An encephalitic illness may accompany a viral illness, for example with mumps, influenza, infectious mononucleosis or herpes simplex, or may follow one by up to a month (post-infectious encephalitis). Fever is more common in the first group, as are vomiting and headache. Patients with post-infectious encephalitis tend to present with seizures, hemiparesis or alteration of consciousness [34].

11.5.1 Investigation

A peripheral leucocytosis is encountered in post-infectious encephalitis but seldom in other forms. In a recent survey, the CSF was normal in 25% of patients with post-infectious encephalitis, but seldom where the encephalitis coincided with a virus infection [34]. The EEG is usually abnormal, irrespective of the type of illness. Non-specific slowing is common, but in herpes simplex encephalitis high voltage periodic sharp waves can be detected over one or other temporal lobe in the majority [35,36]. The advent of effective therapy for herpes simplex cases has led to a considerable literature on methods of early diagnosis.

In the absence of a CT scanning facility, technetium scanning can be of value, demonstrating uptake in one or both temporal lobes, typically between 10 and 21 days from the onset of the illness [37]. In one study of 113 biopsy proven cases of herpes encephalitis, the mean CSF protein concentration was 0.8 g/l with 18% having normal values [38]. The mean white cell count was 130/mm^3, the majority being lymphocytes. Rarely, there are more than 1000 cells/mm^3, or there is no increase in the cell count. An increased red cell count in the CSF, reflecting the haemorrhagic nature of the encephalitis, is found in the majority [38]. The CSF pleocytosis can persist for months [36]. In the study of 113 biopsy proven cases, three had completely normal CSF.

The hope that the diagnosis of herpes simplex encephalitis could be readily confirmed by identification, using an indirect immunofluorescent technique, of viral antigen in CSF lymphocytes was stimulated by a report suggesting that nearly all patients with encephalitis due to herpes simplex had positive findings [39]. Further experience has refuted this conclusion; identification of viral antigen from CSF lymphocytes could be achieved in only 4% of patients in a recent series [40].

Detection of viral antibodies in the CSF is a well-proven method of diagnosis but suffers from the disadvantage of delay before significant levels appear. A variety of techniques has been described, including the formulation of a ratio which allows for alteration of the blood: CSF barrier. By this method, a ratio exceeding the normal was detectable in only 50% of proven cases when tested in the first 10 days of the illness[41]. Overall, diagnosis based on rising CSF antibody levels achieves a sensitivity between 70 and 90% and a specificity between 81 and 88%[40]. IgG ratios in the CSF are elevated in the majority of patients[42].

Radiological techniques for assisting diagnosis, prior to the introduction of CT scanning, principally concentrated on angiography. CT scanning is a more effective tool, demonstrating attenuation in one or both temporal lobes sometimes with enhancement and mass effect[43]. However, a normal scan does not exclude the diagnosis and in the experience of some, the EEG provides more accurate localization[38]. Indeed this group recorded 23 patients with herpes simplex encephalitis and a normal scan in whom localization was achieved by either EEG or technetium scanning.

Definitive diagnosis rests with the results of brain biopsy, when the findings of intranuclear inclusions is suggestive (achieving a specificity of 86%[40]) and isolation of the virus conclusive.

CT scanning assists the diagnosis of post-infectious encephalitis. In an analysis of 11 patients, seven had a combination of brain stem oedema, low density areas in the basal ganglia and deep white matter with cortical enhancing lesions[44].

11.5.2 Recommendation

Diagnosis of acute encephalitis on clinical grounds alone is prone to error, and the results of investigation may be misleadingly normal. Urgency in diagnosis relates to the availability of partially effective treatment for herpes simplex infection. Inevitably, therefore, investigation is directed to exclude or confirm that diagnosis.

EEG, examination of CSF and CT scanning are necessary. EEG is most likely to localize the predominant site of involvement, relevant if biopsy is to be pursued. A combination of lymphocytic pleocytosis with an excess of red cells in the CSF is suggestive. Search for viral antigen in the spinal fluid is unrewarding. Viral antibody studies are valuable but frequently fail to establish the diagnosis in the first ten days of the illness. CT scanning sometimes reveals pathognomonic changes but can be normal in proven cases. Definitive early diagnosis still requires virus isolation by brain biopsy.

11.6 STATUS EPILEPTICUS

Status epilepticus is defined as a single seizure persisting for more than 30 minutes, or a succession of two or more fits without recovery of consciousness. Tonic–clonic, focal motor, absence and complex partial forms are described. The incidence in epileptic patients lies between 1 and 5% with a mortality reported between 3 and 20%. In adults, status epilepticus is rarely, if ever, the first manifestation of cryptogenic epilepsy [45]. In one study, the condition was symptomatic in 63% of cases, the commonest pathologies being tumour, cerebrovascular disease, infection and trauma [45]. In patients presenting with status who are found to have an underlying tumour, localization is most commonly to the frontal lobes. In a study of 98 patients with status, some 50% had had no previous seizures [46]. Non-compliance in the taking of anticonvulsants was the commonest cause. Other factors included alcohol withdrawal, focal pathology and metabolic disorders. Focal features in the seizures are just as likely in patients with a metabolic derangement as in those with structural lesions.

Focal motor status is usually confined to the face and eyes, or the face and arm. The responsible EEG focus lies in the contralateral frontal, central or anterior temporal region. Absence and complex partial status are uncommon and difficult to diagnose. The former results in an acute confusional state sometimes accompanied by myoclonic jerks of the eyes and hands, the latter in a fluctuating state of arousal periodically interspersed with typical attacks.

11.6.1 Investigations

Metabolic studies are essential in the investigation of patients with status. Factors sometimes incriminated include hyponatraemia, hypo- or hypercalcaemia, hypoglycaemia, hypo- or hyperthyroidism, hypoxia, hepatic encephalopathy and hyperosmolar states [46]. The peripheral white count is often elevated, whether or not there is an underlying infection. Non-specific changes in the CSF include a moderately elevated cell count and protein concentration.

The EEG is particularly helpful in the diagnosis of absence [47] and complex partial status [48] (Fig. 11.4). Where status occurs in the setting of established epilepsy, CT scanning is unlikely to reveal any fresh pathological change. If there is no previous history of epilepsy, CT scanning is essential.

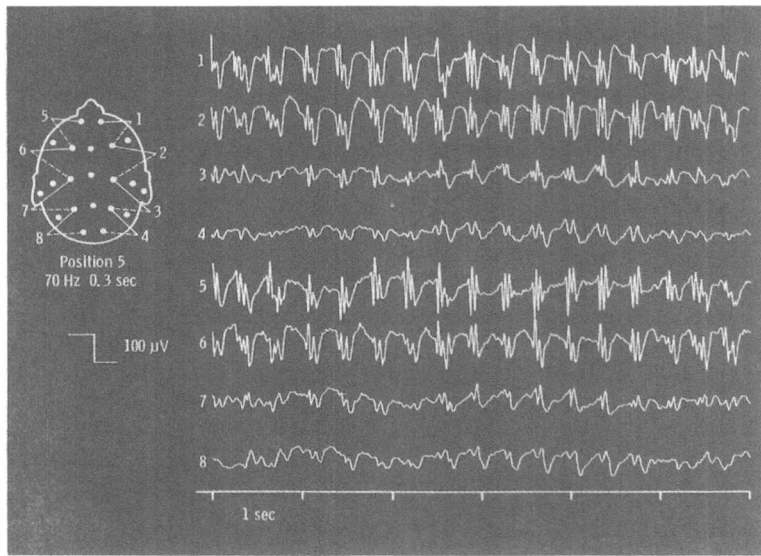

Fig. 11.4 EEG showing minor status. The patient, aged 46, had presented with a confusional state associates with twitching of the mouth

11.6.2 Recommendation

Metabolic screening should be performed immediately to exclude potential triggering factors. The EEG is particualry helpful if either absence or complex partial status is considered a possible diagnosis. CT scanning is performed if the status has arisen *de novo*.

REFERENCES

1. Carpenter, R.B. and Petersdorf, R.G. (1962) The clinical spectrum of bacterial meningitis. *Am. J. Med.,* 33, 262–75.
2. Swartz, M.N. and Dodge, P.R. (1965) Bacterial meningitis – A review of selected aspects. 1. General clinical features, special problems and unusual meningeal reactions mimicking bacterial meningitis. *N. Engl. J. Med.,* 272, 725–31.
3. Bohr, V., Rasmussen, N., Hansen, B. *et al.* (1983) 875 cases of bacterial meningitis: diagnostic procedures and the impact of preadmission antibiotic therapy. Part III of a three-part series. *J. Infect.,* 7, 193–202.
4. Swartz, M.N. and Dodge, P.R. (1965) Bacterial meningitis – A review of selected aspects. 1. General clinical features, special problems and

unusual meningeal reactions mimicking bacterial meningitis (continued). *N. Engl. J. Med.,* **272,** 779–87.

5. Coonrod, J.D. and Rytel, M.W. (1972) Determination of aetiology of bacterial meningitis by counter immunoelectrophoresis. *Lancet,* i, 1154–7.

6. Whittle, H.C., Tugwell, P., Egler, L.J. and Greenwood, G.M. (1974) Rapid bacteriological diagnosis of pyogenic meningitis by latex agglutination. *Lancet,* ii, 619–21.

7. Curtis, G.D.W., Slack, M.P.E. and Tompkins, D.S. (1981) Cerebrospinal fluid lactate and the diagnosis of meningitis. *J. Infect.,* 3, 159–65.

8. Corston, R.N., McGale, E.H.F., Tonier, C.S. *et al.* (1981) Cerebrospinal fluid amino acid concentrations in patients with viral and tuberculous meningitis. *J. Neurol. Neurosurg. Psychiatry,* **44,** 791–5.

9. Peltola, H.O. (1982) C-reactive protein for rapid monitoring of infections of the central nervous system. *Lancet,* i, 980–3.

10. Dodge, P.R. and Swartz, M.N. (1965) Bacterial meningitis – A review of selected aspects II. Special neurological problems, postmeningitic complications and clinicopathological correlations. *N. Engl. J. Med.,* **272,** 954–60.

11. Durack, D.T. and Spanos, A. (1982) End-of-treatment spinal tap in bacterial meningitis. Is it worthwhile? *J. Am. Med. Assoc.,* **248,** 75–8.

12. Weisberg, L.A. (1980) Cerebral computerized tomography in intracranial inflammatory disorders. *Arch. Neurol.,* 37, 137–42.

13. Swartz, M.N. and Dodge, P.R. (1965) Bacterial meningitis – A review of selected aspects 1. General clinical features, special problems and unusual meningeal reactions mimicking bacterial meningitis (continued). *N. Engl. J. Med.,* **272,** 842–8.

14. Kaseff, L.G., Nieberding, P.H., Shorago, G.W. and Huertas, G. (1980) Fistula between the middle ear and subarachnoid space as a cause of recurrent meningitis: detection by means of thin-section, complex motion tomography. *Radiology,* **135,** 105–8.

15. Lepow, M.L., Coyne, N., Thompson, L.B. *et al.* (1962) A clinical, epidemiologic and laboratory investigation of aseptic meningitis during the four-year period 1955–1958. II. The clinical disease and its sequelae. *N. Engl. J. Med.,* **266,** 1188–93.

16. Meyer, H.M. Jr, Johnson, R.T., Crawford, I.P. *et al.* (1960) Central nervous system syndromes of 'viral' etiology. *Am. J. Med.,* **29,** 334–47.

17 Chonmaitree, T., Menegus, M.A. and Powell, K.R. (1982) The clinical relevance of 'CSF viral culture'. A two-year experience with aseptic meningitis in Rochester, NY. *J. Am. Med. Assoc.,* **247,** 1843–7.

18. Feigin, R.D. and Shackelford, P.G. (1973) Value of repeat lumbar puncture in the differential diagnosis of meningitis. *N. Engl. J. Med.,* **289,** 571–4.

19. Swart, S., Briggs, R.S. and Millac, P.A. (1981) Tuberculous meningitis in Asian patients. *Lancet,* ii, 15–16.

20. Taylor, K.B., Smith, H.V. and Vollum, R.L. (1955) Tuberculous meningitis of acute onset. *J. Neurol. Neurosurg. Psychiatry*, 18, 165–73.
21. Kennedy, D.H. and Fallon, R.J. (1979) Tuberculous meningitis. *J. Am. Med. Assoc.*, 241, 264–8.
22. Roberts, F.J. (1981) Problems in the diagnosis of tuberculous meningitis. *Arch. Neurol.*, 38, 319–20.
23. Stockstill, M.T. and Kauffman, C.A. (1983) Comparison of cryptococcal and tuberculous meningitis. *Arch. Neurol.*, 40, 81–5.
24. Sada, E., Ruiz-Palacios, G.M., Lopez-Vidal, Y. and Ponce de Leon, S. (1983) Detection of mycobacterial antigens in cerebrospinal fluid of patients with tuberculous meningitis by enzyme-linked immunosorbent assay. *Lancet*, ii, 651–2.
25. Krambovitis, E., McIllmurray, M.B., Lock, P.E. *et al.* (1984) Rapid diagnosis of tuberculous meningitis by latex particle agglutination. *Lancet*, ii, 1229–31.
26. Mårdh, P-A., Larsson, L., Høiby, N. *et al.* (1983) Tuberculostearic acid as a diagnostic marker in tuberculous meningitis. *Lancet*, i, 367.
27. Weinberg, J.R. and Coppack, S.P. (1985) Positive bromide partition test in the absence of tuberculous meningitis. *J. Neurol. Neurosurg. Psychiatry*, 48, 278–80.
28. Mandal, B.K., Evans, D.I.K., Ironside, A.G. and Pullan, B.R. (1972) Radioactive bromide partition test in differential diagnosis of tuberculous meningitis. *Br. Med. J.*, 4, 413–15.
29. Bullock, M.R.R. and Welchman, J.M. (1982) Diagnostic and prognostic features of tuberculous meningitis on CT scanning. *J. Neurol. Neurosurg. Psychiatry*, 45, 1098–101.
30. Lees, A.J., MacLeod, A.F. and Marshall, J. (1980) Cerebral tuberculomas developing during treatment of tuberculous meningitis. *Lancet*, i, 1208–11.
31. Edwards, V.E., Sutherland, J.M. and Tyrer, J.H. (1970) Cryptococcosis of the central nervous system. Epidemiological, clinical, and therapeutic features. *J. Neurol. Neurosurg. Psychiatry*, 33, 415–25.
32. Tjia, T.L., Yeow, Y.K. and Tan, C.B. (1985) Cryptococcal meningitis. *J. Neurol. Neurosurg. Psychiatry*, 48, 853–8.
33. Miller, J.D. and Ross, C.A.C. (1968) Encephalitis. A four-year survey. *Lancet*, i, 1121–6.
34. Kennard, C. and Swash, M. (1981) Acute viral encephalitis. Its diagnosis and outcome. *Brain*, 104, 129–48.
35. Ch'ien, L.T., Boehm, R.M., Robinson, H. *et al.* (1977) Characteristic early electroencephalographic changes in herpes simplex encephalitis. Clinical and virologic studies. *Arch. Neurol.*, 34, 361–4.
36. Koskiniemi, M., Vaheri, A., Manninen, V. *et al.* (1980) Herpes simplex virus encephalitis. New diagnostic and clinical features and results of therapy. *Arch. Neurol.*, 37, 763–7.
37. Karlin, C.A., Robinson, R.G., Hinthorn, D.R. and Liu, C. (1978) Radionuclide imaging in herpes simplex encephalitis. *Radiology*, 126, 181–4.

38. Whitley, R.J., Soong, S-J., Linneman, C. Jr *et al.* (1982) Herpes simplex encephalitis. Clinical assessment. *J. Am. Med. Assoc.,* **247**, 317–20.
39. Dayan, A.D. and Stokes, M.I. (1973) Rapid diagnosis of encephalitis by immunofluorescent examination of cerebrospinal fluid cells. *Lancet,* i, 177–9.
40. Nahmias, A.J., Whitley, R.J., Visintine, A.N. *et al.* (1982) Herpes simplex virus encephalitis: laboratory evaluations and their diagnostic significance. *J. Infect. Dis.,* **145**, 829–36.
41. Klapper, P.E., Laing, I. and Longson, M. (1981) Rapid non-invasive diagnosis of herpes encephalitis. *Lancet,* ii, 607–9.
42. Koskiniemi, M.-L. and Vaheri, A. (1982) Diagnostic value of cerebrospinal fluid antibodies in herpes simplex virus encephalitis. *J. Neurol. Neurosurg. Psychiatry,* **45**, 239–42.
43. Kaufman, D.M., Zimmerman, R.D. and Leeds, N.E. (1979) Computed tomography in herpes simplex encephalitis. *Neurology,* **29**, 1392–6.
44. Lukes, S.A. and Norman, D. (1983) Computed tomography in acute disseminated encephalomyelitis. *Ann. Neurol.,* **13**, 567–72.
45. Oxbury, J.M. and Whitty, C.W.M. (1971) Causes and consequences of status epilepticus in adults. A study of 86 cases. *Brain,* **94**, 733–44.
46. Aminoff, M.J. and Simon, R.P. (1980) Status epilepticus. Causes, clinical features and consequences in 98 patients. *Am. J. Med.,* **69**, 657–66.
47. Schwartz, M.S. and Scott, D.F. (1971) Isolated petit-mal status presenting *de novo* in middle age. *Lancet,* ii, 1399–401.
48. Engel, J. Jr, Ludwig, B.I. and Fetell, M. (1978) Prolonged partial complex status epilepticus: EEG and behavioral observations. *Neurology,* **28**, 863–9.

12

Neurological emergencies – 2

12.1 SUBARACHNOID HAEMORRHAGE

Subarachnoid haemorrhage represents 8% of all cerebrovascular events. Up to 25% of patients are dead within 24 hours, the figure rising to perhaps 50% by three months[1]. Subarachnoid haemorrhage from aneurysmal rupture reaches a peak incidence in the early fifties, some 20 years later than for cases due to arteriovenous malformation[2]. Anterior communicating aneurysms are the commonest source of subarachnoid bleeding, followed by posterior communicating then middle cerebral aneurysms. Vertebrobasilar aneurysms account for some 5% of the total[2]. Aneurysmal rupture is more common in women, except for the anterior communicating group. Some 20% of patients have more than one aneurysm. Other sources of subarachnoid haemorrhage include primary haemorrhage into the brain substance with subsequent rupture into the subarachnoid space or ventricular system, and bleeding due to a disorder of haemostasis.

The symptomatology of subarachnoid haemorrhage includes headache, vomiting, and an altered level of consciousness. Seizures may occur. Focal neurological signs are usually the consequence of concomitant parenchymal haemorrhage or vasospasm. Rebleeding causes a high mortality rate and though reaching a maximum in the first two weeks after the initial haemorrhage is not confined to that period. The rebleeding rate in non-surgically treated aneurysm, once patients have survived beyond six months, is estimated to be around 3% per annum[3].

A number of indirect effects following subarachnoid haemorrhage can cause diagnostic confusion. Fever occurs in the majority of patients and some develop a disturbance of electrolyte or fluid balance. A number of ECG abnormalities are described including ST segment changes, a prolonged QT interval and altered configuration of the T wave. The changes may be accompanied by a moderate rise in the level of cardiac enzymes [4].

12.1.1 Investigations

Though the EEG may show changes which suggest the possible site of aneurysmal rupture leading to subarachnoid haemorrhage [5], it is now rarely performed as part of the investigation of this condition. It has been established that cerebral blood flow values correlate with the level of consciousness, the presence of vasospasm and focal neurological deficit. Furthermore, blood flow levels, measured within two weeks of onset, appear to correlate with eventual outcome. It has been suggested that, if mean cortical flow is below a certain level (60 ml/100 g/min), operative intervention should be deferred [6]. At present, however, the main investigative techniques employed in patients with suspected subarachnoid haemorrhage are lumbar puncture, CT scanning and cerebral angiography.

Rarely, normal CSF has been reported soon after the onset of subarachnoid haemorrhage [7], but in general, the development of blood-stained fluid with a xanthochromic supernatant is almost inevitable. The rate of haemolysis of red cells after subarachnoid bleeding varies considerably and is unrelated to the number of red cells in the initial specimen [8]. It is generally stated that haemolysis reaches a maximum about five days after onset. In one study, the mean duration of persisting red cells after subarachnoid haemorrhage was 9 days, though with a range from 4 to 19 days [9]. Rarely, red cells can persist for 30 days [8], though in such cases a contribution from further small, clinically undetected, bleeds would be difficult to exclude.

Though haemolysis has been reported to begin within four hours of haemorrhage, most authors have suggested it appears after about 12 hours. Rarely it may be delayed for up to 4 days [9]. Mean duration of xanthochromia after subarachnoid haemorrhage was 20 days in one study [9]. Experimental evidence suggests that bleeding provokes activity of haem-oxygenase in the arachnoid and choroid plexuses leading to the conversion of haem into bilirubin. Peak activity of this enzyme, in experimental animals, is reached some 12 hours after the subarachnoid injection of blood [10]. In distinguishing traumatic from subarachnoid bleeding, successive clearing of the specimen in the former case is stressed, along with an absence of xanthochromia. If, however, the fluid contains over 12 000 red cells, oxyhaemoglobin will stain the supernatant within 30 minutes of the puncture, whereas if the red cells exceed 150 000 enough serum chromogens are present to produce xanthochromia[11]. Delay in performing lumbar puncture after subarachnoid haemorrhage can result in the discovery of other changes in the CSF which may then cause diagnostic confusion. An increase in mononuclear cells is likely two to four weeks after the ictus[9], whereas even within the first week, a moderate depression of glucose concentration can be found[12].

Although CSF examination has been the cornerstone of diagnosis in the past, it is now recognized that the procedure is not without risk in the patient with subarachnoid haemorrhage. In one study, seven of 55 patients deteriorated after lumbar puncture, resulting in death in four of them[13]. Post-mortem examination in three of these patients showed tentorial and tonsillar coning. Of 12 patients with intracerebral clot and ventricular displacement on CT scanning, five had lumbar puncture performed. Three of these patients deteriorated.

CT scanning is now firmly established as being of major importance in the investigation of suspected subarachnoid haemorrhage. A recent publication of the cooperative aneurysm study in the United States summarized the results of 1378 CT scans in 1412 patients with subarachnoid haemorrhage[1]. CT scanning demonstrated subarachnoid blood in 90.5% of patients scanned with 24 hours of onset. The yield fell to 66.7% if three days had elapsed. The study indicated that the scan was more often normal in the alert patient. Other findings included intracerebral or intraventricular haemorrhage (each in about one-sixth of the studies) and hydrocephalus in 16%. An aneurysm was located by scanning in 5.5%, though contrast studies were not routine. The demonstration of infarcted areas was not common when scanning was performed in the first few days after onset. In an earlier study[14], some correlation had been found between the amount of subarachnoid blood, as assessed by CT scanning, the patient's neurological status and the presence of spasm at angiography. In the cooperative study it was shown that the finding of a thin collection of subarachnoid blood was more common in patients in Grade I of the Botterell scale (i.e. those least affected) whereas the presence of diffuse blood, or local thick clots carried a worse prognosis[1]. Measurement of the largest clot in the subarachnoid cisterns and cerebral fissues indicates that those

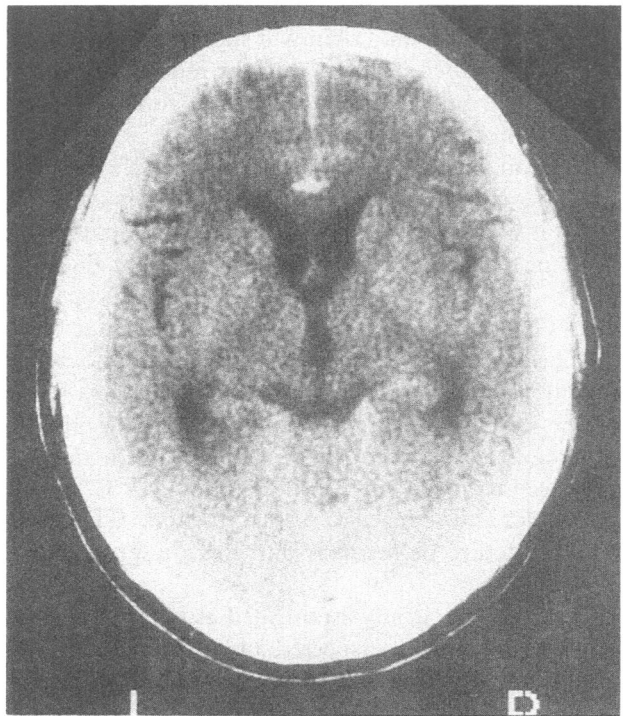

Fig. 12.1 CT demonstrating blood in the anterior interhemispheric fissure following rupture of an anterior communicating aneurysm

patients with the largest clots are most at risk from developing focal ischaemic neurological deficit[15]. Poor outcome also correlates with the presence of post-contrast enhancement[16]. Though loosely described as being subarachnoid in distribution, it has been suggested that the enhancement is gyral, reflecting increased blood volume in small cortical vessels.

Other authors have reported a higher yield for the detection of an aneurysm. For example, in one study of anterior cerebral or anterior communicating aneurysm, an enhancing lesion, of 10–16 mm in diameter, compatible with an aneurysm was found in 26% of cases scanned within three days of onset[17]. An additional benefit from CT scanning is the ability to predict the likely source of subarachnoid bleeding from the scan appearance. For example, following rupture of an anterior cerebral or anterior communicating aneurysm, subarachnoid blood may be confined to the pericallosal or anterior

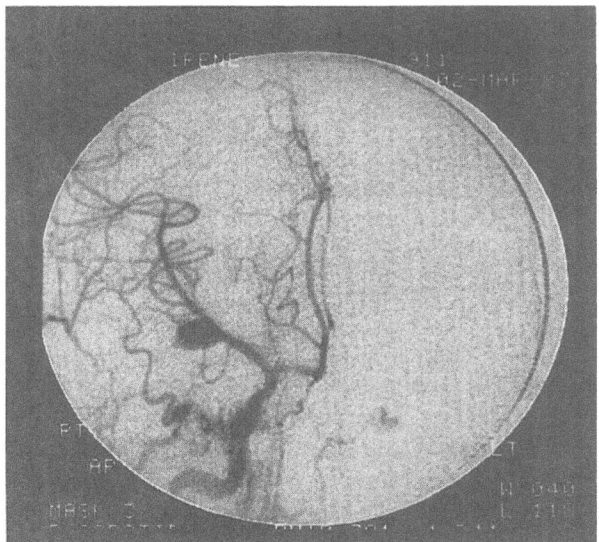

Fig. 12.2 Angiogram demonstrating middle cerebral aneurysm

interhemispheric fissure, or there may be an isolated caval–septal haematoma[17] (Fig. 12.1). The finding of blood in the basal cisterns is almost inevitably associated with the detection of an aneurysm at angiography[18]. The detection, by CT scanning, of focal subarachnoid blood is particularly valuable when the angiogram subsequently demonstrates multiple aneurysms.

Angiography remains the definitive investigation in subarachnoid haemorrhage.

In one study of patients with subarachnoid haemorrhage who had come to autopsy, where one or more aneurysms were demonstrated, a retrospective analysis of the angiographic findings was performed[19]. All the patients had had bilateral carotid angiography succeeded after 48 hours by vertebral angiography if the initial study had been negative. The responsible aneurysm was demonstrated in 89% of the patients (Fig. 12.2). If patients having an inadequate examination, or who had had an aneurysm which, though present in retrospect, was missed at the initial assessment were excluded, the yield rose to 93.5%. Reasons for negative angiography include vasospasm, disintegration of the aneurysm at the time of rupture and an aneurysm too small to be detected. Little benefit accrues from repeating angiography in patients with subarachnoid haemorrhage

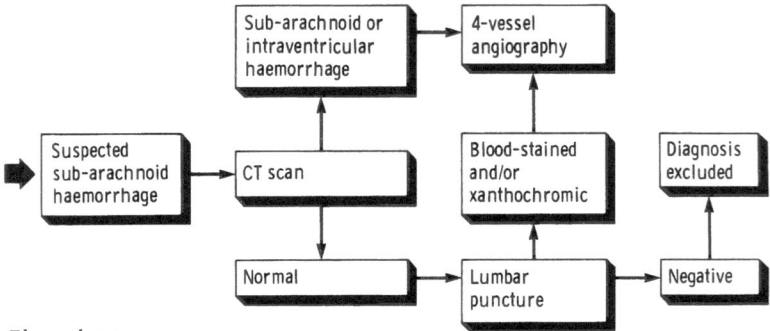

Flow chart

and initial negative angiography [20]. The finding of vasospasm is of some value, since its distribution tends to follow the area of aneurysmal rupture. There is some evidence to suggest that the presence of vasospasm increases the risk of early surgical intervention, so that its presence is a relative criterion for deferring surgery. There is no uniformity of opinion regarding the need for further angiography after surgery. It is particularly indicated where there has been some doubt regarding the success of the operation in terms of total occlusion of the aneurysm.

12.1.2 Recommendation (see flow chart)

In patients with suspected subarachnoid haemorrhage, CT scanning is the initial investigation of choice. Demonstration of subarachnoid, intracerebral or intraventricular blood obviates the need for lumbar puncture. Scanning should be performed as soon as possible, since the yield falls rapidly as time elapses from the onset. If the scan is negative, or if there is likely to be a substantial delay before CT scanning can be performed, then lumbar puncture is performed. Though the diagnosis is thereby almost always established, it must be recognized that the procedure is not without risk.

If the diagnosis has been confirmed then, providing the patient's condition is satisfactory, early four vessel angiography is necessary. Management subsequently depends on the findings and the patient's clinical status.

12.2 STROKE-IN-EVOLUTION

Discussion of the appropriate investigation for stroke-in-evolution is hindered by the lack of accepted criteria for making the diagnosis.

Clearly progression of disability after onset of stroke is implied, but how long that period should be and whether immediate or delayed has not been established. In some cases the progression is smooth, in others there is an episodic quality (stuttering hemiplegia). In one study, 26% of cases of acute infarction in carotid territory had a progressive course, compared to 54% of infarcts in vertebrobasilar territory[21]. Though it has been generally assumed that the majority of patients with stroke-in-evolution harbour thrombus in large arteries, it is now appreciated that a similar presentation can occur with an embolus derived from a cardiac source. Furthermore, as many as one-third of cases of lacunar infarction show a stepwise progression, and as many as two-thirds of cases of intracerebral haematoma display a gradual onset[21]. When investigating a potential cardiac source for a cerebral embolus, echocardiography and prolonged ECG monitoring has proved disappointing. Echocardiography can fail to recognize intracardiac thrombus and may fail to display valvular vegetations in patients with clinically obvious infective endocarditis[22]. In one study of patients with cerebral infarction, clinical examination proved as valuable for the detection of a significant cardiac source for an embolus as did echocardiography. Cross-sectional echocardiography appears more sensitive for this purpose than M-mode echocardiography (see Chapter 3).

12.2.1 Recommendation

CT scanning is mandatory for the investigation of patients with a progressing stroke. Patients with a lacunar infarct, or with an intracerebral haemorrhage, are unlikely to require angiography. If the scan is normal, or reveals an infarct in carotid territory, and clinical assessment has revealed no cardiological abnormality, then urgent carotid angiography is appropriate for patients whose ischaemic event is in carotid territory. Patients demonstrated to have a carotid stenosis will be candidates for endarterectomy.

REFERENCES

1. Adams, H.P. Jr, Kassell, N.F., Torner, J.C. and Sahs, A.L. (1983) CT and clinical correlations in recent aneurysmal subarachnoid hemorrhage: A preliminary report of the cooperative aneurysm study. *Neurology*, 33, 981–8.
2. Locksley, H.B. (1966) Natural history of subarachnoid hemorrhage, intracranial aneurysms and arteriovenous malformations. Based on 6368 cases in the cooperative study. *J. Neurosurg.*, 25, 219–39.

3. Winn, H.R., Richardson, A.E. and Jane, J.A. (1977) The long-term prognosis in untreated cerebral aneurysms. 1. A 10-year evaluation of 364 patients. *Ann. Neurol.*, 1, 358–70.

4. Stober, T. and Kunze, K. (1982) Electrocardiographic alterations in subarachnoid haemorrhage. Correlation between spasm of the arteries of the left side of the brain and T inversion and QT prolongation. *J. Neurol.*, 227, 99–113.

5. Margerison, J.H., Binne, C.D. and McCaul, I.R. (1970) Electroencephalographic signs employed in the location of ruptured intracranial arterial aneurysms. *Electroencephalogr. Clin. Neurophysiol.*, 28, 296–306.

6. Géraud, G., Tremoulet, M., Guell, A. and Bes, A. (1984) The prognostic value of noninvasive CBF measurement in subarachnoid hemorrhage. *Stroke*, 15, 301–5.

7. Adams, H.P. Jr, Jergenson, D.D., Kassell, N.F. and Sahs, A.L. (1980) Pitfalls in the recognition of subarachnoid hemorrhage. *J. Am. Med. Assoc.*, 244, 794–6.

8. Tourtellotte, W.W., Metz, L.N., Bryan, E.R. and De Jong, R.N. (1964) Spontaneous subarachnoid hemorrhage. Factors affecting the rate of clearing of the cerebrospinal fluid. *Neurology*, 14, 301–6.

9. Richardson, J.C. and Hyland, H.H. (1941) Intracranial aneurysms. A clinical and pathological study of subarachnoid and intracerebral haemorrhage caused by berry aneurysms. *Medicine (Baltimore)*, 20, 1–83.

10. Roost, K.T., Pimstone, N.R., Diamond, I. and Schmid, R. (1972) The formation of cerebrospinal fluid xanthochromia after subarachnoid hemorrhage. Enzymatic conversion of hemoglobin to bilirubin by the arachnoid and choroid plexus. *Neurology*, 22, 973–7.

11. Petito, F. and Plum, F. (1974) The lumbar puncture. *N. Engl. J. Med.*, 290, 225–7.

12. Vincent, F.M. (1981) Hypoglycorrhachia after subarachnoid hemorrhage. *Neurosurgery*, 8, 7–9.

13. Duffy, G.P. (1982) Lumbar puncture in spontaneous subarachnoid haemorrhage. *Br. Med. J.*, 285, 1163–4.

14. Davis, J.M., Davis, K.R. and Crowell, R.M. (1980) Subarachnoid hemorrhage secondary to ruptured intracranial aneurysm: prognostic significance of cranial CT. *Am. J. Roentgenol.*, 134, 711–15.

15. Gurusinghe, N.T. and Richardson, A.E. (1984) The value of computerized tomography in aneurysmal subarachnoid hemorrhage. The concept of the CT score. *J. Neurosurg.*, 60, 763–70.

16. Doczi, T., Ambrose, J. and O'Laoire, S. (1984) Significance of contrast enhancement in cranial computerized tomography after subarachnoid hemorrhage. *J. Neurosurg.*, 60, 335–42.

17. Weisberg, L.A. (1985) Ruptured aneurysms of anterior cerebral or anterior communicating arteries: CT patterns. *Neurology*, 35, 1562–6.

18. Van Gijn, J. and Van Dongen, K.J. (1980) Computerized tomography in subarachnoid hemorrhage: difference between patients with and

without an aneurysm on angiography. *Neurology,* **30**, 538–9.
19. Perrett, L.V. and Bull, J.W.D. (1959) Some aspects of subarachnoid haemorrhage – a symposium III. The accuracy of radiology in demonstrating ruptured intracranial aneurysms. *Br. J. Radiol.,* **32**, 85–92.
20. Forster, D.M.C., Steiner, L., Hakanson, S. and Bergvall, U. (1978) The value of repeat pan-angiography in cases of unexplained subarachnoid hemorrhage. *J. Neurosurg.,* **48**, 712–16.
21. Gautier, J.C. (1985) Stroke-in-evolution. *Stroke,* **16**, 729–33.
22. Come, P.C., Riley, M.F. and Bivas, N.K. (1983) Roles of echocardiography and arrhythmia monitoring in the evaluation of patients with suspected systemic embolism. *Ann. Neurol.,* **13**, 527–31.

13

Neurological
emergencies – 3

13.1 HEAD INJURY

In patients with head injury, radiological investigation is primarily
aimed at establishing which individuals have evidence of intracranial
haemorrhage and might, therefore, respond to surgical intervention.
The necessity for screening patients with a mild head injury by
radiological procedures, remains controversial. In one study, the risk
of developing an intracranial haematoma where orientation was
preserved and no skull fracture visible was of the order of 1 in 6000,
rising to a 1 in 4 risk if consciousness was impaired and a fracture
present[1]. CT scanning of patients with disorientation and a
fracture following head injury will allow early detection of two-
thirds of all traumatic intracranial haemorrhage[1] (Fig. 13.1a,b).
MRI scanning has some advantage over CT in the detection of
post-traumatic cerebral contusion[2]. Whereas CT detects parenchymal, non-haemorrhagic lesions only in those with severe injury
and persistent coma, MRI reveals white matter changes even where
consciousness has been regained after 5 minutes[3]. T_2-weighted
images have proved most sensitive in detecting parenchymal abnormalities, the lesions appearing as areas of increased signal[3,4].
Indeed MRI detected brain abnormalities in 88% of patients with
recent head injury in one series[3]. The final outcome in these
individuals was not discussed and correlations between MRI change
and sequelae from head injury have not yet been determined.

Other investigative techniques have been used in attempting
predictions of outcome after head injury. Serum levels of brain
creatine kinase (CK-BB) rise after head injury, correlating with its
severity, but overlap between patient groups is considerable[5]. The
EEG is commonly abnormal within the first few days of a head injury
sufficient to cause coma, displaying either generalized or focal

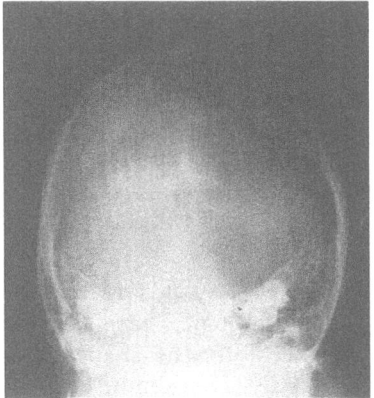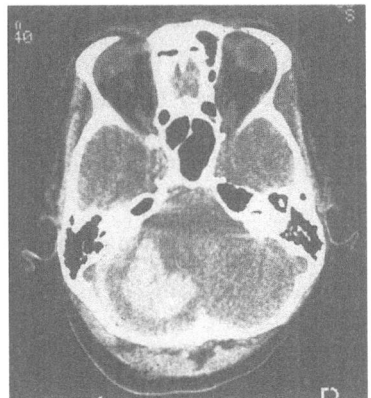

Fig. 13.1 (a) Skull X-ray showing left occipital fracture. (b) CT scan showing left cerebellar haematoma and left sided subdural haematoma in the posterior fossa with evidence of external swelling at site of occipital injury

slow-wave activity[6]. The predictive value for the later development of epilepsy of a localized electrophysiological abnormality is, however, limited, unless this consists of spike and wave activity. Where EEGs are performed several years after injury, epileptiform activity correlates both with the degree of brain volume loss (as measured by CT) and the incidence of post-traumatic epilepsy[7].

Evoked responses have been studied as a guide to the integrity of ascending pathways within the brain stem following head injury. Following concussion, delay of the auditory N1 and N3 waves has been reported compared to controls[8]. In patients with more substantial trauma, sufficient to disturb consciousness for at least 24 hours, outcome was related to the presence or absence of waves I to V. Absence of V alone, or its prolongation was associated with a relatively good recovery, whereas disappearance of waves III to V was associated with death or the development of a vegetative state[9]. Comparison of auditory and somatosensory potentials as a guide to outcome has been made[10]. Normal auditory responses did not reliably predict a favourable outcome. Unilateral or bilateral absence of the cortical (N20) somatosensory responses within the first four days of injury predicted an unfavourable result. Transit time within the central somatosensory pathways increases after head injury, the delay being proportional to the severity of the injury[10].

13.1.1 Extradural haematoma

The vast majority of extradural haematomas result from bleeding from a lacerated middle meningeal artery. Skull X-ray detects a fracture in this area. CT scanning demonstrates a biconvex hyperdense mass with compression of underlying brain [11].

13.1.2 Subdural haematoma

Although subdural haematomas are conventionally divided into acute, subacute and chronic forms, no chronological basis exists for such a clear-cut distinction [12]. Furthermore, the shape of the haematoma, as defined pathologically, or by CT scanning, does not allow a confident prediction of chronicity. A crescentic haematoma, conventionally regarded as being of recent origin, may represent a chronic lesion, whereas a biconvex shape cannot be correlated with a more protracted history [13]. The diagnosis of subdural haematoma remains difficult, not assisted by the fact that a history of trauma is lacking in at least 25% of cases [12].

Plain skull X-ray revealed abnormalities in 39 and 50% of patients in two large series [14,15]. Displacement of a calcified pineal gland is more common than detection of a skull fracture. CSF examination, at least if conventional tests are used, is of limited value in diagnosis. The pressure is elevated in no more than a third, and the protein concentration in a similar proportion. Xanthochromia is detected in less than half, though if spectrophotometry is used, the yield has been reported to rise to 100% [16].

Early papers suggested a particular EEG appearance in subdural haematoma, combining focal suppression with superimposed slow wave activity. Others have concluded that there is no characteristic pattern. A normal recording was reported in 13 and 19% in two studies [15,17]. A unilateral abnormality usually accurately predicts the side of the lesion [17] but most commonly is interpreted as the consequence of a tumour [15].

Technetium scanning provides a higher diagnostic yield than EEG. In one study, of 32 patients, the scan was abnormal in 30. The characteristics of the scan did not allow prediction of the age of the haematoma, nor did the intensity of the abnormality correlate with the size of the lesion [18]. Both false positive and negative studies occur.

Prior to the introduction of CT scanning, angiography provided

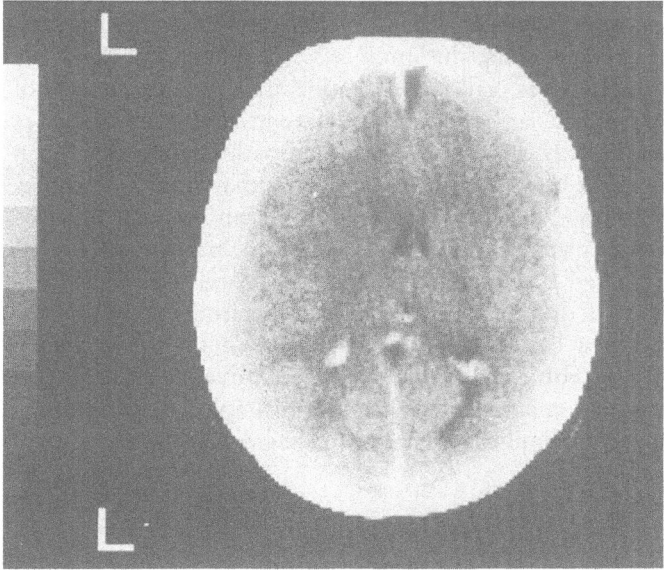

Fig. 13.2 CT scan showing left sided isodense subdural haematoma

the most accurate means for defining the presence of a subdural collection[14]. Shift of the anterior cerebral artery and internal cerebral vein was an almost universal finding in unilateral acute subdurals[19]. Comparison of angiography and technetium scanning indicates that the latter technique is likely to fail to reveal collections less than 1 cm in depth[18].

In an early account of CT scanning in subdural haematoma, scans showing high density areas were associated with a short history and the presence of blood clot at surgery[11]. Hyperdense, isodense and hypodense patterns are described, and may coincide in the same patient. Ventricular displacement is more likely where the scan is hyperdense[20]. False positive and false negative diagnoses in this study each amounted to 4%. Detection of isodense subdurals poses particular problems (Fig. 13.2). The diagnosis is suggested by medial displacement of the cortical sulci, and, on contrast studies, medial displacement of cortical veins from the inner table. Where bilateral isodense subdurals exist, the ventricles become small and compressed[21]. MRI can demonstrate isodense subdurals where CT scanning has been negative or equivocal[22].

Increasingly, a proportion of patients with subdural haematomas are managed without recourse to surgery. In a follow-up of 21 unoperated patients, the number with abnormal EEGs, 17 at the time of diagnosis, had fallen to nine after a mean interval of three weeks[17]. In an analysis of eleven, angiographically proven, subdurals, only three were associated with abnormal EEGs at three to six weeks after diagnosis, though ten had had abnormal recordings initially[23]. Positive technetium scans persisted at this stage but had returned to normal, except in one patient (whose subdural had resolved on angiographic criteria) three years later[23]. The position of the deep cerebral veins, determined by angiography, represents a better guide to resolution than displacement of the anterior cerebral artery[24]. With the advent of the CT scanner, non-surgical management has been simplified, resolution being appraised by diminishing size of the haematoma.

13.2 SPINAL INJURY

In patients with spinal injury, fracture can usually be detected by plain X-rays, abetted, if necessary, by tomography. Plain films underestimate the presence of spinal fracture, and the investigation of choice in spinal injury is plain CT, supported by metrizamide studies if neurological deficit is suspected. Urological involvement in conus medullaris and cauda equina injury results in an absent or depressed bulbucavernous reflex, detruser areflexia on cystometrography, neuropathic changes on perineal floor EMG and evidence of bethanechol chloride supersensitivity (indicated by a rise in intravesical pressure above baseline values at a standard filling volume)[25].

13.3 ACUTE SPINAL CORD COMPRESSION

13.3.1 Metastatic disease

In a survey of 235 cases of epidural spinal cord compression from a metastatic tumour, breast, lung, prostate and kidney accounted for almost half the primary sources[26]. Among 131 cases, 47% had an ESR exceeding 30, and 22% an elevated alkaline phosphatase level[27]. Abnormalities on plain X-ray were found in 57 and 84% of patients in two series[28,27]. The findings, in order of frequency, include collapse of the vertebral body, pedicle erosion and crush

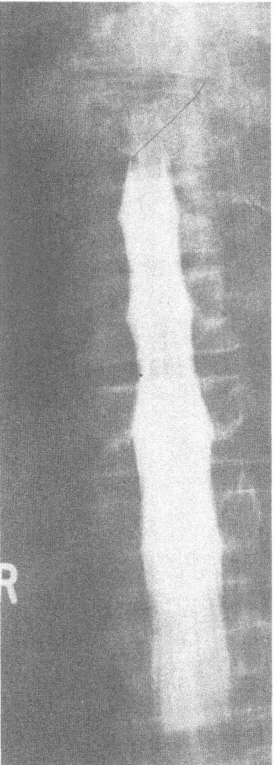

Fig. 13.3 Myelogram showing complete block of the contrast column by a metastasis from carcinoma of the prostate

fractures. An elevated CSF protein is very common but a pleocytosis is unusual and malignant cells are seldom recovered[27]. Myelography is inevitably abnormal, the vast majority of patients showing a complete block of the contrast column (Fig. 13.3)[26–28]. Multiple levels of obstruction are found in 10% overall, but in 29% of cases where the primary tumour originates in the breast[27]. Both technetium scans using radiolabelled polyphosphate and plain CT are more successful than plain X-rays in detecting spinal metastatic disease[29]. Indeed, plain CT, in one series of 50 patients, achieved an accuracy of 96% in the diagnosis of cord compression[30]. CT with metrizamide achieves the same degree of diagnostic accuracy as conventional myelography, and has the advantage of usually being

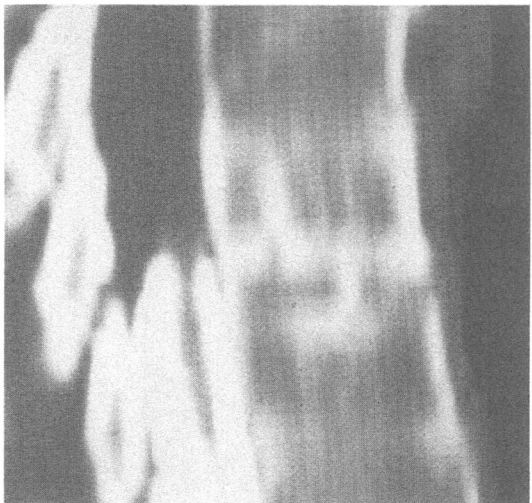

Fig. 13.4 CT with metrizamide. Sagittal reconstruction demonstrating complete block of the contrast column caused by an extradural lymphoma

capable of defining the upper limit of an extradural mass even where complete block to the flow of contrast is apparent on myelography[31] (Fig. 13.4).

13.3.2 Subdural and epidural haematoma

CT provides specific data in patients with cord compression which allows differentiation of epidural from subdural haematoma. The former appears as a well-defined, biconvex high-density mass lying posteriorly or posterolaterally against the inner border of the bony spinal canal with obliteration of the epidural fat. The latter has a concave or straight margin and appears as a dense band separated from the bony wall by epidural fat[32].

13.3.3 Epidural empyema

In patients with epidural abscess, evidence pointing to the presence of an infective process depends on the duration of symptoms. In a group of patients with an acutely evolving picture (onset to surgery being less than two weeks), the mean peripheral white cell count was 16 700, falling to normal values in those with a longer history[32]. The CSF is almost inevitably abnormal, showing an elevated protein concentration and a moderate pleocytosis[33]. Plain X-rays of the spine commonly reveal evidence of osteomyelitis, whereas myelography, inevitably abnormal, usually demonstrates a complete block. Subdural abscess is less common, less often associated with vertebral osteomyelitis, but otherwise presents in a similar fashion [34].

The advent of CT scanning has encouraged conservative management of epidural abscess, utilizing serial scans, for poor surgical-risk patients. CT changes (incorporating studies after intravenous contrast) include loss of the epidural fat shadow and fixation of contrast in the dura surrounded by a higher density area between the dural sheath and bone[35].

CT is undoubtedly the investigation of choice for the detection of infection in the vertebral body or disc space. In osteomyelitis of the spine, plain X-rays may reveal erosion of the cortex of the vertebral body and of the end plate, but only some two to six weeks after the development of infection. Bone scanning is positive in the majority of patients with osteomyelitis of the spine but CT both detects bone lesions earlier, and is accurate in defining the presence of a paraspinal mass[36]. In infectious spondylitis, the CT changes may not be distinguishable from those produced by tumour. Plain X-rays remain of value here, most commonly demonstrating erosion of the adjacent endplate[37].

Tuberculosis of the spine presents less abruptly than infections triggered by pyogenic organisms. CT is more accurate than plain X-rays or bone scanning in establishing the extent of bony damage. Compared to pyogenic collections, tuberculous abscesses show a more irregular rim, are more frequently multilocular, more often calcified and more liable to spread to the superficial dorsal soft tissues[38].

13.3.4 Transverse myelitis

Whilst transverse myelitis can hardly be regarded as a cause of spinal cord compression, it undoubtedly figures in the list of differential diagnoses when the clinician is faced with an acutely evolving cord syndrome. Certain clinical features may suggest the diagnosis, including the history of an antecedent viral or bacterial infection. The conditions, and infectious illnesses, associated with the disorder are legion, including herpes, ECHO virus, Epstein–Barr virus and mycoplasma[39]. The CSF is liable to show a pleocytosis together with an elevated protein concentration but is sometimes normal [40]. Myelography is either normal or shows a degree of cord swelling at the relevant level. Although somatosensory responses from the lower limb are abnormal, those from the upper limb, and their visual and auditory counterparts are likely to be normal [41]. Later evidence of MS is found in only a small minority of these patients.

REFERENCES

1. Mendelow, A.D., Teasdale, G., Jennett, B. *et al.* (1983) Risks of intracranial haematoma in head injured adults. *Br. Med. J.*, **287**, 1173–6.
2. Gandy, S.E., Snow, R.B., Zimmerman, R.D. and Deck, M.D.F. (1984) Cranial nuclear magnetic resonance imaging in head trauma. *Ann. Neurol.*, **16**, 254–7.
3. Jenkins, A., Teasdale, G., Hadley, M.D.M. *et al.* (1986) Brain lesions detected by magnetic resonance imaging in mild and severe head injuries. *Lancet*, **ii**, 445–6.
4. Han, J.S., Kaufman, B., Alfidi, R.J. *et al.* (1984) Head trauma evaluated by magnetic resonance and computed tomography: a comparison. *Radiology*, **150**, 71–7.
5. Phillips, J.P., Jones, H.M., Hitchcock, R. *et al.* (1980) Radioimmuno-assay of serum creatine kinase BB as index of brain damage after head injury. *Br. Med. J.*, **281**, 777–9.
6. Courjon, J. (1970) A longitudinal electro-clinical study of 80 cases of post-traumatic epilepsy observed from the time of the original trauma. *Epilepsia*, **11**, 29–36.
7. Jabbari, B., Vengrow, M.I., Salazar, A.M. *et al.* (1986) Clinical and radiological correlates of EEG in the late phase of head injury: a study of 515 Vietnam veterans. *Electroencephalogr. Clin. Neurophysiol.*, **64**, 285–93.
8. Noseworthy, J.H., Miller, J., Murray, T.J. and Regan, D. (1981) Auditory brain stem responses in post concussion syndrome. *Arch. Neurol.*, **38**, 275–8.
9. Tsubokawa, T., Nishimoto, H., Yamamoto, T. *et al.* (1980) Assessment of brainstem damage by the auditory brainstem response in acute severe head injury. *J. Neurol. Neurosurg. Psychiatry*, **43**, 1005–11.
10. Cant, B.R., Hume, A.L., Judson, J.A. and Shaw, N.A. (1986) The assessment of severe head injury by short-latency somatosensory and brain-stem auditory evoked potentials. *Electroencephalogr. Clin. Neurophysiol.*, **65**, 188–95.
11. Svendsen, P. (1976) Computer tomography of traumatic extracerebral lesions. *Br. J. Radiol.*, **49**, 1004–12.
12. Wintzen, A.R. (1980) The clinical course of subdural haematoma. A retrospective study of aetiological, chronological and pathological

features in 212 patients and a proposed classification. *Brain*, **103**, 855–67.

13. Radcliffe, W.B., Guinto, F.C. Jr, Adcock, D.F. and Krigman, M.R. (1972) Subdural hematoma shape. A new look at an old concept. *Am. J. Roentgenol.*, **115**, 72–7.
14. McKissock, W., Richardson, A. and Bloom, W.H. (1960) Subdural haematoma. A review of 389 cases. *Lancet*, i, 1365–9.
15. Luxon, L.M. and Harrison, M.J.G. (1979) Chronic subdural haematoma. *Q. J. Med.*, **189**, 43–53.
16. Kjellin, K. G. and Steiner, L. (1974) Spectrophotometry of cerebrospinal fluid in subacute and chronic subdural haematomas. *J. Neurol. Neurosurg. Psychiatry*, **37**, 1121–7.
17. Jaffe, R., Librot, I.E. and Bender, M.B. (1968) Serial EEG studies in unoperated subdural hematoma. *Arch. Neurol.*, **19**, 325–30.
18. Gilday, D.L., Coates, G. and Goldenberg, D. (1973) Subdural hematoma – what is the role of brain scanning in its diagnosis? *J. Nucl. Med.*, **14**, 283–7.
19. Ferris, E.J., Lehrer, H. and Shapiro, J.H. (1967) Pseudo-subdural hematoma. *Radiology*, **88**, 75–84.
20. Forbes, G.S., Sheedy, P.F. II, Piepgras, D.G. and Houser, O.W. (1978) Computed tomography in the evaluation of subdural hematomas. *Radiology*, **126**, 143–8.
21. Kim, K.S., Hemhati, M. and Weinberg, P.E. (1978) Computed tomography in isodense subdural hematoma. *Radiology*, **128**, 71–4.
22. Moon, K.L. Jr, Brant-Zawadzki, M., Pitts, L.H. and Mills, C.M. (1984) Nuclear magnetic resonance imaging of CT-isodense subdural hematomas. *Am. J. Neuroradiol.*, **5**, 319–22.
23. Lusins, J., Jaffe, R. and Bender, M.B. (1976) Unoperated subdural hematomas. Long-term follow-up study by brain scan and electroencephalography. *J. Neurosurg.*, **44**, 601–7.
24. Fogel, L.M., Capesius, P., Ludwiczak, R. *et al.* (1975) Postoperative angiographic control of chronic subdural hematomas in adults. *Neuroradiology*, **10**, 155–8.
25. Pavlakis, A.J., Siroky, M.B., Goldstein, I. and Krane, R.J. (1983) Neurourologic findings in conus medullaris and cauda equina injury. *Arch. Neurol.*, **40**, 570–3.
26. Gilbert, R.W., Kim, J.-H. and Posner, J.B. (1978) Epidural spinal cord compression from metastatic tumor: diagnosis and treatment. *Ann. Neurol.*, **3**, 40–51.
27. Stark, R.J., Henson, R.A. and Evans, S.J.W. (1982) Spinal metastases: a retrospective survey from a general hospital. *Brain*, **105**, 189–213.
28. Auld, A.W. and Buerman, A. (1966) Metastatic spinal epidural tumors. An analysis of 50 cases. *Arch. Neurol.*, **15**, 100–8.
29. Redmond, J. III, Spring, D.B., Munderloh, S.H. *et al.* (1984) Spinal computed tomography scanning in the evaluation of metastatic disease. *Cancer*, **54**, 253–8.
30. Wang, A.-M., Lewis, M.L., Rumbaugh, C.L. *et al.* (1984) Spinal cord or

nerve root compression in patients with malignant disease: CT evaluation. *J. Comp. Assist. Tomogr.*, 8, 420–8.

31. Fink, I.J., Garra, B.S., Zabell, A. and Doppman, J.L. (1984) Computed tomography with metrizamide myelography to define the extent of spinal canal block due to tumor. *J. Comp. Assist. Tomogr.*, 8, 1072–5.
32. Tantana, S., Pilla, T.J. and Luisiri, A. (1986) Computed tomography of acute spinal subdural hematoma. *J. Comp. Assist. Tomogr.*, 10, 891–2.
33. Baker, A.S., Ojemann, R.G., Swartz, M.N. and Richardson, E.P. Jr (1975) Spinal epidural abscess. *N. Engl. J. Med.*, 293, 463–8.
34. Fraser, R.A.R., Ratzan, K., Wolpert, S.M. and Weinstein, L. (1973) Spinal subdural empyema. *Arch. Neurol.*, 28, 235–8.
35. Leys, D., Lesoin, F., Viaud, C. *et al.* (1985) Decreased morbidity from acute bacterial spinal epidural abscesses using computed tomography and nonsurgical treatment in selected patients. *Ann. Neurol.*, 17, 350–5.
36. Golimbu, C., Firooznia, H. and Rafii, M. (1983) CT of osteomyelitis of the spine. *Am. J. Neuroradiol.*, 4, 1207–11.
37. Hermann, G., Mendelson, D.S., Cohen, B.A. and Train, J.S. (1983) Role of computed tomography in the diagnosis of infectious spondylitis. *J. Comp. Assist. Tomogr.*, 7, 961–8.
38. Whelan, M.A., Naidich, D.P., Post, J.D. and Chase, N.E. (1983) Computed tomography of spinal tuberculosis. *J. Comp. Assist. Tomogr.*, 7, 25–30.
39. Westenfelder, G.O., Akey, D.T., Corwin, S.J. and Vick, N.A. (1981) Acute transverse myelitis due to *Mycoplasma pneumoniae* infection. *Arch. Neurol.*, 38, 317–18.
40. Acute transverse myelopathy (1986). *Lancet*, i, 20–1.
41. Ropper, A.H., Miett, T. and Chiappa, K.H. (1982) Absence of evoked potential abnormalities in acute transverse myelopathy. *Neurology*, 32, 80–2.

14

Cranial nerve disorders

14.1 THE FIRST CRANIAL NERVE

Patients complaining solely of altered olfaction are encountered infrequently in neurological practice. Transient alteration of smell is common after upper respiratory tract infection but sometimes, though the infection appears banal, the impairment of olfaction persists. A similar, chronic, impairment of smell can follow head injury. Olfactory meningiomas represent less than 10% of all intracranial meningiomas and are, therefore, seldom seen, but typically they present as unilateral or bilateral impairment of smell, eventually leading to anosmia, without, at least initially, evidence of frontal lobe or optic nerve disturbance. CT scanning will detect all such tumours, even at this early stage[1].

14.1.1 Recommendation

CT scanning should be performed in all patients with impaired smell, particularly if progressive, unless there is firm evidence for the causative agent, for example head injury.

14.2 THE SECOND CRANIAL NERVE

14.2.1 Acute unilateral visual failure

Rapid visual loss in a young individual which can not be attributed to retinal disease is most often the result of optic nerve demyelination (see Chapter 6). In the older patient, anterior ischaemic optic neuropathy is a common cause of this presentation. The condition can be the manifestation of a more generalized vascular disorder, or be secondary to cranial arteritis. When anterior ischaemic optic neuropathy is diagnosed, estimation of the ESR is mandatory. The vast majority of patients with cranial arteritis will have a markedly elevated level. If a normal value is obtained, but the diagnosis is still suspected, the patients should be given a trial of steroids whilst temporal artery biopsy is performed.

14.2.2 Subacute unilateral visual failure

Most patients with a slowly progressive visual failure, confined to one eye, are likely to have a lesion compressing the optic nerve, though a similar presentation can occur with multiple sclerosis, and with various inflammatory disorders, for example sarcoid. Optic nerve compression within the orbit usually leads to a combination of visual failure, proptosis, and disc swelling. Pre-chiasmatic optic nerve compression results in visual failure, an afferent pupillary defect, impaired colour vision, but, at least initially, a normal optic disc.

Recommendation

High resolution CT scanning of the orbit and chiasmatic region is required but may not detect all meningiomas[2]. In some cases, exploration of the orbit or optic canal is required, either to exclude a meningioma, or to confirm the presence of a granulomatous lesion. Sarcoid granuloma can affect the optic nerve without associated features of systemic sarcoidosis[3].

14.2.3 Bilateral visual failure

There are numerous causes of bilateral visual failure though many of these will declare themselves either from associated symptomatology, for example evidence of a cord lesion in a case of multiple sclerosis, or from the setting in which the visual failure occurs, for example in a patient being treated with ethambutol.

Recommendation

Initial investigations should include standard tests for syphilis, and estimation of serum vitamin B_{12} levels. Either computerized tomography or magnetic resonance imaging will be necessary to exclude compressive lesions causing bilateral visual failure.

14.2.4 Lesions of the chiasm or post-chiasmatic visual pathway

Chiasmatic visual field defects are usually the result of compression by pituitary tumour, craniopharyngioma, meningioma or aneurysm. Investigation includes plain skull X-rays, CT or MRI scanning and, where necessary, angiography if aneurysm is suspected. Isolated optic tract lesions, typically producing a markedly incongruous homonymous hemianopia, are rare. In one series of 21 cases, 15 were due to tumour[4]. Clearly scanning is required for such cases. Isolated homonymous hemianopia is more commonly the result of a lesion affecting the optic radiation or visual cortex[5]. In one series of 104 cases, 89% were considered to have a vascular basis, generally occlusion of the calcarine or posterior cerebral artery. The investigation of completed stroke is considered in Chapter 3. Where isolated homonymous hemianopia results from tumour, clinical re-appraisal is likely to see the early emergence of other neurological signs, or extension of the visual field defect.

14.3 PUPILLARY SYNDROMES

14.3.1 Horner's syndrome

Interruption of the sympathetic outflow to the eye results in meiosis and ptosis. Involvement of fibres to the sweat glands of the face produces anhidrosis. A central Horner's syndrome is the consequence of a disruption of sympathetic fibres between the hypothalamus and the upper thoracic spinal cord. Pre- and post-ganglionic Horner's syndrome result from interruption of extra-axial fibres before or beyond the superior cervical ganglion respectively.

Simple anisocoria, where the pupil sizes differ by more than 0.4 mm, is see in as many as 30% of normal individuals. The pupillary asymmetry does not increase in the dark. Although most patients with a combination of meiosis and ptosis have Horner's syndrome, pharmacological testing of the pupil in some cases reveals intact sympathetic innervation[6]. In one analysis of 450 cases of Horner's syndrome, the cause could not be identified in 40% [7]. Of the remainder, over half were due to tumour, migrainous neuralgia or the consequence of carotid angiography or neck trauma. Where an analysis of Horner's syndrome has been performed by a neurologist rather than ophthalmologist, central rather than peripheral forms have predominated, typically the consequence of cerebrovascular disease [8].

(a) Investigations

Since the combination of ptosis and meiosis is not always the consequence of interruption of sympathetic fibres to the eye, pharmacological testing of the pupil is appropriate if the diagnosis of Horner's syndrome is to be established with certainty. For this purpose, cocaine (usually in a concentration of 4%) is applied to both eyes. The pupil affected by Horner's syndrome dilates poorly or not at all. For further localization of the site of involvement, 1% hydroxyamphetamine is used. This dilates central and preganglionic Horner's pupils, but has no effect on a post-ganglionic lesion. In reality, failure to dilate the pupil of a post-ganglionic lesion is not invariable [9]. Analysis of facial sweating has been advocated to assist localization. In post-ganglionic Horner's syndrome, impairment of facial sweating is confined to the side of the nose and the medial aspect of the forehead. If there is facial hemi-anhidrosis, the lesion is pre-ganglionic [10].

In many patients with Horner's syndrome, the aetiological agent is apparent from accompanying signs. Enthusiasm for extensive investigation of an isolated Horner's syndrome has been based on the desire to exclude an underlying neoplasm. In one series, less than 3% of isolated Horner's syndrome were due to neoplasm, the vast majority of which were located at the pulmonary apex.

(b) Recommendation

For isolated Horner's syndrome, the diagnosis should be preferably confirmed by pharmacological testing, using 4% cocaine. Chest radiography suffices as the sole investigation unless other complaints emerge.

14.3.2 The Holmes–Adie pupil

In the Holmes–Adie, or tonic pupil syndrome, the pupil is dilated, responds poorly to light but tonically to a near stimulus. Following relaxation of a near effort, dilatation of the affected pupil is typically prolonged. The responsible lesion is thought to lie in the ciliary ganglion or distally in the short ciliary nerves. The pupil typically shows denervation hypersensitivity, constricting with the installation of 2.5% methacholine, but the specificity of this test has been questioned. In one study, only 64% of patients with a tonic pupil syndrome showed constriction with 2.5% methacholine, compared to 80% when 0.125% pilocarpine was used[11]. In another report, though supersensitivity to methacholine was almost inevitable, it was also found in patients with pre-ganglionic third nerve lesions[12].

The tonic pupil syndrome can follow trauma to the eye, certain viral infections or may be associated with a more generalized neurological disorder, for example autonomic failure. In practice, however, it is usually seen in isolation sometimes associated with depression of the deep tendon reflexes. The isolated syndrome predominates in women, is usually unilateral, and tends to present in the 20–50 age group.

Recommendation

An isolated tonic pupil syndrome does not require investigation. Confirmation of denervation hypersensitivity aids diagnosis, but is not essential to it.

14.3.3 The Argyll Robertson pupil

The Argyll Robertson pupil is small, irregular, shows a depressed or absent light reaction, but an intact near response. The condition is usually bilateral. Vision is not affected. Although light–near dissociation occurs in a number of circumstances, for example in an eye with impaired vision, or secondary to diabetes, a pupil which fulfils the above criteria is almost always the result of neurosyphilis.

Recommendation

The standard tests for neurosyphilis should be performed in both the serum and CSF. The CSF criteria indicating active syphilitic infection are detailed in Chapter 6.

14.4 THE THIRD CRANIAL NERVE

Lesions of the third cranial nerve within the brain stem, particularly of a vascular nature, are likely to be accompanied by long tract signs. Nuclear lesions are uncommon, often incomplete, and sometimes the consequence of a mid-brain metastasis (Fig.14.1). Peripheral third nerve palsies are usually due to diabetes, vascular disease, for example that associated with cranial arteritis, or posterior communicating aneurysm. The palsy associated with diabetes is often, but

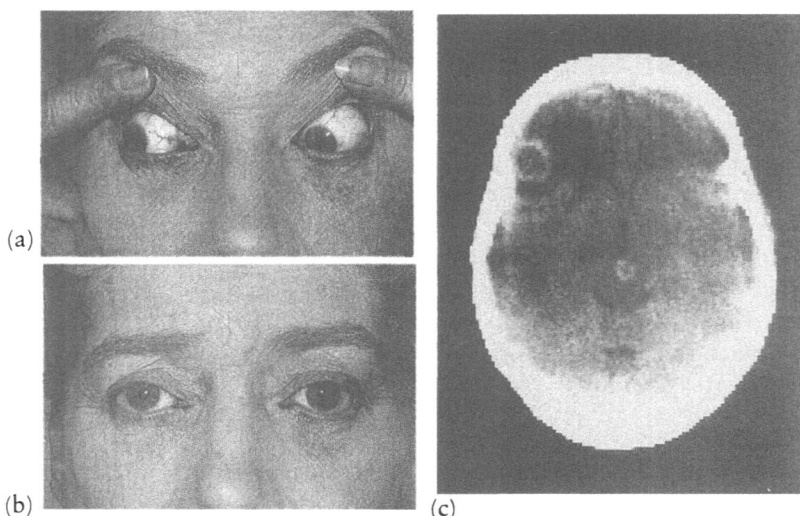

Fig. 14.1 Partial third nerve palsy, particularly affecting inferior rectus (a,b) with CT scan showing mid-brain metastasis (c). (There is also a left frontal metastasis.)

not always, pupil sparing, a finding which is rare when a posterior communicating aneurysm is responsible, unless the palsy is incomplete.

Oculomotor palsy secondary to aneurysm may be due to direct compression or the consequence of pressure effects from an associated subarachnoid haemorrhage[13].

In one study of 1000 cases of third, fourth and sixth nerve paralysis, the oculomotor nerve was affected alone in 290 cases[14]. Nearly a quarter of the patients were undiagnosed in terms of pathogenesis. Aneurysm, vascular disease, neoplasm and head injury accounted for 62.4% of the total. None of the cases were due to syphilis.

14.4.1 Recommendation

The flow-chart indicates the investigative methods used in third nerve palsy according to the pupillary findings.

14.5 THE FOURTH CRANIAL NERVE

Palsies of the fourth cranial nerve are rarer than those of the third or sixth nerves (172 v 290 v 419 in one series)[14]. In the same study, 36% of cases were undiagnosed, and 32% attributed to trauma.

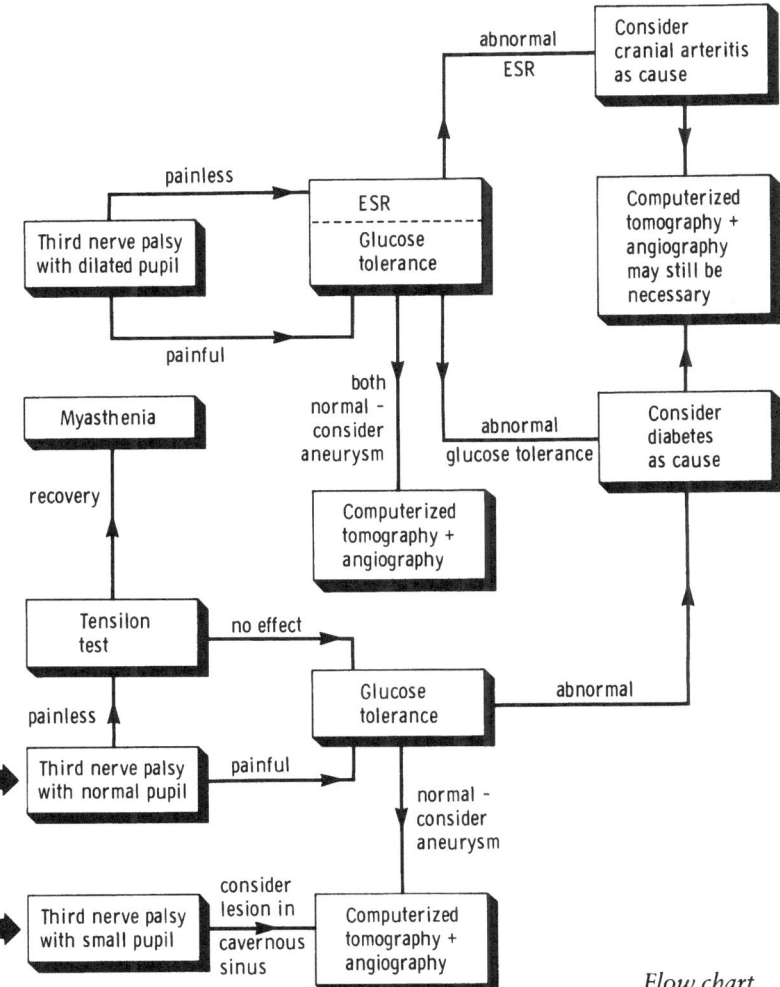

Flow chart

Whilst the nerve can be damaged at any point of its course, involvement in the subarachnoid space is most common. Close to the brain stem both fourth nerves are usually affected while distally, in the cavernous sinus, other cranial nerve signs are likely.

14.5.1 Recommendation

In a patient with an isolated fourth nerve palsy, a tensilon test should be performed, and diabetes excluded. Despite an apparent neurogenic basis for the palsy, dysthyroid eye disease can present in this fashion. If other neurological signs remain absent, further investigation is not justified.

14.6 THE SIXTH CRANIAL NERVE

Nuclear sixth nerve lesions produce a conjugate gaze paresis whereas peripheral lesions result in an isolated weakness of the lateral rectus muscle. Sixth nerve palsies are the commonest of the ocular motor nerve palsies. In the series already referred to [14], 29.6% of abducens nerve palsies were undiagnosed. Trauma, neoplasia and vascular disease accounted for 49% of the total. Many disorders can produce this lesion, including aneurysm, meningitis, myasthenia and elevated intracranial pressure. In Gradenigo's syndrome, mastoiditis causes inflammatory reaction in the petrous apex which in turn affects the sixth, and often the fifth and seventh, cranial nerves.

14.6.1 Recommendation

A tensilon test should be performed to exclude myasthenia and a forced duction test is of value in an attempt to exclude dysthyroid eye disease. The ESR should be estimated and a glucose tolerance test carried out. Radiological studies are probably not justified unless accompanying pain is particularly prominent or persistent.

14.7 COMBINED OCULAR MOTOR PALSIES

The presence of multiple ocular motor palsies can often allow localization of the causative lesion. Those in the orbit usually result in proptosis and are most often the consequence of inflammatory or metastatic disease. A parasellar syndrome can occur with neoplasm, aneurysm or inflammatory disease. Neither the mode of onset nor evolution of the syndrome confidently predict its basis [15]. The CSF changes in the various parasellar syndromes are non-specific. Naso-pharyngeal tumours account for 20% of the cases. Radiological investigation, including plain skull radiographs and CT or MRI is mandatory [16] (Fig. 14.2). If the pareses are painless and the pupils

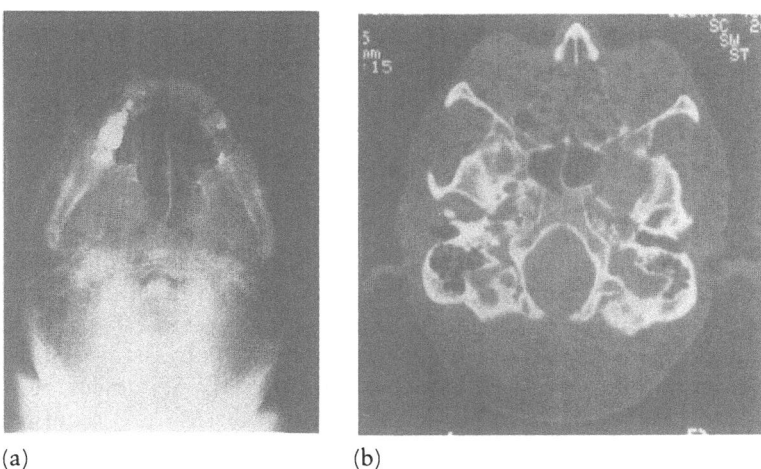

(a)   (b)

Fig. 14.2 Plain skull radiograph (a) and CT scan of skull base (b) showing bone erosion due to cavernous aneurysm

spared, myasthenia gravis and dysthyroid eye disease require exclusion.

14.8 THE FIFTH CRANIAL NERVE

Lesions isolated to the fifth cranial nerve are decidedly uncommon, though malignant invasion of the skull base, for example from nasopharyngeal tumour, may present with trigeminal involvement. Malignant invasion of the Gasserian ganglion is usually painful, the pain sometimes resembling that of trigeminal neuralgia. Trigeminal neurinoma can arise from the main trunk of the nerve or one of its branches. When the lesion is proximal, motor involvement usually accompanies the sensory deficit. Rarely, facial numbness may be the presenting feature of such diverse conditions as leprosy, syphilis and sarcoidosis. Facial numbness is not uncommon in multiple sclerosis, but the progression from isolated facial numbness to trigeminal neuralgia and thence to evidence of disseminated disease is decidedly rare [17]. Isolated trigeminal neuropathy is a condition of unknown aetiology in which a sensory neuropathy afflicts one or more branches of the trigeminal nerve [18]. In a review of 64 patients presenting with facial numbness [19], 29 proved to have a tumour, 16 arising from the cerebellopontine angle and 11 from the skull base. Six patients had an acute illness with additional involvement of the sixth or seventh cranial nerves, often accompanied by a CSF pleocytosis. It is now recognized that either unilateral or bilateral trigeminal neuropathy may be the first manifestation of a connective tissue disorder, for example Sjogren's disease or systemic lupus erythematosus[20].

14.8.1 Recommendation

Even where facial numbness is painless, and unaccompanied by motor involvement, the possibility of underlying tumour must be seriously considered. Plain skull radiographs and CT or MRI scanning is appropriate, with particular attention to changes in the configuration of the skull base and exit foramina. Serological tests looking for evidence of collagen vascular disease are required, including antibody to ribonucleoprotein (RNP). A prolonged period of follow-up is needed before the diagnosis of isolated trigeminal neuropathy can be accepted.

14.9 THE SEVENTH CRANIAL NERVE

Whilst an acutely evolving unilateral lower motor neurone facial weakness is generally an isolated, and non-recurrent, disorder (Bell's palsy), it is recognized that a similar clinical presentation may reflect a pathological process having more widespread implications, for example sarcoidosis or multiple sclerosis (Fig. 14.3).

The aetiology of Bell's palsy is unknown, though various viral agents have been implicated in its pathogenesis. The evidence for an increased occurrence of Bell's palsy in diabetic patients is not conclusive. Perhaps around 70% of patients may be expected to show a complete recovery.

Various electrophysiological tests have been used to allow prediction of outcome, though, since there is no firmly established treatment for this condition, a greater knowledge of severity of involvement serves merely to enhance the physician's sense of impotence. The presence of fibrillation in muscles supplied by the facial nerve implies denervation and a correspondingly worse prognosis. Inexcitability of muscle to peripheral facial nerve stimulation is also associated with a poor outcome. The earliest prediction of outcome is achieved by assessing threshold to galvanic stimulation of the tongue[21]. An increased threshold is closely correlated with subsequent evidence of denervation.

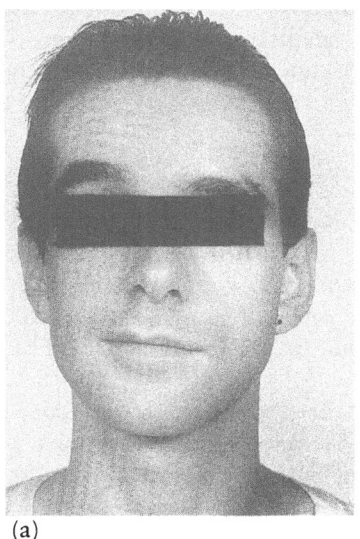
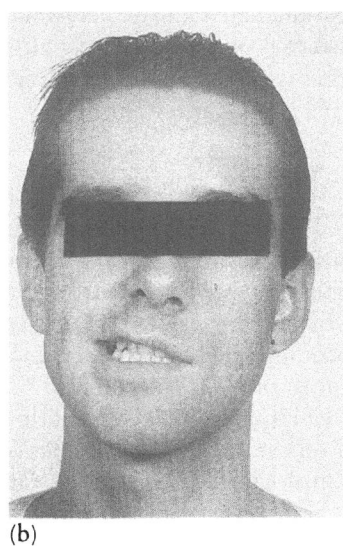

(a)   (b)

Fig. 14.3 (a and b) Lower motor neurone facial weakness in patient with multiple sclerosis

14.9.1 Recommendation

In patients with a typical Bell's palsy, chest radiography is appropriate, and, perhaps, a glucose tolerance test. Extensive investigation for an underlying systemic disorder is not justified unless additional neurological symptoms or signs appear.

14.10 THE EIGHTH CRANIAL NERVE

Isolated sensori-neural deafness is rarely the province of the neurologist. In practice, only some 5–10% of patients with progressive, unilateral, hearing loss prove to have an acoustic neuroma. Though acoustic neuromas typically present with a combination of hearing loss, tinnitus and dizziness, in some patients hearing loss is initially the sole complaint, whereas in others the tumour presents atypically with headache, dizziness or facial numbness [22].

Audiometry is abnormal in some 95% of patients, particularly for high-frequency. The stapedial reflex is abnormal in about 85% of patients. Brain-stem auditory evoked responses (BAER) are particularly valuable in diagnosing acoustic neuroma. Plain skull radiography and tomography of the internal auditory meatus often fails to reveal small acoustic neuroma. CT scanning with air introduced by cisternal puncture detects all but the smallest tumours. The most-sensitive technique for the diagnosis of intracanalicular tumours is MRI (see Chapter 7).

14.10.1 Recommendation

The most valuable screening procedure in the investigation of patients with progressive unilateral deafness is BAER. If this suggests a possible acoustic neuroma, and routine CT scanning is negative, then either cisternal CT scanning with air, or MRI are the recommended procedures. Larger tumours are readily detected by conventional CT scanning.

Isolated tinnitus is similarly seldom seen in neurological practice. In one study of 121 patients[23], 21% were considered to have a neurological disease responsible, though it is apparent that in almost all these cases the neurological disease could be diagnosed on the basis of the examination. Though, in one case, tinnitus was the sole manifestation of an acoustic neuroma, radiological investigation of patients with isolated tinnitus, and a normal neurological examin-ation, hardly appears justified.

14.11 THE LOWER CRANIAL NERVES

Isolated palsies of the ninth, tenth, eleventh and twelfth cranial nerves are very uncommon, though malignant invasion of the skull base in the region of the occipital condyle produces a characteristic picture of severe unilateral occipital pain associated with a unilateral twelfth nerve paresis[24]. The jugular foramen syndrome involves disruption of the glossopharyngeal, vagus and accessory nerves. Tumour is the commonest cause and is more likely to be metastatic than primary. Glomus jugulare tumours tend to involve other cranial nerves besides those issuing from the jugular foramen, particularly the hypoglossal nerve[25]. Various other eponymous lower cranial nerve syndromes are described, some with additional involvement of oculosympathetic fibres. Where they are unaccompanied by long tract signs, tumour invasion of the skull base is the likeliest cause.

14.11.1 Recommendation

Isolated or multiple lower cranial nerve lesions require radiological investigation. Plain skull radiographs, supplemented by tomography

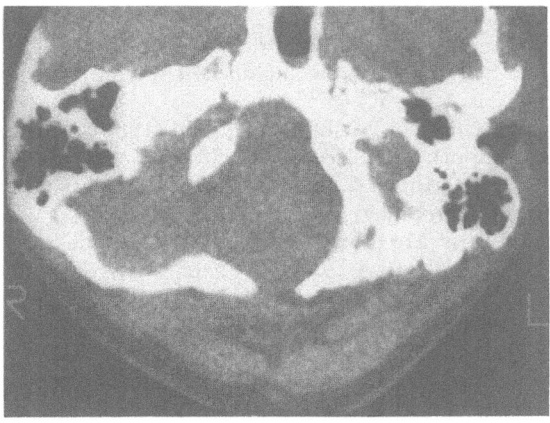

Fig. 14.4 CT scan of the skull base in a patient with a glomus jugulare tumour, showing bone erosion

of areas suggested by the constellation of signs is the first step. If necessary, CT scan of the skull base will help to identify tumour masses and bone erosion (Fig. 14.4).

14.12 MULTIPLE CRANIAL NERVE PALSIES

If the combination of multiple cranial nerve palsies is such that a single lesion is likely to be responsible, then radiological investigation as already detailed will be necessary to establish its pathological basis. In some instances, however, the cranial nerve involvement is more diffuse, and cannot be attributed to a single lesion. Where this presentation occurs in the setting of an overt basal meningitis, there can be little difficulty in establishing the diagnosis. In some patients, however, multiple cranial nerve palsies are the first manifestation of either skull metastases or carcinomatous meningitis[26]. Multiple, relapsing cranial nerve palsies have been described in sarcoidosis, or as a syndrome of uncertain aetiology[27].

14.12.1 Recommendation

Skull radiography and bone scanning should be performed followed by CT scanning, including basal skull views. If these are non-contributory, then CSF examination is required.

REFERENCES

1. Bakay, L. (1984) Olfactory meningiomas. The missed diagnosis. *J. Am. Med. Assoc.*, **251**, 53–5.
2. Ebers, G.C., Girvin, J.P. and Canny, C.B. (1980) A 'possible' optic nerve meningioma. *Arch. Neurol.*, **37**, 781–3.
3. Gudeman, S.K., Selhorst, J.B., Susac, J.O. and Waybright, E.A. (1982) Sarcoid optic neuropathy. *Neurology*, **32**, 597–603.
4. Savino, P.J., Paris, M., Schatz, N.J. *et al.* (1978) Optic tract syndrome: A review of 21 patients. *Arch. Ophthalmol.*, **96**, 656–63.
5. Trobe, J.D., Lorber, M.L. and Schlezinger, N.S. (1973) Isolated homonymous hemianopia: A review of 104 cases. *Arch. Ophthalmol.*, **89**, 377–81.
6. Thompson, B.M., Corbett, J.J., Kline, L.B. and Thompson, S. (1982) Pseudo-Horner's syndrome. *Arch. Neurol.*, **39**, 108–11.
7. Maloney, W.F., Younge, B.R. and Moyer, N.J. (1980) Evaluation of the causes and accuracy of pharmacologic localization in Horner's syndrome. *Am. J. Ophthalmol.*, **90**, 394–402.
8. Keane, J.R. (1979) Oculosympathetic paresis: Analysis of 100 hospitalized patients. *Arch. Neurol.*, **36**, 13–16.
9. van der Wiel, H.L. and van Gijn, J. (1983) Localization of Horner's syndrome. Use and limitations of the hydroxyamphetamine test. *J. Neurol. Sci.*, **59**, 229–35.
10. Morris, J.G.L., Lee, J. and Lim, C.L. (1984) Facial sweating in Horner's syndrome. *Brain*, **107**, 751–8.
11. Bourgon, P., Pilley, S.F.J. and Stanley Thompson, H. (1978) Cholinergic supersensitivity of the iris sphincter in Adie's tonic pupil. *Am. J. Ophthalmol.*, **85**, 373–7.
12. Ponsford, J.R., Bannister, R. and Paul, E. (1982) Methacholine pupillary responses in third nerve palsy and Adie's syndrome. *Brain*, **105**, 583–97.
13. Hyland, H.H. and Barnett, H.J.M. (1954) The pathogenesis of cranial nerve palsies associated with intracranial aneurysms. *Proc. R. Soc. Med.*, **47**, 141–6.
14. Rush, J.A. and Younge, B.R. (1981) Paralysis of cranial nerves III, IV and VI. Cause and prognosis in 1,000 cases. *Arch. Ophthalmol.*, **99**, 76–9.
15. Thomas, J.E. and Yoss, R.E. (1970) The parasellar syndrome: Problems in determining etiology. *Proc. Mayo Clin.*, **45**, 617–23.
16. Kattah, J.C., Silgals, R.M., Manz, H. *et al.* (1985) Presentation and management of parasellar and suprasellar metastatic mass lesions. *J. Neurol. Neurosurg. Psychiatry*, **48**, 44–9.
17. Harris, W. (1950) Rare forms of paroxysmal trigeminal neuralgia, and their relation to disseminated sclerosis. *Br. Med. J.*, **2**, 1015–19.
18. Spillane, J.D. and Wells, C.E.C. (1959) Isolated trigeminal neuropathy: A report of 16 cases. *Brain*, **82**, 391–416.
19. Horowitz, S.H. (1974) Isolated facial numbness: Clinical significance

and relation to trigeminal neuropathy. *Ann. Intern. Med.*, **80**, 49–53.
20. Searles, R.P., Mladinich, E.K. and Messner, R.P. (1978) Isolated trigeminal sensory neuropathy: Early manifestation of mixed connective tissue disease. *Neurology*, **28**, 1286–9.
21. Peiris, O.A. and Miles, D.W. (1965) Galvanic stimulation of the tongue as a prognostic index in Bell's palsy. *Br. Med. J.*, **2**, 1162–3.
22. Hart, R.G., Gardner, D.P. and Howieson, J. (1983) Acoustic tumors: Atypical features and recent diagnostic tests. *Neurology*, **33**, 211–21.
23. Lechtenberg, R. and Shulman, A. (1984) The neurologic implications of tinnitus. *Arch. Neurol.*, **41**, 718–21.
24. Greenberg, H.S., Deck, M.D.F., Vikram, B. *et al.* (1981) Metastasis to the base of the skull: Clinical findings in 43 patients. *Neurology*, **31**, 530–7.
25. Siekert, R.G. (1956) Neurologic manifestations of tumors of the glomus jugulare. *Arch. Neurol. Psychiatry*, **76**, 1–13.
26. Olson, M.E., Chernik, N.L. and Posner, J.B. (1974) Infiltration of the leptomeninges by systemic cancer. A clinical and pathologic study. *Arch. Neurol.*, **30**, 122–37.
27. Symonds, C. (1958) Recurrent multiple cranial nerve palsies. *J. Neurol. Neurosurg. Psychiatry*, **21**, 95–100.

15

Cerebellar and spinal cord syndromes

Although disease of the cerebellum, or the spinocerebellar pathways, produces easily recognizable clinical features, it is seldom that the manifestations are sufficiently distinctive to establish an exact diagnosis without recourse to neurological investigation. The tempo and distribution of the disorder may allow some specification. An acutely evolving cerebellar syndrome is generally vascular in origin, and, since the advent of CT scanning, is recognized to be a more common form of stroke than was previously considered likely. The cerebellar disturbance due to primary or secondary tumour, when affecting one or other hemisphere, is predominantly unilateral, a feature which seldom occurs in degenerative disease of the cerebellum. Cerebellar signs are common in multiple sclerosis but rarely as isolated features.

15.1 FAMILIAL CEREBELLAR DISORDERS

A confined symmetrical cerebellar syndrome is likely to have a degenerative basis though in many of the familial cerebellar disorders other neurological findings coexist. Many of the familial conditions, particularly those inherited on an autosomal recessive basis, present in the first two decades of life, and their investigation will not be considered further. There are, however, a number, some associated with metabolic dysfunction, which present beyond the age of 20. A group of intermittent cerebellar ataxias is described, some of which are secondary to a specific metabolic disorder such as Hartnup disease[1]. In most of them, onset is in childhood, and the patient is asymptomatic between attacks. In other families, however, intermittent cerebellar symptoms, with onset in early adult life, have been followed by evidence of progressive cerebellar degeneration. Inheritance in these cases is on an autosomal dominant basis[2].

Metabolic disorders associated with cerebellar symptomatology, for example abeta-lipoproteinaemia, are likely to present in childhood. Familial hypo-beta-lipoproteinaemia can, however, present in adult life with ataxia and pyramidal features [3]. Patients have depressed cholesterol and beta-lipoprotein concentrations in the serum. In familial cerebrotendinous xanthomatosis, cerebellar ataxia may emerge after the age of 20, but by then most patients display other features of the disease, including swelling of the Achilles tendons and cataracts [4]. Tissue and serum levels of cholestanol are elevated. A condition with some similarities to Friedreich's ataxia can result from a partial deficiency of β-hexosaminidase A but cases generally present before the age of 20, at least in terms of their cerebellar deficiency, though evidence of neuropathy and dementia may emerge later [5].

Familial cerebellar disorders presenting beyond the age of 20 are usually inherited on an autosomal dominant basis. In some cases, the condition is that of a pure cerebellar degeneration, with pathological changes predominantly affecting the superior and anterior vermis and the cerebellar hemispheres [6]. In others, the pathological changes are those of olivo-ponto-cerebellar atrophy (OPCA). The clinical and genetic features of the latter are complex [7]. Classification (based on autopsy proven cases) into five categories has been suggested, all but one inherited as a dominant trait. Associated conditions occurring with some of the subgroups include ophthalmoplegia and atypical retinitis pigmentosa. A condition also inherited as an autosomal dominant has been described in Portuguese individuals or in descendants from Azorean Portuguese. The condition results in ataxia, pyramidal and extra-pyramidal signs and ophthalmoplegia [8]. Similar cases have recently been reported in non-Portuguese individuals resident in India [9] and Japan [10]. Onset of ataxia has generally been in the third or fourth decades of life. There are pathological distinctions from OPCA [10]. A proportion of patients with OPCA have been found to have depressed glutamate dehydrogenase activity in cultured fibroblasts or leucocytes. In an initial report, depressed levels were found in two siblings with features of type IV OPCA, though inheritance in this family suggested a recessive rather than dominant condition [11]. Subsequently, attempts have been made to define a subgroup of patients with OPCA in whom certain clinical or electrophysiological abnormalities predict the likelihood of finding evidence of glutamate dehydrogenase deficiency. It has been suggested that those patients with GDH deficiency have evidence of abnormal peripheral sensory-motor conduction, particularly sensory, together with prolongation of brain-stem auditory evoked responses (BAER)[12]. Glutamate dehydrogenase deficiency has been found in both non-dominant and dominant forms of OPCA. In some cases, whilst GDH levels have been found to be normal, the catalytic activity of the enzyme has not been stimulated by ADP[13].

Friedreich's ataxia rarely presents after the age of 20, and probably never after 25[14]. Soon after presentation, diagnostic features include areflexia in the lower limbs with limb and truncal ataxia. EMG examination reveals depressed or absent sensory action potentials in virtually all patients and appears to be an early feature, detectable in the youngest patients[15]. Neuro-otological abnormalities on the other hand, including altered BAER, are less consistent[16]. ECG changes are common in Friedreich's ataxia, though the changes are non-specific and seldom include evidence of conduction abnormalities[14]. A condition with some similarities to Friedreich's ataxia, but with preservation of the knee jerks has been described[17]. It is inherited as an autosomal recessive trait. Sensory action potentials are preserved whereas cardiomyopathy is lacking. Like patients with Friedreich's ataxia, onset is generally before the age of 20 years.

15.1.1 Investigation

The role of evoked potentials in distinguishing the various inherited ataxias has been discussed[18]. Abnormal visual evoked responses have been found in up to two-thirds of patients with Friedreich's ataxia, consisting of depressed amplitude, dispersion and increased latency. Similar changes occur in the other ataxias. BAER findings have been reported variously in Friedreich's ataxia. They are commonly abnormal in OPCA but usually normal in the other inherited ataxias. Somatosensory responses tend to be abnormal in Friedreich's ataxia (prolongation and abnormal shape of N20) but normal in the other groups.

15.1.2 Recommendation

A detailed discussion of the investigation of those inherited ataxias presenting before the age of 20 will not be attempted. The majority of these conditions are inherited as a recessive trait, and many have a metabolic basis. Later appearance of ataxia is sometimes found in hypo-beta-lipoproteinaemia and cholestanolosis, requiring, for diagnosis, the study of cholesterol and lipoprotein levels, and measurement of serum cholestanol levels respectively.

The diagnosis of Friedreich's ataxia is suggested by a particular clinical picture. Support for the diagnosis can be obtained by measurement of sensory action potentials and evoked responses. Slightly atypical features, for example delayed appearance of the lower motor neurone signs, or the presence of dementia, suggest the possibility of chronic G_{M2} gangliosidosis and necessitates measurement of β-hexosaminidase A activity.

Familial ataxias presenting after the age of 20 usually show dominant inheritance. Where the pattern suggests one of the variants of OPCA, electrophysiological investigation is appropriate, including nerve conduction studies and measurement of brain stem auditory evoked responses. Estimates of platelet glutamate dehydrogenase activity may serve to delineate certain subgroups of the disorder with greater accuracy. The investigation should include the effects of activation by ADP.

15.2 NON-FAMILIAL CEREBELLAR
   SYNDROMES

A non-familial, slowly evolving, cerebellar syndrome is relatively rare in neurological practice. Perhaps the commonest single cause of this presentation is alcoholism[19]. The ataxia predominantly affects the lower limbs and nystagmus is seldom prominent. A sub-acute cerebellar degeneration occurs in association with carcinoma. Involvement is generally symmetrical and usually affects all four limbs. Dysarthria is common but nystagmus not conspicuous in the majority of cases[20]. An association between myxoedema and cerebellar ataxia is recognized[21]. Generally manifestations of hypothyroidism antedate the ataxia which typically mainly affects gait. Nystagmus is lacking. It is recognized that vitamin E deficiency, secondary to chronic fat malabsorption, can result in neurological disability including ataxia and neuropathic changes. Recently a case of ataxia associated with areflexia and impaired proprioception was found to have absent levels of vitamin E in the absence of any evidence of fat malabsorption. Depressed vitamin E levels were found in several members of the patient's family[22].

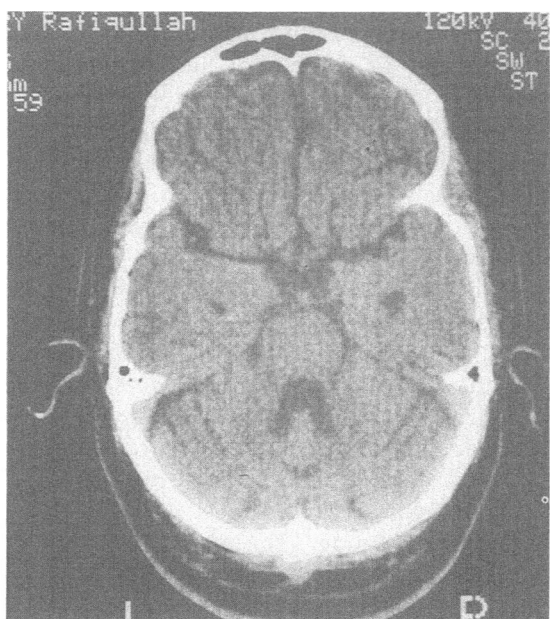

Fig. 15.1 CT scan demonstrating cerebellar atrophy with a dilated fourth ventricle

15.2.1 Investigation

CSF examination is of very limited value in the investigation of a chronic cerebellar syndrome. The protein concentration may be moderately elevated in patients with alcoholic cerebellar degeneration or in those cases associated with hypothyroidism. In carcinomatous cerebellar degeneration an elevated lymphocyte count may be found in addition. Radiological investigation is of limited value. In alcoholic cerebellar degeneration, atrophy is prominent in the superior vermis and, to a lesser extent, in the hemispheres [23]. In the cerebellar atrophy associated with carcinoma, prominence of the cerebellar folio is an early feature (Fig. 15.1).

15.2.2 Recommendation

In a slowly evolving cerebellar syndrome CT or MRI scanning should be performed, largely to exclude non-degenerative pathologies, for example neoplasm. A detailed drug history is necessary with particular emphasis on the possibility of acohol abuse. Thyroid function tests should be performed. Estimation of serum vitamin E levels should be considered where a spinocerebellar syndrome appears in childhood or early adult life. The possibility of an occult neoplasm (particularly of bronchus or ovary) should be considered and excluded, where possible, though the cerebellar syndrome may antedate the declaration of the causative cancer by up to two years, and possibly for longer.

15.3 SUB-ACUTE SPINAL CORD SYNDROMES

The time course of an evolving spinal cord disturbance can give some indication of its underlying pathogenesis. A rapidly developing condition can be a feature of multiple sclerosis, of transverse myelitis, of acute cord compression from tumour or infection, or from the effects of a vascular lesion of the cord. These are considered elsewhere. The differential diagnosis of a more slowly evolving cord syndrome is equally wide and for most patients with this clinical picture, extensive investigation is often required to establish a specific diagnosis. Some patients with multiple sclerosis have a progressive paraparesis without clinical involvement of other parts of the nervous system. Their investigation is considered in Chapter 6.

An extensive group of patients presenting with a spastic paraplegia – paraparesis has been analysed[24]. In 77.3%, the diagnosis was readily apparent without recourse to extensive investigation. In 108 patients, more detailed investigation was necessary, resulting in a diagnosis, other than MS, which included tumour and arteriovenous malformation, in 78. In 44 patients no cause for the spastic paraplegia was discovered. None had evidence of MS (though neither oligoclonal studies nor evoked responses were performed) and in all myelography was normal, or showed minor degenerative changes only. The concept of primary lateral sclerosis, a degenerative disorder confined to the pyramidal tracts of the spinal cord is of long standing[25]. The criteria for making such a diagnosis have been defined as the insidious onset of a slowly progressive pyramidal tract syndrome, where signs are confined to pyramidal tract dysfunction and where follow up has failed to establish any alternative diagnosis. Pathological studies in such cases have seldom been available. Familial forms of such a syndrome are well recognized, with both recessive and dominant inheritance. How strictly the boundaries of the condition should be defined has been debated.

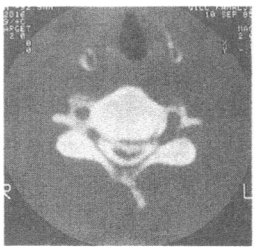 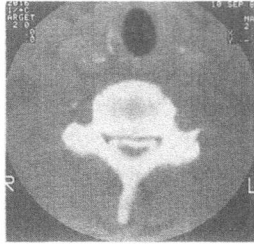 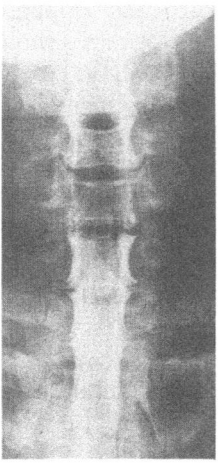

Fig. 15.2 (l & r) CT and myelogram showing narrowing of the C5/6 disc space with posterior protrusion of the disc associated with cord flattening

Dominant inheritance outweighs recessive [26], though the clinical features of the two subgroups are similar [27]. Posterior column degeneration is a prominent feature at post-mortem examination and some patients have abnormal somatosensory evoked responses, though with normal peripheral sensory conduction [28]. In general, patients displaying recessive inheritance present before the age of 10, whereas patients in families with a dominant inheritance can present beyond the age of 30 years. Familial forms of spastic paraplegia with prominent involvement of other neurological systems virtually always present in the first two decades of life [29]. A picture of progressive spastic paraplegia with sex-linked recessive inheritance should alert the physician to the possibility of adrenoleukodystrophy [30]. There may be an associated neuropathy, determined by EMG examination. The paraplegia is liable to present in the third decade of life and adrenal function tests are not inevitably altered. In one family, where the disease affected two brothers, onset was at the ages of 40 and 50 respectively [31]. A similar spastic paraparesis may be found in symptomatic female carriers. Typically, patients display abnormal levels of saturated very long-chain fatty acids in plasma and fibroblasts.

A common cause of slowly progressive non-familial paraplegia is cervical myelopathy secondary to spondylitic disease. Plain X-rays of the spine are inevitably abnormal in such cases, though the changes correlate poorly with the degree or duration of spinal cord disease[32]. There is, however, a close correlation between the sagittal diameter of the cervical canal, as measured from plain X-rays and the presence or absence of signs of myelopathy[33]. In one study, 86% of those patients shown at operation to have evidence of cord compression had a neural canal (measured from a spondylotic bar to the nearest point on the posterior wall of the canal) of less than or equal to 12 mm[34]. Measurement of the antero-posterior diameter of the cord, and its area, based on CT analysis, gives the most sensitive measure of cord compression, whereas the nature of the cord deformity relates well with the distribution and severity of the patient's symptoms[35] (Fig. 15.2). Thoracic disc herniation is considerably rarer than its cervical counterpart, and is principally confined to the lower segments.

A slowly evolving cord syndrome can occur in association with an intramedullar or extramedullar tumour. Intramedullary tumours include astrocytomas and ependymomas. Metastases to the spinal cord are rare. Myelography in the case of an intramedullar tumour displays a uniformly expanded cord which, if sufficiently large, may suffice to block the flow of contrast medium (Fig. 15.3). Most extramedullary but intradural tumours are either meningiomas or neurofibromas. The shape of the tumour is usually at least partly visible with conventional myelography. In the case of extradural tumours, displacement of the contrast column away from the site of compression occurs with a serrated pattern to the margin of the medium in the antero-posterior projection.

Angiomas of the spinal cord may present abruptly, with an acute cord syndrome, but on other occasions produce a slowly evolving picture, sometimes interspersed with brief exacerbations, the picture then resembling multiple sclerosis. Radiation myelopathy usually affects the cervical cord and results in a progressive paraplegia, sometimes asymmetrical, and typically delayed for several months to years after radiotherapy has been completed. A brief, reversible cord syndrome may follow radiotherapy, its most prominent feature being a positive Lhermitte phenomenon. Many bone or joint disorders primarily affecting the spinal column, for example Paget's disease and rheumatoid arthritis, may have secondary effects on cord function. In rheumatoid arthritis the degree of atlanto-axial subluxation on plain X-ray is not closely related to the presence or absence of myelopathy, though CT scanning of the cervical region with intrathecal metrizamide suggests that the mobility of any

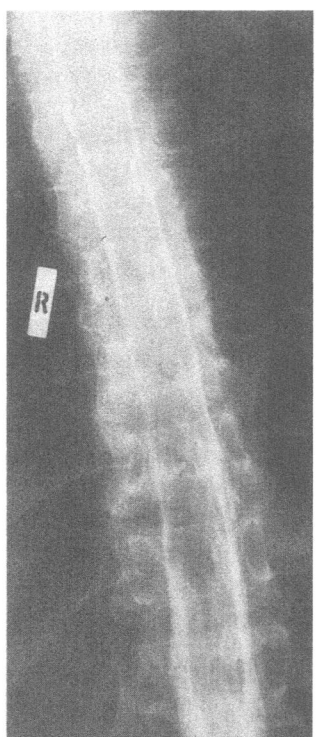

Fig. 15.3 Myelogram displaying uniform expansion of the thoracic cord due to an ependymoma

atlanto-axial subluxation is related to the severity of the adjacent cord deformity[36]. Subacute combined degeneration of the spinal cord is rare. Whereas most cases display typical haematological changes in blood and bone marrow, the cord syndrome can emerge when such changes are lacking[37]. An association between folate deficiency and a spinal cord syndrome has been less convincingly established[38].

15.3.1 Investigation

Examination of the cerebrospinal fluid is of rather limited value in the investigation of a slowly evolving spinal cord syndrome, assuming that cases due to multiple sclerosis have already been excluded. In primary lateral sclerosis the protein concentration may be elevated[39], as it may be in patients with cervical myelopathy due to disc disease[32]. Abnormal protein concentrations are frequent in the presence of tumour, and values rise as the degree of obstruction increases. In general, values are higher with the intradural, extramedullar tumours and more so for neurofibroma than meningioma. Manometric studies have been made redundant by the introduction of more sophisticated techniques for the detection of obstruction of the subarachnoid space.

Plain X-ray changes, although of considerable use in the assessment of patients with cervical myelopathy due to disc disease, play a small role in the appraisal of patients with suspected tumour. Bone erosion is not uncommon in cases of neurofibroma, whereas widening of the spinal canal may be evident in extensive spinal tumours, for example ependymoma[40]. Paget's disease typically results in widening and flattening of the vertebral body, with alteration of its trabecular pattern.

Myelography has been the principal method of investigation of suspected cord compression for many years. Its value, compared to CT scanning of the spine with intrathecal metrizamide, or MRI of the spine, has been critically appraised. The degree of cord deformity resulting from cervical disc protrusion can be more accurately predicted from CT scanning than by conventional myelography[35], and the same superiority holds for the investigation of the myelopathy related to rheumatoid arthritis[36]. The indications for computer-assisted myelography have been discussed[41]. Where CT scanning followed conventional myelography, additional data on the nature of the lesion were obtained in two-thirds of the cases. The role of MRI in the diagnosis of spinal cord disease is still being explored[42]. In general spin echo sequences are more valuable than inversion recovery, with short TR and TE providing the best differentiation between the spinal cord and surrounding structures.

Angiography of the spinal cord is largely confined to the diagnosis of angiomatous malformations. Myelography often, but not inevitably, detects abnormal vessels, but requires prone and supine films with a large volume of contrast. For definitive diagnosis, and in the appraisal prior to surgical intervention, aortography with selective catheterization of the individual feeders remains essential[43].

Electrophysiological studies can provide further information regarding the nature of a spinal cord disturbance. Whilst early reports of somatosensory responses in cervical spondylosis concentrated on the abnormalities found in association with radiculopathy [44], an increasingly sophisticated recording technique has allowed identification of postsynaptic cervical cord potentials, thought to correspond to activity in the central grey matter, which are most consistently abnormal in the presence of cervical cord lesions [45]. Abnormalities, however, are less likely to be found in the evanescent myelopathy following spinal irradiation [46].

Electrophysiological investigation reveals a number of abnormalities in subacute combined degeneration of the spinal cord. EEG changes [47], reversing after treatment, and altered latencies of the visual evoked responses [48] can be found in the absence of overt cerebral or optic nerve symptomatology. Peripheral nerve dysfunction is detectable by measurement of lower limb motor conduction velocity [49], or sensory action potential amplitude [50]. Somatosensory evoked responses, particularly those from the leg, are delayed [50].

Serological studies are of some value in patients with tropical spastic paraplegia, since the condition is thought to be the result of infection with human T-lymphotropic virus type 1 (HTLV-1) [51].

15.3.2 Recommendation

Though radiological investigation is often required in the investigation of a slowly evolving spinal cord syndrome, the diagnosis of multiple sclerosis (discussed in Chapter 6) can generally be achieved without recourse to myelography. Familial spastic paraplegias do not require further investigation unless the pattern suggests sex-linked inheritance, in which case plasma or fibroblast very-long-chain fatty acids should be measured to exclude adrenoleukodystrophy.

The exclusion of a compressive lesion affecting spinal cord function will require specialized radiological investigation. Plain X-rays should be performed initially and are particularly valuable in the evaluation of cervical myelopathy due to spondylitic disease. The comparative role of myelography, computerized tomography and magnetic resonance imaging in the evaluation of spinal cord disease remains unsettled. At present, with the limited availability of magnetic resonance imaging, at least in the United Kingdom, myelography remains the investigation of choice, followed, in certain circumstances, by computerized tomography, particularly where further information is required regarding the type and degree of cord deformity. Angiography is limited to the investigation of suspected cord angioma.

Electrophysiological investigation has a limited role in the routine evaluation of a spinal cord syndrome. The diagnosis of subacute combined degeneration is readily achieved by measurement of serum B_{12} levels, rather than depending on relatively subtle changes in peripheral or central conduction times. CSF evaluation provides little specific diagnostic data other than for cases of multiple sclerosis.

REFERENCES

1. Hill, W. and Sherman, H. (1968) Acute intermittent familial cerebellar ataxia. *Arch. Neurol.*, **18**, 350–7.
2. Parker, H.L. (1946) Periodic ataxia. *Collected Papers of the Mayo Clinic*, **38**, 642–5.
3. Mars, H., Lewis, L.A., Robertson, A.L. Jr *et al.* (1969) Familial hypo-betalipoproteinaemia. *Am. J. Med.*, **46**, 886–900.
4. Farpour, H. and Mahloudji, M. (1975) Familial cerebrotendinous xanthomatosis. Report of a new family and review of the literature. *Arch. Neurol.*, **32**, 223–5.
5. Willner, J.P., Grabowski, G.A., Gordon, R.E. *et al.* (1981) Chronic G_{M2} gangliosidosis masquerading as atypical Friedreich ataxia: Clinical, morphologic, and biochemical studies of nine cases. *Neurology*, **31**, 787–98.
6. Hoffman, P.M., Stuart, W.H., Earle, K.M. and Brody, J.A. (1971) Hereditary late-onset cerebellar degeneration. *Neurology*, **21**, 771–7.
7. Konigsmark, B.W. and Weiner, L.P. (1970) The olivopontocerebellar atrophies: A review. *Medicine (Baltimore)*, **49**, 227–41.
8. Woods, B.T. and Schaumburg, H.H. (1972) Nigro-spino-dentatal degeneration with nuclear ophthalmoplegia. A unique and partially treatable clinico-pathological entity. *J. Neurol. Sci.*, **17**, 149–66.
9. Bharucha, N.E., Bharucha, E.P. and Bhabha, S.K. (1986) Machado–Joseph–Azorean disease in India. *Arch. Neurol.*, **43**, 142–5.
10. Yuasa, T., Ohama, E., Harayama, H. *et al.* (1986) Joseph's disease: Clinical and pathological studies in a Japanese family. *Ann. Neurol.*, **19**, 152–7.
11. Plaitakis, A., Nicklas, W.J. and Desnick, R.J. (1980) Glutamate dehydrogenase deficiency in three patients with spinocerebellar syndrome. *Ann. Neurol.*, **7**, 297–303.
12. Chokroverty, S., Duvoisin, R.C., Sachdeo, R. *et al.* (1985) Neurophysiologic study of olivopontocerebellar atrophy with or without glutamate dehydrogenase deficiency. *Neurology*, **35**, 652–9.
13. Sorbi, S., Tonini, S., Giannini, E. *et al.* (1986) Abnormal platelet glutamate dehydrogenase activity and activation in dominant and

nondominant olivopontocerebellar atrophy. *Ann. Neurol.,* **19,** 239–45.
14. Harding, A.E. (1981) Friedreich's ataxia: A clinical and genetic study of 90 families with an analysis of early diagnostic criteria and intrafamilial clustering of clinical features. *Brain,* **104,** 589–620.
15. Ouvrier, R.A., McLeod, J.G. and Conchin, T.E. (1982) Friedreich's ataxia: Early detection and progression of peripheral nerve abnormalities. *J. Neurol. Sci.,* **55,** 137–45.
16. Ell, J., Prasher, D. and Rudge, P. (1984) Neuro-otological abnormalities in Friedreich's ataxia. *J. Neurol. Neurosurg. Psychiatry,* **47,** 26–32.
17. Harding, A.E. (1981) Early onset cerebellar ataxia with retained tendon reflexes: A clinical and genetic study of a disorder distinct from Friedreich's ataxia. *J. Neurol. Neurosurg. Psychiatry,* **44,** 503–8.
18. Nuwer, M.R., Perlman, S.L., Packwood, J.W. and Kark, R.A.P. (1983) Evoked potential abnormalities in the various inherited ataxias. *Ann. Neurol.,* **13,** 20–7.
19. Victor, M., Adams, R.D. and Mancall, E.L. (1959) A restricted form of cerebellar cortical degeneration occuring in alcoholic patients. *Arch. Neurol.,* **1,** 579–688.
20. Lord Brain and Wilkinson, M. (1965) Subacute cerebellar degeneration associated with carcinoma. *Brain,* **88,** 465–78.
21. Cremer, G.M., Goldstein, N.P. and Paris, J. (1969) Myxedema and ataxia. *Neurology,* **19,** 37–46.
22. Harding, A.E., Matthews, S., Jones, S. *et al.* (1985) Spinocerebellar degeneration associated with a selective defect of vitamin E absorption. *N. Engl. J. Med.,* **313,** 32–5.
23. Hillbom, M., Muuronen, A., Holm, L. and Hindmarsh, T. (1986) The clinical versus radiological diagnosis of alcoholic cerebellar degeneration. *J. Neurol. Sci.,* **73,** 45–53.
24. Ungar-Sargon, J.Y., Lovelace, R.E. and Brust, J.C.M. (1980) Spastic paraplegia – paraparesis. A reappraisal. *J. Neurol. Sci.,* **46,** 1–12.
25. Stark, F.M. and Moersch, F.P. (1945) Primary lateral sclerosis. A distinct clinical entity. *J. Nervous Mental Dis.,* **102,** 332–7.
26. Holmes, G.L. and Shaywitz, B.A. (1977) Strumpell's pure familial spastic paraplegia: Case study and review of the literature. *J. Neurol. Neurosurg. Psychiatry,* **40,** 1003–8.
27. Harding, A.E. (1981) Hereditary 'pure' spastic paraplegia: A clinical and genetic study of 22 families. *J. Neurol. Neurosurg. Psychiatry,* **44,** 871–83.
28. Thomas, P.K., Jefferys, J.G.R., Smith, I.S. and Loulakakis, D. (1981) Spinal somatosensory evoked potentials in hereditary spastic paraplegia. *J. Neurol. Neurosurg. Psychiatry,* **44,** 243–6.
29. Harding, A.E. (1983) Classification of the hereditary ataxias and paraplegias. *Lancet,* i, 1151–5.
30. O'Neill, B.P., Moser, H.W., Saxena, K.M. and Marmion, L.C. (1984) Adrenoleukodystrophy: Clinical and biochemical manifestations in carriers. *Neurology,* **34,** 798–801.

31. O'Neill, B.P., Swanson, J.W., Brown, F.R. III *et al.* (1985) Familial spastic paraparesis: An adrenoleukodystrophy phenotype? *Neurology,* **35**, 1233–5.
32. Clarke, E. and Robinson, P.K. (1956) Cervical myelopathy: A complication of cervical spondylosis. *Brain,* **79**, 483–510.
33. Burrows, E.H. (1963) The sagittal diameter of the spinal canal in cervical spondylosis. *Clin. Radiol.,* **14**, 77–86.
34. Symon, L. and Lavender, P. (1967) The surgical treatment of cervical spondylotic myelopathy. *Neurology,* **17**, 117–27.
35. Yu, Y.L., Stevens, J.M., Kendall, B. and du Boulay, G.H. (1983) Cord shape and measurements in cervical spondylotic myelopathy and radiculopathy. *Am. J. Neuroradiol.,* **4**, 839–42.
36. Stevens, J.M., Kendall, B.E. and Crockard, H.A. (1986) The spinal cord in rheumatoid arthritis with clinical myelopathy: A computed myelographic study. *J. Neurol. Neurosurg. Psychiatry,* **49**, 140–51.
37. Jewesbury, E.C.O. (1954) Subacute combined degeneration of the cord and achlorhydric peripheral neuropathies without anaemia. *Lancet,* **ii**, 307–12.
38. Reynolds, E.H., Rothfeld, P. and Pincus, J.H. (1973) Neurological disease associated with folate deficiency. *Br. Med. J.,* **2**, 398–400.
39. Russo, L.S. Jr (1982) Clinical and electrophysiological studies in primary lateral sclerosis. *Arch. Neurol.,* **39**, 662–4.
40. Fearnside, M.R. and Adams, C.B.T. (1978) Tumours of the cauda equina. *J. Neurol. Neurosurg. Psychiatry,* **41**, 24–31.
41. Barrow, D.L., Wood, J.H. and Hoffman, J.C. Jr (1983) Clinical indications for computer-assisted myelography. *Neurosurgery,* **12**, 47–56.
42. Aichner, F., Poewe, W., Rogalsky, W. *et al.* (1985) Magnetic resonance imaging in the diagnosis of spinal cord diseases. *J. Neurol. Neurosurg. Psychiatry,* **48**, 1220–9.
43. Di Chiro, G., Doppman, J. and Ommaya, A.K. (1967) Selective arteriography of arteriovenous aneurysms of spinal cord. *Radiology,* **88**, 1065–77.
44. Ganes, T. (1980) Somatosensory conduction times and peripheral, cervical and cortical evoked potentials in patients with cervical spondylosis. *J. Neurol. Neurosurg. Psychiatry,* **43**, 683–9.
45. Emerson, R.G. and Pedley, T.A. (1986) Effect of cervical spinal cord lesions on early components of the median nerve somatosensory evoked potential. *Neurology,* **36**, 20–6.
46. Lecky, B.R.F., Murray, N.M.F. and Berry, R.J. (1980) Transient radiation myelopathy: Spinal somatosensory evoked responses following incidental cord exposure during radiotherapy. *J. Neurol. Neurosurg. Psychiatry,* **43**, 747–50.
47. Walton, J.N., Kiloh, L.G., Osselton, J.W. and Farrall, J. (1954) The electroencephalogram in pernicious anaemia and subacute combined degeneration of the cord. *Electroencephalogr. Clin. Neurophysiol.,* **6**, 45–64.

48. Troncoso, J., Mancall, E.L. and Schatz, N.J. (1979) Visual evoked responses in pernicious anaemia. *Arch. Neurol.* **36**, 168–9.
49. Cox-Klazinga, M. and Endtz, L.J. (1980) Peripheral nerve involvement in pernicious anaemia. *J. Neurol. Sci.,* **45**, 367–71.
50. Fine, E.J. and Hallet, M. (1980) Neurophysiological study of subacute combined degeneration. *J. Neurol. Sci.,* **45**, 331–6.
51. Román, G.C. (1987) Retrovirus-associated myelopathies. *Arch. Neurol.,* **44**, 659–63.

Index